Review Questions & Answers for Veterinary Technicians

Review Questions & Answers for Veterinary Technicians

second edition

Thomas P. Colville, DVM, MSc
Department of Veterinary and Microbiological Sciences
North Dakota State University
Fargo, North Dakota

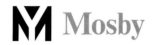 Mosby

St. Louis Baltimore Boston Carlsbad Chicago Naples New York Philadelphia Portland
London Madrid Mexico City Singapore Sydney Tokyo Toronto Wiesbaden

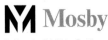

Dedicated to Publishing Excellence

A Times Mirror
Company

Publisher: Don Ladig
Executive Editor: Paul W. Pratt, VMD
Senior Developmental Editor: Jolynn Gower
Project Manager: Dana Peick
Book Design: Reed Technology and Information Services, Inc.
Manufacturing Supervisor: Tony McAllister
Composition by: Reed Technology and Information Services, Inc.
Printing/binding by: Maple-Vail Book Manufacturing Group

Printed in the United States of America

Mosby-Year Book, Inc.
11830 Westline Industrial Drive
St. Louis, Missouri 63146

Library of Congress Cataloging-in-Publication Data

Review questions and answers for veterinary technicians/edited
  by Thomas P. Colville—2nd ed.
    1. Animal health technicians—United States—Examinations,
questions, etc. 2. Animal health technology—United States—
Examinations, questions, etc. I. Colville, Thomas P.
SF774.4.R48   1995
6336.089'076—dc20

95-44415
CIP

98 99 / 9 8 7 6 5 4 3 2

Contributors

Douglas E. N. Bach, DVM
Lecturer
Veterinary Technology
Ridgetown College
Ridgetown, Ontario, Canada

Marta M. Bates, CAHT
Operating Room Nurse
University of Pennsylvania
Kennett Square, Pennsylvania

Robert "Pete" Bill, DVM, PhD
Veterinary Technology Program
School of Veterinary Medicine
Purdue University
West Lafayette, Indiana

Kerry L. Coombs, DVM
Program Director
Omaha College of Health Careers
Omaha, Nebraska

Patricia Creamer, CAHT
ICU Supervisor
University of Pennsylvania
School of Veterinary Medicine
Kennett Square, Pennsylvania

Kimberly S. Cullen, CAHT
Operating Room Nurse
University of Pennsylvania
Kennett Square, Pennsylvania

Shannon M. Dowie, CAHT
Operating Room Nurse
University of Pennsylvania
Kennett Square, Pennsylvania

Robin E. Duntze, DVM
Director of Veterinary Technology
Jefferson College
Hillsboro, Missouri

Edward I. Gordon, DVM
Professor and Director
Veterinary Science Technology
   Program
State University of New York
College of Technology
Canton, New York

Connie Han, RVT
Veterinary Technology Program
School of Veterinary Medicine
Purdue University
West Lafayette, Indiana

Beth Harries, MEd, LVT
Program Coordinator
Veterinary Technology Program
Wayne County Community College
Detroit, Michigan

Eloyes Hill, MT
Research Specialist II
Veterinary Science and
   Microbiology Department
North Dakota State University
Fargo, North Dakota

Jean Holtzen, CVT
Omaha College of Health Careers
Omaha, Nebraska

Anne D. Hope, CAHT
Operating Room Supervisor
University of Pennsylvania
Kennett Square, Pennsylvania

Karen Hrapkiewicz, DVM
Program Director
Veterinary Technology Program
Wayne County Community College
Detroit, Michigan

Cheryl Hurd, RVT
Veterinary Technology Program
School of Veterinary Medicine
Purdue University
West Lafayette, Indiana

Henry J. Kagerer, DVM
Professor of Veterinary Technology
Colorado Mountain College
Spring Valley Campus
Glenwood Springs, Colorado

Kay Knox
Veterinary Technology Program
School of Veterinary Medicine
Purdue University
West Lafayette, Indiana

Barb Lewis, BA, MA, CVT
Assistant Professor
Veterinary Technology Program
Morehead State University
Morehead, Kentucky

Marsha E. Madsen, MS, RVT
Instructor
Veterinary Technology Program
Brigham Young University
Provo, Utah

Diane McKelvey, DVM
Lecturer
Centralia College
Huron Park, Ontario, Canada

Sarah McLaughlin, DVM
Professor
Health Sciences
St. Lawrence College
Kingston, Ontario, Canada

Marilyn L. Meyers, RVT, LATG
Operating Room Supervisor
Small Animal Surgery
Veterinary Teaching Hospital
Veterinary Technology Program
School of Veterinary Medicine
Purdue University
West Lafayette, Indiana

Karl M. Peter, DVM
Professor of Veterinary Technology
Foothill College
Los Altos Hills, California

Stuart L. Porter, VMD
Professor and Director
Veterinary Technology Program
Blue Ridge Community College
Weyers Cave, Virginia

Paul W. Pratt, VMD
Executive Editor
Mosby-Year Book, Inc.
Santa Barbara, California

Teri Raffel, CVT, AAS
Instructional Assistant
Veterinary Technician Program
Madison Area Technical College
Madison, Wisconsin

Lori Renda-Francis, LVT
Lab Supervisor and Instructor
Veterinary Technician Program
Macomb Community College
Clinton Township, Michigan

Nancy Robinson, RVT
Veterinary Medical Technology
   Program
Central Carolina Community
   College
Sanford, North Carolina

Contributors

Blaine R. Russell, CVM
Director of Veterinary Technology
Yuba College
Marysville, California

Pam Schendel, BS, RVT
Laboratory Technologist
Veterinary Teaching Hospital
School of Veterinary Medicine
Purdue Unversity
West Lafayette, Indiana

Mary Lou Shea, CAHT
Director of Nursing
University of Pennsylvania
School of Veterinary Medicine
Kennett Square, Pennsylvania

Randal M. Shirbroun, DVM
Coordinator
Veterinary Technology Program
Nebraska College of Technical
   Agriculture
Curtis, Nebraska

Teresa F. Sonsthagen, BS, CVT
Veterinary Technology Program
Department of Veterinary and
   Microbiological Sciences
North Dakota State University
Fargo, North Dakota

Richard N. Thwaits, DVM, PhD
Director of Veterinary Technology
Animal Science Department
Brigham Young University
Provo, Utah

C. Lee Tyner, DVM
Coordinator
Veterinary Technology Program
Morehead State University
Morehead, Kentucky

S. Randall Vanderhurst, DVM
Professor of Veterinary Technology
Veterinary Technology Program
Colorado Mountain College
Spring Valley Campus
Glenwood Springs, Colorado

Paula J. Voglewede, BS, RVT, AAS
Chief Intensive Care Technologist
Small Animal Hospital
Veterinary Technology Program
School of Veterinary Medicine
Purdue University
West Lafayette, Indiana

Mary K. Walsh
Operating Room Nurse
University of Pennsylvania
Kennett Square, Pennsylvania

Christee Williams, CVT
Instructor
Veterinary Technology Department
Tri-County Technical College
Pendleton, South Carolina

George W. Younger, DVM
Director of Veterinary Technology
Veterinary Technology Program
Tomball College
Tomball, Texas

Preface

This book is the result of the collaboration of 40 veterinary technician educators representing 22 educational institutions in the United States and Canada. They responded to the need for a resource that would help veterinary technician students and graduate veterinary technicians review for academic course examinations, as well as for national, state, and provincial credentialing examinations. This text is the first resource of its kind to be authored entirely by veterinary technician educators.

The questions in *Review Questions & Answers for Veterinary Technicians, second edition* were carefully constructed, specifically for this book, to test factual knowledge, reasoning skills, and clinical judgment. No question has been knowingly "recycled" from any previous or current credentialing examination, but when properly used, the questions can help identify subject areas of strength and weakness.

Acknowledgments

A great deal of work on the part of a group of dedicated people went into producing this book. I am honored to have been able to work with these skilled professionals, and I am pleased to acknowledge the vital contributions they have made.

I am grateful to the 40 veterinary technician educators who took time out of their busy schedules to create the questions for this book; as a veterinary technician educator myself, I know how difficult it is to find time for "extra" projects. It is a tribute to the commitment of these individuals that they took the time to write such an excellent assemblage of challenging questions.

The staff of Mosby–Year Book provided much appreciated guidance and encouragement through the gestation and birth of this book. Dr. Paul Pratt initiated the original concept and edited the book's first edition. He has been a leader in recruiting veterinary technician educators to author and edit books for veterinary technicians. Jolynn Gower took stacks of question-and-answer manuscripts and skillfully assembled them into this superb educational resource.

On behalf of all the veterinary technician educators who authored this book, I would like to acknowledge our students and graduates. They are pioneers in this young profession. Their hard work and devotion to their profession is inspiring and gratifying. It is for them that this book exists, and it is to them that it is dedicated.

Finally, I would like to gratefully acknowledge the support and help I received from my personal and professional partner, Dr. Joann Colville. She not only tolerated the weekends and evenings I spent working on this book but also gave excellent guidance and suggestions on many aspects of the book's organization and content.

Thomas P. Colville, DVM, MSc

Credentialing of Veterinary Technicians

To work as a veterinary technician in most states, individuals must pass a "credentialing" examination administered by an appropriate regulatory agency to confirm that each candidate possesses sufficient veterinary technology-related knowledge and skills. Successful completion of this credentialing process generally confers the title of Certified Veterinary Technician (CVT), Registered Veterinary Technician (RVT), or Licensed Veterinary Technician (LVT) on the individual, depending on the terminology used in that state. Candidates should contact the appropriate regulatory agency in the state or province in which they desire credentialing to obtain information on the specific processes and requirements. Contact information is provided below.

Many states use the Veterinary Technician National Examination (VTNE) as all or part of their credentialing process. The VTNE is prepared by the Professional Examination Service and consists of 200 multiple-choice questions in 7 primary areas: Pharmacy & Pharmacology; Surgical Preparation & Assisting; Laboratory Procedures; Animal Nursing; Radiology, Ultrasound and Other Electronic Imaging; Anesthesia; and Office & Hospital Procedures. The examination is designed to assess essential job-related knowledge at the entry level.

Candidates moving from one state to another can pay a fee and have their VTNE test score reported to their new state by contacting the Interstate Reporting Service, Professional Examination Service, 475 Riverside Drive, New York, NY 10115-0089; telephone (212) 870-3149.

United States

For the convenience of technicians seeking information on credentialing; the addresses of state regulatory agencies follow:

Alabama
Executive Officer
State Board of Veterinary Medical Examiners
P.O. Box 1767
Decatur, AL 35602

Alaska
Executive Officer
Division of Occupational Licensing
Department of Commerce and Economic Development
P.O. Box 110806
Juneau, AK 99811-0800

Arizona
Executive Director
Veterinary Medical Examining Board
1645 West Jefferson
Room 410
Phoenix, AZ 85007

Arkansas
Executive Secretary
Arkansas Veterinary Medical Examining Board
#1 Natural Resources Drive
P.O. Box 5497
Little Rock, AR 72215

California
Executive Officer
Board of Examiners in Veterinary Medicine
Suite 6
1420 Howe Ave.
Sacramento, CA 95825

Colorado
Veterinary Association
Suite 701
1780 S. Bellaire
Denver, Colorado 80222

Connecticut
Connecticut Association of Animal Health Technicians
2500 Black Road Turnpike
Fairfield, CT 06430

Delaware
Administrative Assistant
Board of Veterinary Medicine
Cannon Building
Suite 203
P.O. Box 1401
Dover, DE 19903

District of Columbia
Executive Officer
Board of Veterinary Examiners
Room 913
614 H St. NW
Washington, DC 20001

Florida
Veterinary Technician Committee
Florida Veterinary Medical Association
P.O. Box 2092
Sebring, FL 33871

Georgia
Executive Director
State Examinings Boards
166 Pryor St. SW
Atlanta, GA 30303

Hawaii
Executive Officer
Board of Veterinary Examiners
Box 3469
1010 Richards St.
Honolulu, HI 96801

Idaho
Executive Officer
Board of Veterinary Medicine
P.O. Box 77249
Boise, ID 83707

Illinois
Executive Officer
Veterinary Licensing and Disciplinary Board
Department of Professional Regulation
320 W. Washington
Springfield, IL 62786

Indiana
Board Director
Health Professions Bureau
Room 041
402 W. Washington St.
Indianapolis, IN 46204

Iowa
Secretary
Board of Veterinary Medicine
2nd Floor
Wallace Building
Des Moines, IA 50319

Kansas
Registration Board
Box 121
Colby, KS 67701

Kentucky
Executive Officer
Board of Veterinary Examiners
P.O. Box 456
Frankfort, KY 40602

Louisiana
Animal Health Technician Certification Committee
Department of Agriculture/Animal Science
Northwestern State University of Louisiana
Natchitoches, LA 71497

Maine
Division of Licensing and Enforcement
Department of Professional and Financial Regulation
State House Station 35
Augusta, ME 04333

Maryland
Secretary
Board of Veterinary Medical Examiners
50 Harry S. Truman Parkway
Annapolis, MD 21401

Massachusetts
Technician Committee
Massachusetts Veterinary Medical Association
200 Westboro Rd.
North Grafton, MA 01536

Michigan
Licensing Administrator
Board of Veterinary Medicine
Department of Commerce
P.O. Box 30018
611 W. Ottawa
Lansing, MI 48909

Minnesota
Veterinary Technician Committee
Minnesota Veterinary Medical Association
2469 University Avenue West
St. Paul, MN 55114

Mississippi
Executive Secretary
Board of Veterinary Medicine
209 S. Lafayette St.
Starkville, MS 39759

Missouri
Executive Director
Veterinary Medical Board
P.O. Box 633
Jefferson City, MO 65102

Montana
Board of Veterinary Medicine
Department of Commerce
Lower Level, Arcade Building
111 N. Last Chance Gulch
Helena, MT 59620

Nebraska
Associate Director
Bureau of Examining Boards
Department of Health
P.O. Box 95007
301 Centennial Mall South
Lincoln, NE 68509

Nevada
Executive Officer
Board of Veterinary Medical Examines
Executive Plaza
Suite 246
1005 Terminal Way
Reno, NV 89502

New Hampshire
Secretary-Treasurer
Board of Veterinary Medicine
P.O. Box 2042
Concord, NH 03302-2042

New Jersey
Board of Veterinary Medical Examiners
P.O. Box 45020
Newark, NJ 07101

New Mexico
Executive Director
Board of Veterinary Examiners
Suite 400-C
1650 University Blvd. NE
Albuquerque, NM 87102

New York
Executive Secretary
Board of Veterinary Medical Examiners
Room 3043
Cultural Education Center
Albany, NY 12230

North Carolina
Executive Director
Veterinary Medical Board
P.O. Box 12587
Raleigh, NC 27605

North Dakota
Executive Secretary
Veterinary Medical Examining Board
c/o North Dakota Board of Animal Health
J-Wing, First Floor
State Capitol
600 E. Boulevard Ave.
Bismarck, ND 58505-0390

Ohio
Executive Secretary
Veterinary Medical Licensing Board
16th Floor
77 S. High St.
Columbus, OH 43266-0116

Oklahoma
Executive Officer
Board of Veterinary Medical Examiners
P.O. Box 54556
Oklahoma City, OK 73154

Oregon
Executive Secretary
Veterinary Medical Examining Board
Suite 407
800 NE Oregon St.
#21
Portland, OR 97232

Pennsylvania
Chairman
Board of Veterinary Medicine
P.O. Box 2649
Harrisburg, PA 17105-2649

Rhode Island
Administrator
Division of Professional Regulation
Department of Health
Room 104
3 Capitol Hill
Providence, RI 02908

South Carolina
Administrator
Board of Veterinary Medical Examiners
P.O. Box 11329
Columbia, SC 29211-1329

South Dakota
Executive Secretary
Board of Veterinary Medical Examiners
411 S. Fort St.
Pierre, SD 57501

Tennessee
Administrator
Board of Veterinary Medical Examiners
283 Plus Park Blvd.
Nashville, TN 37217

Texas
Executive Director
Board of Veterinary Medical Examiners
Suite 306
1946 South IH-35
Austin, TX 78704-3644

Utah
Assistant Director
Division of Occupational and Professional Licensing
P.O. Box 45805
160 East 300 South
Salt Lake City, Utah 84145-0805

Vermont
State Veterinary Board
Office of Professional Regulations
109 State St.
Montpelier, VT 05609-1106

Virginia
Executive Officer
Board of Veterinary Medicine
Fourth Floor
6606 W. Broad St.
Richmond, VA 23230-1717

Washington
Program Manager
Veterinary Board of Governors
1300 SE Quince
Olympia, WA 98504-7866

West Virginia
Executive Secretary
Board of Veterinary Medicine
1900 Kanawha Blvd.
East Charleston, WV 25303-0119

Wisconsin
Bureau Director
Veterinary Examining Board
P.O. Box 8935
Madison, WI 53708

Wyoming
Executive Officer
Board of Veterinary Medicine
Herschler Building
Cheyenne, WY 82002

Canada

Technicians interested in practicing in Canadian provinces should contact the following regulatory agencies:

Alberta
Sectetary-Treasurer and Registrar
Board of Veterinary Medical Examiners
#100
8615 149th St.
Edmonton, Alberta T5R 1B3

British Columbia
Board of Veterinary Medical Examiners
Suite 155
1200 W. 73rd Ave.
Vancouver, British Columbia V6P 6G5

Manitoba
Registrar
Veterinary Medical Board
Agricultural Services Complex
545 University Crescent
Winnipeg, Manitoba R3T 5S6

New Brunswick
Secretary-Treasurer and Registrar
Board of Veterinary Medical Examiners
P.O. Box 1065
Moncton, New Brunswick E1C 8P2

Nova Scotia
Executive Officer
15 Cobe Quid Rd.
Lower Sackville, Nova Scotia B4C 2M9

Ontario
Registrar
College of Veterinarians
RR3
2106 Gordan St.
Guelph, Ontario N1H 6H9

Quebec
General Director and Secretary
Board of Veterinary Medical Examiners
Suite 200
795 Avenue du Palais
St. Hyacinthe, Quebec J2S 5C6

Saskatchewan
Secretary-Treasurer and Registrar
Board of Veterinary Medical Examiners
Unit 104
112 Research Dr.
Saskatoon, Saskatchewan S7N 3R3

Introduction

Review Questions & Answers for Veterinary Technicians, second edition covers every major aspect of veterinary technology. Over 2,400 multiple-choice questions, nearly all of which are new since the first edition, are divided into 13 general subject areas.

Subjects covered

Anatomy and physiology questions take a system-oriented approach to the structure and function of the bodies of common domestic animal species. Topics include cells and tissues; the skeletal, integumentary, circulatory, respiratory, digestive, nervous, muscular, sensory, endocrine, urinary, and reproductive systems; and the mammary glands and lactation.

The **anesthesiology** section includes questions on preanesthetic and anesthetic drugs, anesthesia machines, endotracheal intubation, patient monitoring, and anesthetic emergencies.

The **animal care** questions cover topics such as restraint and handling, housing, exercise, nutrition, and sanitation.

The **clinical laboratory** section covers topics that relate to the many laboratory analyses and examinations commonly performed in veterinary medicine. Topics include collection, handling, and storage of laboratory samples, hematology, parasitology, urinalysis, blood chemistry, microbiology, cytology, immunology, and quality control.

The **dentistry** section includes questions on dental instrument identification and handling, patient preparation, normal dentition, and dental prophylaxis and treatment.

Emergency care topics include emergency assessment, first aid, and critical care principles and procedures.

The section on **hospital management** includes questions on record keeping and filing systems, as well as ethics and jurisprudence.

Medical mathematics cover calculations common to veterinary technology. Subjects include the metric system, weights and measures, and solution preparation.

Topics included in the **medical nursing** section are animal breeds, normal physiologic values, drug administration, fluid therapy, bandaging and splints, inflammation and wound healing, disease control, physical examination, and public health and zoonoses.

Medical terminology questions cover the language of medicine including prefixes, suffixes, and combining forms.

The **pharmacology** section covers drug-related topics such as dose calculations, classifications, handling, dispensing, and adverse reactions.

Radiography topics include x-ray machines, equipment, and film; imaging principles and procedures; safety, animal-positioning, darkroom, and special radiographic procedures; and quality control.

The **surgical nursing** section includes questions on surgical instruments, suture materials and needles, basic suturing, surgical terminology, and aseptic technique.

How to use this book

The primary intent of this book is to help technicians prepare for examinations—either in academic programs or, after graduation, for credentialing (certification, licensing) purposes. Before beginning a section, review texts and course notes pertaining to that subject area; then approach each section as though it were an actual examination.

> *Carefully read each question.* Look for key words such as "most," "best," "least," "always," "never," and "except." Consider only the facts presented in the question. Do not make assumptions and inferences that may not be true.

> *Carefully evaluate each answer choice.* Each question has only one correct answer. The other three answers are incorrect "distractors." If more than one answer choice appears to be correct, closely examine each one for clues that would eliminate it as incorrect.

> *Select an answer for each question.* Circle the letter preceding your answer choice. If you do not wish to mark in the book, use the blank answer sheets in the back of the book for practice tests.

> *Compare your answers with the correct answers.* The correct answers are listed at the end of each section. Many are accompanied by an explanation.

> *Identify "weak" areas.* Subject areas with many incorrect answers may indicate the need for further review. References in the recommended reading lists at the beginning of each section may be helpful starting points.

Contents

Anatomy and Physiology

Thomas Colville, DVM, MSc
Kerry L. Coombs, DVM
Patricia Creamer, CAHT

Jean Holtzen, CVT
Mary Lou Shea, CAHT
George W. Younger, DVM

Recommended Reading

Cullor JS, Tyler JW, Smith BP: Disorders of the mammary gland. In Smith BP, editor: *Large animal internal medicine*, St Louis, 1990, Mosby.

Cunningham JG: *Textbook of veterinary physiology*, Philadelphia, 1992. WB Saunders.

Dyce KM, Sack WO, Wensing CJG: *Textbook of veterinary anatomy*, Philadelphia, 1987, WB Saunders.

Frandson RD: *Anatomy and physiology of farm animals*, ed 5, Philadelphia, 1992, Lea & Febiger.

Getty R, editor: *Sisson and Grossman's The anatomy of the domestic animals*, ed 5, Philadelphia, 1975, WB Saunders.

Guyton AC: *Textbook of medical physiology*, ed 7, Philadelphia, 1986, WB Saunders.

McCurnin DM: *Clinical textbook for veterinary technicians*, ed 3, Philadelphia, 1994, WB Saunders.

Nicpone–Marieb E: *Human anatomy and physiology*, ed 2, Redwood City Calif, 1992, Benjamin/Cummings

Pasquini C, Spurgeon T: *Anatomy of domestic animals: systemic and regional approach*, Pilot Point Tex, 1992, Sudz Publishing.

Reece O: *Physiology of domestic animals*, Philadelphia, 1991, Lea & Febiger.

Smallwood J: *A guided tour of veterinary anatomy*, Philadelphia, 1992, WB Saunders.

Swenson MJ, editor: *Duke's Physiology of domestic animals*, ed 10, Ithaca NY, 1984, Cornell University Press.

Stashak TS, editor: *Adams' Lameness in horses*, Philadelphia, 1987, Lea & Febiger.

Practice answer sheet is on page 313.

Correct answers are on pages 32–43.

Questions

Cells and Tissues

1. The nucleus is an essential component of all body cells *except* for
   a. Liver cells
   b. Immature red blood cells
   c. Kidney cells
   d. Mature red blood cells

2. The cell membrane that surrounds tissue cells is made up of
   a. Two lipid layers surrounding a protein layer
   b. Two protein layers surrounding a lipid layer
   c. An outer protein layer and an inner lipid layer
   d. An outer lipid layer and an inner protein layer

For questions 3 through 6, select the cell component listed below that is primarily responsible for the function described in the question.

   a. Golgi apparatus
   b. Mitochondria
   c. Nucleolus
   d. Granular (rough) endoplasmic reticulum

3. Protein synthesis

4. Energy supply for various cell processes

5. Concentration and packaging of secretory products

6. Ribonucleic acid (RNA) production

7. Which of the following functions of the epithelium is indicated when stratified squamous epithelium is highly keratinized?
   a. Absorption
   b. Secretion
   c. Excretion
   d. Protection

8. The lining epithelium of blood vessels is called
   a. Mesothelium
   b. Myoepithelium
   c. Endothelium
   d. Exothelium

9. Which type of epithelium lines the upper portion of the respiratory system and plays an important role in the body's defense mechanism?
   a. Pseudostratified ciliated columnar epithelium
   b. Stratified columnar epithelium
   c. Simple cuboidal epithelium
   d. Stratified squamous epithelium

10. The type of epithelial cell capable of significant variation in shape, depending on changes in the size of the organ that it lines, is called a
   a. Squamous epithelium
   b. Columnar epithelium
   c. Transitional epithelium
   d. Cuboidal epithelium

11. The mineral *most* important for normal contraction of striated muscle fibers is
   a. Phosphorus
   b. Iron
   c. Calcium
   d. Magnesium

12. Cardiac muscle fibers can be identified by
   a. The presence of cross striations and peripheral nuclei
   b. The absence of cross striations and the presence of central nuclei
   c. The absence of cross striations and the presence of peripheral nuclei
   d. The presence of cross striations and central nuclei

13. The junctions between adjacent cardiac muscle fibers are called
    a. Terminal bars
    b. Intercalated disks
    c. Motor end plates
    d. Synapses

14. Regeneration of cardiac muscle fibers following injury
    a. Is possible when the nucleus and part of the cytoplasm are preserved
    b. Occurs through mitotic division of fibers
    c. Does not occur
    d. Occurs from perivascular connective tissue cells

15. Peritoneum, pleura, and pericardium consist of a flattened arrangement of
    a. Adipose tissue covered by a layer of mesothelium
    b. Hyaline cartilage covered by a layer of endothelium
    c. Loose connective tissue covered by a layer of endothelium
    d. Loose connective tissue covered by a layer of mesothelium

CIRCULATORY SYSTEM

16. The apex of the heart is normally positioned
    a. Caudal and to the left
    b. Caudal and to the right
    c. Cranial and to the left
    d. Cranial and to the right

17. Which cardiac chamber receives blood from the systemic veins?
    a. Left atrium
    b. Left ventricle
    c. Right atrium
    d. Right ventricle

18. The valve that prevents blood from flowing back into the left atrium during ventricular systole is the
    a. Aortic
    b. Mitral
    c. Pulmonary
    d. Tricuspid

19. The cardiac chamber that pumps blood into the pulmonary artery is the
    a. Left atrium
    b. Left ventricle
    c. Right atrium
    d. Right ventricle

20. The valve that prevents blood from flowing back into the left ventricle during ventricular diastole is the
    a. Aortic
    b. Mitral
    c. Pulmonary
    d. Tricuspid

21. The second heart sound is produced by
    a. Closure of the aortic and pulmonary valves
    b. Closure of the mitral and tricuspid valves
    c. Closure of the aortic and mitral valves
    d. Closure of the mitral and pulmonary valves

22. Which vessel normally carries carbon dioxide–rich blood?
    a. Aorta
    b. Pulmonary vein
    c. Umbilical vein
    d. Vena cava

23. Which of the following organs is *not* essential to life?
    a. Heart
    b. Liver
    c. Pancreas
    d. Spleen

24. The most numerous type of blood cell is the
    a. Basophil
    b. Monocyte
    c. Neutrophil
    d. Red blood cell

25. Which of the following white blood cells is *not* a granulocyte?
    a. Basophil
    b. Eosinophil
    c. Monocyte
    d. Neutrophil

Correct answers are on pages 32–43.

26. For which blood cell is phagocytosis the main function?
    a. Basophil
    b. Eosinophil
    c. Monocyte
    d. Red blood cell

27. Chordae tendineae are present on which valve?
    a. Aortic
    b. Lymphatic
    c. Mitral
    d. Pulmonary

28. The mitral valve of the heart is the
    a. Left atrioventricular valve
    b. Left ventricular outflow valve
    c. Right atrioventricular valve
    d. Right ventricular outflow valve

29. The valve that prevents blood from flowing back into the right ventricle at the end of ventricular systole is the
    a. Aortic
    b. Mitral
    c. Pulmonary
    d. Tricuspid

30. Which blood vessel normally carries oxygen-rich blood?
    a. Aorta
    b. Pulmonary artery
    c. Umbilical artery
    d. Vena cava

31. Which lymphoid organ normally is prominent *only* in young animals?
    a. Gut-associated lymphatic tissue
    b. Spleen
    c. Thymus
    d. Tonsil

32. The least numerous type of blood cell is normally the
    a. Basophil
    b. Eosinophil
    c. Lymphocyte
    d. Monocyte

33. Blood vessels that are the site of transfer of nutrients between the blood and tissues are the
    a. Arteries
    b. Arterioles
    c. Capillaries
    d. Veins

34. The circulatory system is lined by what kind of epithelium?
    a. Simple columnar
    b. Simple squamous
    c. Stratified squamous
    d. Transitional

35. Which vessels contain valves?
    a. Arterioles
    b. Capillaries
    c. Lymph capillaries
    d. Medium-sized veins

36. The heart chamber that pumps blood to the lungs is the
    a. Left atrium
    b. Left ventricle
    c. Right atrium
    d. Right ventricle

37. The heart chamber that receives blood from the pulmonary veins is the
    a. Left atrium
    b. Left ventricle
    c. Right atrium
    d. Right ventricle

38. The heart chamber that pumps blood through the aorta is the
    a. Left atrium
    b. Left ventricle
    c. Right atrium
    d. Right ventricle

39. The valve between the right atrium and right ventricle of the heart is the
    a. Aortic
    b. Mitral
    c. Pulmonary
    d. Tricuspid

40. The valve at the outflow tract of the right ventricle is the
    a. Aortic
    b. Mitral
    c. Pulmonary
    d. Tricuspid

41. The right atrioventricular valve is the
    a. Aortic
    b. Mitral
    c. Pulmonary
    d. Tricuspid

42. The left ventricular outflow valve is the
    a. Aortic
    b. Mitral
    c. Pulmonary
    d. Tricuspid

43. The first heart sound is produced by
    a. Closure of the left and right atrioventricular valves
    b. Closure of the pulmonary and aortic valves
    c. Contraction of the left and right atria
    d. Contraction of the left and right ventricles

44. The bundle of His is located in what part of the heart?
    a. Interventricular septum
    b. Left and right ventricular walls
    c. Right atrial wall
    d. Apex of the heart

45. The blood vessel that shunts blood from the pulmonary artery to the aorta in a fetus is the
    a. Ductus arteriosus
    b. Foramen ovale
    c. Umbilical artery
    d. Umbilical vein

46. The main component of the tunica media of muscular arteries is
    a. Cardiac muscle fibers
    b. Elastic fibers
    c. Skeletal muscle fibers
    d. Smooth muscle fibers

47. The pulmonary valve prevents blood from flowing back into the
    a. Left atrium
    b. Right atrium
    c. Left ventricle
    d. Right ventricle

48. The mitral valve prevents blood from flowing back into the
    a. Left atrium
    b. Right atrium
    c. Left ventricle
    d. Right ventricle

49. The aortic valve prevents blood from flowing back into the
    a. Left atrium
    b. Right atrium
    c. Left ventricle
    d. Right ventricle

50. The tricuspid valve prevents blood from flowing back into the
    a. Left atrium
    b. Right atrium
    c. Left ventricle
    d. Right ventricle

51. Each cardiac cycle in a normal heart results from an impulse that is initiated in the
    a. Atrioventricular node
    b. Bundle of His
    c. Purkinje fibers
    d. Sinoatrial node

52. The ductus arteriosus in a fetus joins the
    a. Aorta and pulmonary artery
    b. Aorta and pulmonary vein
    c. Vena cava and pulmonary artery
    d. Vena cava and pulmonary vein

53. The valve that prevents blood from flowing back into the left ventricle at the end of ventricular systole is the
    a. Aortic
    b. Mitral
    c. Pulmonary
    d. Tricuspid

Correct answers are on pages 32–43.

54. The Purkinje fibers in the heart are located in the
    a. Interventricular septum
    b. Left and right ventricular walls
    c. Right atrial wall
    d. Apex of the heart

55. Blood that has returned to the heart through the cranial and caudal venae cavae passes through which heart valve first?
    a. Aortic
    b. Mitral
    c. Pulmonary
    d. Tricuspid

56. The right atrium receives blood from which blood vessel?
    a. Aorta
    b. Pulmonary artery
    c. Pulmonary vein
    d. Vena cava

57. Which heart chamber pumps blood to the systemic circulation?
    a. Left atrium
    b. Left ventricle
    c. Right atrium
    d. Right ventricle

58. The left atrium receives blood from which blood vessel?
    a. Aorta
    b. Pulmonary artery
    c. Pulmonary vein
    d. Vena cava

59. Which structure of the fetal heart largely allows blood to bypass the pulmonary circulation?
    a. Foramen magnum
    b. Foramen ovale
    c. Nutrient foramen
    d. Obturator foramen

60. The large lymphoid organ that stores blood but is *not* essential to life is the
    a. Kidney
    b. Liver
    c. Pancreas
    d. Spleen

61. Which blood cell is most important in plugging leaks in damaged blood vessels?
    a. Lymphocyte
    b. Neutrophil
    c. Platelet
    d. Red blood cell

62. Which of the following is *not* a feature of the right side of the heart?
    a. Atrium
    b. Chordae tendineae
    c. Pulmonary valve
    d. Mitral valve

63. The first cardiac chamber that blood enters after returning from the lungs is the
    a. Left atrium
    b. Left ventricle
    c. Right atrium
    d. Right ventricle

64. What are the effects of parasympathetic nervous system stimulation on the heart?
    a. Decreased rate and decreased force of contractions
    b. Decreased rate and increased force of contractions
    c. Increased rate and decreased force of contractions
    d. Increased rate and increased force of contractions

65. The foramen ovale in the developing fetus allows blood to flow
    a. From the left atrium to the right atrium
    b. From the right atrium to the left atrium
    c. From the left ventricle to the right ventricle
    d. From the right ventricle to the left ventricle

66. Which body fluid *cannot* clot?
    a. Plasma
    b. Serum
    c. Whole blood
    d. All of these can clot

67. Which blood cell normally contains red-staining granules in its cytoplasm?
    a. Basophil
    b. Eosinophil
    c. Monocyte
    d. Neutrophil

68. Which blood cell normally has a single large nucleus that occupies most of the cell and is important in immunity production?
    a. Eosinophil
    b. Lymphocyte
    c. Monocyte
    d. Neutrophil

69. Which structures are listed in the order in which encountered by a blood cell?
    a. Arteries, veins, capillaries, heart
    b. Capillaries, veins, heart, arteries
    c. Heart, veins, capillaries, arteries
    d. Veins, capillaries, arteries, heart

70. Which vessel brings freshly oxygenated blood from the placenta to a developing fetus?
    a. Ductus arteriosus
    b. Pulmonary vein
    c. Umbilical artery
    d. Umbilical vein

71. Which blood cell normally has a multi-lobed nucleus?
    a. Eosinophil
    b. Lymphocyte
    c. Platelet
    d. Red blood cell

DIGESTIVE SYSTEM

72. Which of the following is *not* one of the main functions of the digestive system?
    a. Absorption
    b. Digestion
    c. Mastication
    d. Secretion

73. The digestive system of herbivores
    a. Contains an enlarged microbial fermentation vat
    b. Is generally simpler and narrower than that of carnivores
    c. Is made to handle both plant and animal food sources
    d. Relies mainly on enzymatic digestion

74. From the stomach to the anus, the digestive tube is lined by what kind of epithelium?
    a. Simple columnar
    b. Simple squamous
    c. Stratified columnar
    d. Stratified squamous

75. Most of a tooth is made up of what connective tissue?
    a. Bone
    b. Cementum
    c. Dentin
    d. Enamel

76. The most rostral teeth in the dental arcade are the
    a. Canines
    b. Incisors
    c. Molars
    d. Premolars

77. The smallest ruminant forestomach, and the one most commonly involved in *hardware disease*, is the
    a. Abomasum
    b. Omasum
    c. Reticulum
    d. Rumen

Correct answers are on pages 32–43.

78. The true stomach of the ruminant is the
    a. Abomasum
    b. Omasum
    c. Reticulum
    d. Rumen

79. The most distal short portion of the small intestine just before it joins the large intestine is the
    a. Duodenum
    b. Ileum
    c. Ilium
    d. Jejunum

80. The longest portion of the large intestine is the
    a. Cecum
    b. Colon
    c. Jejunum
    d. Rectum

81. The root of a tooth is normally covered by
    a. Cartilage
    b. Cementum
    c. Dentin
    d. Enamel

82. The most caudal teeth are the
    a. Canines
    b. Incisors
    c. Molars
    d. Premolars

83. The surface area of the small intestinal lining is increased by
    a. Gyri
    b. Papillae
    c. Rugae
    d. Villi

84. The organ that has endocrine functions and also produces many digestive enzymes is the
    a. Liver
    b. Pancreas
    c. Spleen
    d. Thymus

85. The largest ruminant forestomach is the
    a. Abomasum
    b. Omasum
    c. Reticulum
    d. Rumen

86. The crown of a tooth is covered by
    a. Cementum
    b. Dentin
    c. Enamel
    d. Serosa

87. The cranial cheek teeth are the
    a. Canines
    b. Incisors
    c. Molars
    d. Premolars

88. The ruminant forestomach that dehydrates and grinds feed is the
    a. Abomasum
    b. Omasum
    c. Reticulum
    d. Rumen

89. The most proximal, short portion of the small intestine is the
    a. Cecum
    b. Duodenum
    c. Ileum
    d. Jejunum

90. The longest portion of the small intestine, where most absorption of nutrients occurs, is the
    a. Cecum
    b. Duodenum
    c. Ileum
    d. Jejunum

91. The opening of the esophagus into the stomach is called the
    a. Cardia
    b. Fundus
    c. Pylorus
    d. Ruga

92. The blind-ended sac that is part of the large intestine is the
    a. Cecum
    b. Colon
    c. Duodenum
    d. Rectum

93. The exocrine secretion of the pancreas contains large amounts of
    a. Bile
    b. Digestive enzymes
    c. Hydrochloric acid
    d. Mucus

94. The largest gland in the normal animal body is the
    a. Liver
    b. Pancreas
    c. Spleen
    d. Thymus

95. The vein that carries nutrient-rich blood from the intestines to the liver is the
    a. Ductus arteriosus
    b. Portal vein
    c. Pulmonary vein
    d. Vena cava

96. The outermost layer of the digestive tube is the
    a. Mucosa
    b. Muscle layer
    c. Serosa
    d. Submucosa

97. Which of the following lists all the digestive structures lined by simple columnar epithelium?
    a. Anus, duodenum, ileum, stomach
    b. Cecum, colon, jejunum, stomach
    c. Colon, esophagus, ileum, stomach
    d. Duodenum, jejunum, ileum, pancreas

98. Which of the following is *not* secreted by gastric glands?
    a. Acid
    b. Chyme
    c. Digestive enzymes
    d. Mucus

99. The process or structure in a newborn ruminant animal that allows milk to bypass the rumen and reticulum and go directly to the omasum is the
    a. Eructation
    b. Esophageal groove
    c. Reticular folds
    d. Rumination

100. Which of the following is *not* part of the large intestine?
    a. Cecum
    b. Colon
    c. Ileum
    d. Rectum

101. Villi are prominent in the lining of which structure?
    a. Esophagus
    b. Large intestine
    c. Small intestine
    d. Stomach

102. Which of the following is *not* a normal function of the liver in an adult animal?
    a. Bile secretion
    b. Blood cell formation
    c. Destruction of old red blood cells
    d. Protein synthesis

103. The correct term for the chewing of food is
    a. Eructation
    b. Mastication
    c. Prehension
    d. Rumination

104. In which animal is microbial fermentation most important in the digestive process?
    a. Cat
    b. Dog
    c. Horse
    d. Pig

105. The inner lining of the digestive tube is called the
    a. Mucosa
    b. Muscularum
    c. Serosa
    d. Submucosa

Correct answers are on pages 32–43.

106. The teeth that are *not* present in all common domestic animals are the
  a. Canines
  b. Incisors
  c. Premolars
  d. Molars

107. The common passageway of the respiratory and digestive systems is the
  a. Esophagus
  b. Larynx
  c. Pharynx
  d. Trachea

108. Which fluid contributes *least* to the process of digestion?
  a. Bile
  b. Pancreatic juice
  c. Saliva
  d. Stomach gland secretions

109. In which structure does *no* significant digestion or absorption take place?
  a. Esophagus
  b. Large intestine
  c. Small intestine
  d. Stomach

110. The periodic elimination of excess gas from the ruminant forestomach is termed
  a. Eructation
  b. Mastication
  c. Prehension
  d. Rumination

111. The portal vein carries nutrient-rich blood from the intestines to the
  a. Liver
  b. Pancreas
  c. Spleen
  d. Stomach

ENDOCRINE SYSTEM

112. What gland is also called the *master gland*?
  a. Thyroid
  b. Adrenal
  c. Pituitary
  d. Thymus

113. The anterior pituitary gland secretes
  a. Antidiuretic hormone (ADH)
  b. Insulin
  c. Oxytocin
  d. Follicle-stimulating hormone (FSH)

114. The adrenal glands produce
  a. Insulin
  b. Glucocorticoids
  c. Parathormone
  d. Calcitonin

115. The pancreas produces
  a. Thyroxine
  b. Prolactin
  c. Insulin
  d. Progesterone

116. Which gland regulates most of the endocrine system?
  a. Thyroid
  b. Pancreas
  c. Thymus
  d. Pituitary

117. What hormones are produced by the thyroid gland?
  a. Thyroxine and insulin
  b. Parahormone and thyroxine
  c. Calcitonin and insulin
  d. Thyroxine and calcitonin

118. What hormone stimulates milk letdown?
  a. Testosterone
  b. Epinephrine
  c. Oxytocin
  d. Relaxin

119. Where is the thyroid gland located?
  a. At the base of the brain
  b. Adjacent to the trachea
  c. Adjacent to the cranial end of each kidney
  d. At the duodenal loop

120. What are exocrine glands?
    a. Glands whose secretory products are transported via ducts
    b. Glands whose secretory products enter the bloodstream
    c. Sweat glands
    d. Salivary glands

121. Hypoadrenocorticism is commonly referred to as
    a. Cushing's disease
    b. Addison's disease
    c. Bang's disease
    d. Carre's disease

122. The adrenal medulla secretes
    a. Thyroxine
    b. Estrogen
    c. Progesterone
    d. Epinephrine

123. Which substance is required for production of thyroid hormones?
    a. Insulin
    b. Epinephrine
    c. Iodine
    d. Sodium

124. Which clinical sign is associated with hyperthyroidism?
    a. Loss of weight, with a normal or increased appetite
    b. Lethargy
    c. Decreased tolerance of cold
    d. Decreased metabolic rate

125. An appreciable enlargement of the thyroid gland is termed
    a. Hypothyroidism
    b. Goiter
    c. Parathyroidism
    d. Hypotropism

126. When one hormone increases the activity of another hormone, the effect is termed
    a. Potentiation
    b. Antagonism
    c. Doubling
    d. Nullification

127. The abbreviation ACTH stands for
    a. Acidic color train hormone
    b. Anterior control trophic hormone
    c. Adrenocorticotropic hormone
    d. Adrenal control trophic hormone

128. The most important function of ADH is to
    a. Assist glucose in crossing into body cells
    b. Stimulate parturition
    c. Increase production of thyroid hormone
    d. Help control water loss from the kidney

129. Following coitus, which hormone (that also aids in fetal expulsion) is believed to stimulate uterine contraction and thereby aid transport of sperm to the oviducts?
    a. Oxytocin
    b. Progesterone
    c. Testosterone
    d. FSH

130. Where are the adrenal glands located?
    a. Base of the brain
    b. In the neck
    c. Near the kidneys
    d. Caudal to the eyes

131. Parathyroid hormone is one of the major factors controlling the blood level of
    a. Iodine
    b. Magnesium
    c. Chloride
    d. Calcium

132. The number of parathyroid glands in all species is
    a. 2
    b. 4
    c. 10
    d. Variable

Correct answers are on pages 32–43.

133. The disease caused by a lack of insulin or the body's inability to use insulin is
    a. Diabetes mellitus
    b. Diabetes insipidus
    c. Addison's disease
    d. Cushing's disease

134. Insulin is produced by the beta cells in the islets of Langerhans. What is produced by the alpha cells?
    a. Thyroxine
    b. Glucagon
    c. Estrogen
    d. Calcium

135. What type of hormone transmission uses interstitial fluid to diffuse the hormone through the body?
    a. Endocrine
    b. Neurocrine
    c. Paracrine
    d. Exocrine

136. Which is *not* a classification of endocrine hormones, either by its chemical structure or by its nature of action?
    a. Pancreatic juice
    b. Polypeptide (protein)
    c. Steroid
    d. Amine

INTEGUMENTARY SYSTEM

137. The epithelium is
    a. Simple squamous, keratinized
    b. Simple squamous, nonkeratinized
    c. Stratified squamous, keratinized
    d. Stratified squamous, nonkeratinized

138. The sweat glands are
    a. Compound alveolar
    b. Compound tubular
    c. Simple alveolar
    d. Simple tubular

139. The wall of the hoof grows distally from the
    a. Coronary band
    b. Chestnut
    c. Frog
    d. Periople

140. Which hoof structure normally has the firmest consistency?
    a. Frog
    b. Periople
    c. Sole
    d. Wall

141. The sebaceous glands of the skin are
    a. Compound alveolar
    b. Compound tubular
    c. Simple alveolar
    d. Simple tubular

142. Which of the following is *not* a skin gland?
    a. Mammary
    b. Salivary
    c. Sebaceous
    d. Sudoriferous

143. Which statement concerning the dermis is most accurate?
    a. It contains blood vessels.
    b. Its deepest layer contains pigment cells.
    c. It is composed of stratified squamous epithelium.
    d. Its surface is keratinized.

144. A hair is produced by the
    a. Bulb
    b. Epidermis
    c. Follicle
    d. Root

145. Which structure is located most proximally on a horse's leg?
    a. Chestnut
    b. Coronary band
    c. Ergot
    d. Frog

146. Which of the following is *not* a function of the integument?
    a. Secretion and excretion
    b. Sensation
    c. Synthesis of vitamin E
    d. Temperature regulation

147. The oil glands of the skin are the
   a. Anal glands
   b. Mammary glands
   c. Sebaceous glands
   d. Sudoriferous glands

148. The portion of a hair that is visible above the skin surface is the
   a. Bulb
   b. Follicle
   c. Root
   d. Shaft

149. If a hair is pigmented, the pigment granules are present in which layer?
   a. Cortex
   b. Cuticle
   c. Medulla
   d. Periople

150. The arrector pili muscles are attached to
   a. Guard hairs
   b. Hair beds
   c. Hair clusters
   d. Wool hairs

151. Which of the following is a sweat gland?
   a. Mammary
   b. Salivary
   c. Sebaceous
   d. Sudoriferous

152. Which statement concerning the epidermis is most accurate?
   a. It contains blood vessels.
   b. Its surface layer contains pigment cells.
   c. It is composed of stratified squamous epithelium.
   d. Its surface layer is made up of living cells.

153. Which statement concerning the skin is *least* accurate?
   a. It is involved in synthesis of vitamin D.
   b. It is the largest organ in the body.
   c. Its underlayer (dermis) consists of epithelial and connective tissues.
   d. The epidermis is its more superficial layer.

154. The portion of a hair beneath the skin surface is called the
   a. Bulb
   b. Follicle
   c. Root
   d. Shaft

155. When a horse is standing on firm ground, the only portion of its hoof that normally contacts the ground is the
   a. Coronary band
   b. Sole
   c. Wall
   d. White line

156. The epidermis of the skin is composed of which kind of epithelium?
   a. Simple squamous, keratinized
   b. Simple squamous, nonkeratinized
   c. Stratified squamous, keratinized
   d. Stratified squamous, nonkeratinized

MAMMARY GLANDS AND LACTATION

Questions 157 through 160

The number of teats on the mammary glands of different animals varies. List the correct number of teats for each species.

   a. 2
   b. 4
   c. 12
   d. 14

157. Mare

158. Cow

159. Sow

160. Rat

161. The suspensory apparatus of the udder includes the
   a. Symphyseal tendon
   b. Urethralis muscle
   c. Deep digital flexor tendon
   d. Proximal digital annular ligament

Correct answers are on pages 32–43.

162. In cows, the "milk vein" is the
    a. External pudendal
    b. Femoral
    c. Lateral thoracic
    d. Subcutaneous abdominal

163. Colostrum provides the neonate with
    a. Immunoglobulins
    b. Erythrocytes
    c. Granulocytes
    d. Glucocorticoids

164. Production of colostrum is initiated by
    a. Specialized endothelial cells
    b. The fetus
    c. A response to hormonal influences
    d. The portal hepatic system

165. Colostrum provides which type of immunity?
    a. Active
    b. Passive
    c. Cellular
    d. Acquired

166. In cows, production of colostrum begins
    a. During the last 2 to 3 weeks of gestation
    b. When the calf suckles
    c. During the first postparturient estrous cycle
    d. During the first trimester of pregnancy

167. The quality of a mare's colostrum can be evaluated by all of the following *except*
    a. Stickiness
    b. Specific gravity
    c. Smell
    d. Direct measurement of IgG in the fluid

168. Agalactia is
    a. A commercially produced milk replacer
    b. A disease or condition that adversely affects the dam's lactation
    c. Rejection of a newborn by the dam
    d. Blood-tinged colostrum

169. A cow with mastitis should be
    a. Milked frequently
    b. Milked from all quarters except the affected one
    c. Not milked at all
    d. Immediately sent to have her teat removed

170. The agent that aids in secretion and release of milk from the mammary gland after parturition is
    a. Oxytetracycline
    b. Progesterone
    c. Oxytocin
    d. Prednisolone

171. Which is *not* a common cause of enlarged mammary glands in horses?
    a. Mastitis
    b. Abscess
    c. Periparturient udder edema (physiologic)
    d. Tuberculosis

MUSCULAR SYSTEM

172. The principal muscle of respiration is the diaphragm. Where is it located?
    a. Between the thorax and abdomen
    b. Between the ribs
    c. At the thoracic inlet
    d. Cranial to the heart

173. In general, muscles are divided into three major groups according to their cellular structure. These are
    a. Striped, skeletal, and visceral
    b. Smooth, unstriped, and visceral
    c. Striated, smooth, and cardiac
    d. Striped, skeletal, and heart

174. What feature is unique to cardiac muscle?
    a. Tone
    b. Muscular fibers
    c. Purkinje fibers
    d. Striations

175. Which word describes the action of a muscle that moves toward the midline?
    a. Flexion
    b. Adduction
    c. Extension
    d. Abduction

176. The function of Purkinje fibers is to
    a. Hold the heart in the proper shape
    b. Maintain proper valve shape during heart contractions
    c. Transmit the signal for ventricular contractions
    d. Maintain ventricular size

177. What is the basic unit of function in a striated muscle?
    a. Dark bands
    b. Light bands
    c. Fiber
    d. Tendon

178. Which muscle is the main extensor of the elbow?
    a. Biceps brachium
    b. Triceps brachium
    c. Trapezius
    d. Brachiocephalicus

179. What is the chief action of the biceps brachium?
    a. Extension of the elbow
    b. Flexion of the elbow
    c. Adduction of the shoulder
    d. Flexion of the neck

180. A hip adductor is found on which side of the femur?
    a. Cranial
    b. Caudal
    c. Lateral
    d. Medial

181. What is the point of insertion for the four heads of the quadriceps femoris?
    a. Tibia
    b. Acetabulum
    c. Hock
    d. Elbow

182. Which abdominal muscle layer is the most superficial?
    a. External oblique
    b. Internal oblique
    c. Rectus
    d. Transversus

183. The maximum amount that a muscle fiber can contract is about what proportion of its resting length?
    a. One fourth
    b. One half
    c. Twice
    d. Four times

184. The *least* movable of the attachments of a muscle to bone is the
    a. Periosteum
    b. Origin
    c. Insertion
    d. Contracture

185. Muscles that tend to pull a limb toward the median plane are termed
    a. Flexors
    b. Extensors
    c. Adductors
    d. Abductors

186. The large muscle in the calf of the leg that flexes the stifle and extends the hock is the
    a. Gastrocnemius
    b. Biceps brachium
    c. Triceps brachium
    d. Sartorius

187. Muscles that attach to the skin and are responsible for skin movement are termed
    a. Flexors
    b. Extensors
    c. Adductors
    d. Cutaneous

188. The spasmodic muscular contractions that produce heat to help maintain normal body temperature are called
    a. Convulsions
    b. Tonus
    c. Shivering
    d. Peristalsis

Correct answers are on pages 32–43.

189. Skeletal muscles that are arranged circularly to constrict a body opening are termed
    a. Sphincters
    b. Flexors
    c. Abductors
    d. Adductors

190. Loss of nerve supply to a muscle results in
    a. Denervation hypertrophy
    b. Disuse hypertrophy
    c. Disuse hypoplasia
    d. Denervation atrophy

191. Which triangular and flat muscle originates along the dorsal midline and inserts mainly on the spine of the scapula?
    a. Biceps brachii
    b. Trapezius
    c. Deltoideus
    d. Triceps brachii

192. What muscle is the main adductor of the shoulder?
    a. Omotransversarius
    b. Brachiocephalicus
    c. Biceps brachii
    d. Pectoralis

193. The biceps femoris, semitendinosus, and semimembranosus are known collectively as the
    a. Hamstring
    b. Calf
    c. Forearm
    d. Dewlap

194. With which type of tissue is muscle attached to bone?
    a. Ligaments
    b. Fat
    c. Cartilage
    d. Tendons

195. Tendons that are flat and usually attach to flat muscles are known as
    a. Diarthroses
    b. Fasciae
    c. Arthroses
    d. Spheroses

Nervous System

196. The central nervous system encompasses which subdivisions?
    a. Brain and spinal cord
    b. Spinal nerves
    c. Sympathetic nerves
    d. All cranial nerves

197. Nerve processes that conduct impulses toward the cell bodies are referred to as
    a. Axons
    b. Cytons
    c. Somas
    d. Dendrites

198. Neurons interposed between afferent and efferent neurons are called
    a. Intercalated
    b. Internuncial
    c. Association
    d. All of these

199. From an evolutionary standpoint, which of the following is one of the oldest parts of the cerebrum? It is associated primarily with the sense of smell and is sometimes called the olfactory brain.
    a. Rhinencephalon
    b. Diencephalon
    c. Longitudinal fissure
    d. Telencephalon

200. Hydrocephalus (water on the brain) causes the cerebrum to become extremely thin and may impair or prevent parturition. The most frequent cause of this abnormality is
    a. Obstruction of the interventricular foramina
    b. Occlusion of the cerebral aquaduct
    c. A porous dura mater
    d. Fetal malpresentation

201. The ventral corticospinal tract connects the motor area of the cerebral cortex with motor cells in the ventral gray horns on the same and opposite sides of the spinal cord. The impulses are associated with
    a. Pain and temperature
    b. Pressure sensations
    c. Voluntary motor activity
    d. Tone of the extensor muscles

202. Each forelimb of animals is innervated by a brachial plexus containing cervical and thoracic nerves. In which species is the brachial plexus *not* comprised of the last 3 cervical nerves and the first thoracic nerve?
    a. Horses
    b. Cattle
    c. Pigs
    d. Dogs

203. Of the following nerves supplied by the brachial plexus, which one does *not* innervate muscles in the shoulder?
    a. Thoracodorsal
    b. Long thoracic
    c. Axillary
    d. Median

204. Which nerve (the largest peripheral nerve in the body) stimulates muscles of the thigh region (e.g., biceps femoris)?
    a. Tibial
    b. Femoral
    c. Sciatic
    d. Ulnar

205. Damage to which nerve, most commonly affected by dystocias, results in the inability to adduct the rear legs in the cow?
    a. Obturator
    b. Tibial
    c. Sciatic
    d. Radial

206. Of the 12 cranial nerves, which is a motor nerve to muscles in the shoulder and neck?
    a. Accessory
    b. Vestibulocochlear
    c. Trochlear
    d. Hypoglossal

207. Which nerve (one of the longest in the body) supplies parasympathetic fibers to the heart and lungs and to nearly all the abdominal viscera?
    a. Glossopharyngeal
    b. Facial
    c. Vagus
    d. Oculomotor

208. The most distal part of the digestive tract and most of the urogenital system are supplied with fibers from which portion of the parasympathetic nervous system?
    a. Sacral
    b. Cervical
    c. Thoracic
    d. Lumbar

209. The plasma membrane of the neuron in the resting state (electrically polarized) is very permeable to K^+ but is almost impermeable to
    a. Na^+
    b. Cl^-
    c. Ca^{++}
    d. Mg^{++}

210. When Na^+ is rushing into a nerve cell, the cell is unable to produce another action potential regardless of how strong a stimulus is applied. This time is called the
    a. Absolute refractory period
    b. Relative refractory period
    c. Threshold stimulus period
    d. Action potential period

Correct answers are on pages 32–43.

211. Which term refers to the fact that a number of axonal endings synapse on a single cell and its dendrites?
    a. Convergence
    b. Propagation
    c. Orthodromic movement
    d. Divergence

212. Cranial nerves are unique in that some are responsible for performing multiple functions. Which cranial nerve has multiple functions?
    a. Trigeminal
    b. Oculomotor
    c. Vestibulocochlear
    d. Optic

213. If an animal loses its balance and develops nystagmus, the nerve most likely to be the cause is the
    a. Abducens
    b. Auditory
    c. Optic
    d. Vagus

214. If an animal is unable to control its fall and cannot right itself, which spinal tract is most likely affected?
    a. Dorsal white columns
    b. Ventral white columns
    c. Lateral white columns
    d. Adjacent white columns

215. The condition referred to as "sweeney" results from damage to the
    a. Axillary nerve
    b. Radial nerve
    c. Suprascapular nerve
    d. Supraspinatus muscle

216. Injury to which nerve is commonly seen with dystocias in cows that have a small or juvenile pelvis?
    a. Pudendal
    b. Obturator
    c. Perineal
    d. Femoral

217. The autonomic nervous system is directly responsible for innervation of
    a. Visceral organs
    b. Lumbar muscles
    c. Triceps muscles
    d. Somatic organs

218. Parasympathetic stimulation is distributed to visceral structures by which four cranial nerves?
    a. III,V,VII,X
    b. I, III, IV, X
    c. III, VII, IX, X
    d. IX, X, XI, XII

219. Which of the following is *not* a result of sympathetic nervous system stimulation?
    a. Decreased blood pressure
    b. Increased heart rate
    c. Increased activity of the respiratory-bronchiole dilator reflex
    d. Decreased gut motility

220. The terminal part of the spinal cord is called the
    a. Tail
    b. Cauda equina
    c. Terminal dendrite
    d. Rumpalis endicus

221. *Soma* is another term for
    a. Cytoplasm
    b. Nerve cell body
    c. Nucleus
    d. Centrosome

222. Which term is applied to inflammation of the covering layers of the spinal cord?
    a. Meningitis
    b. Encephalitis
    c. Myelitis
    d. Encephalomyelitis

223. Which of the following correctly lists the number of cervical nerves and corresponding number of cervical vertebrae?
   a. 7, 8
   b. 8, 7
   c. 7, 9
   d. 9, 7

224. Which structure, whose Latin name means "little brain," is located at the caudal part of the brain and contains over half of the brain's nerves?
   a. Cerebral cortex
   b. Brainstem
   c. Medulla oblongata
   d. Cerebellum

225. Injury to which nerve results in knuckling of the forepaw onto its dorsal aspect?
   a. Median
   b. Musculocutaneous
   c. Axillary
   d. Radial

226. Complex reflexes are mediated through certain centers in the brain. The medulla oblongata contains reflex centers for all of the following *except*
   a. Heart contractions
   b. Swallowing
   c. Vomiting
   d. Knee jerk

227. Raising a horse's head prevents kicking by extending the neck, which increases the tone of the extensor muscles of the forelimbs and decreases the tone of the extensors in the hind limbs. This postural reaction is referred to as the
   a. Tonic eye reflex
   b. Extensor postural thrust
   c. Tonic neck reflex
   d. Auditory obtundation

228. Which morphine-like substance found in the thalamus and hypothalamus acts as a natural analgesic?
   a. Endorphin
   b. Epinephrine
   c. Nonepinephrine
   d. Acetylcholine

229. Any change in a nerve's environment that depolarizes the resting potential and leads to production of a nerve impulse is called
   a. An action potential
   b. The relative refractory period
   c. Repolarization
   d. A stimulus

230. What specialized structure of a neuron conducts impulses away from the cell body?
   a. Neurolemma
   b. Axon
   c. Dendrite
   d. Neuroglia

REPRODUCTIVE SYSTEM

231. What is the normal average gestation period of horses?
   a. 63 days
   b. 148 days
   c. 285 days
   d. 336 days

232. What is an ectopic pregnancy?
   a. Fetus that is born dead
   b. Short-term pregnancy
   c. Pregnancy that takes place outside the uterus
   d. Pregnancy that exists beyond the normal term

233. What two hormones influence the growth of lactating tissue?
   a. Estrogen and progesterone
   b. Estrogen and oxytocin
   c. Progesterone and oxytocin
   d. Testosterone and oxytocin

Correct answers are on pages 32–43.

234. Where is the ovum fertilized?
    a. Uterus
    b. Oviducts
    c. Vagina
    d. Cervix

235. The correct order for the stages of the estrous cycle is
    a. Proestrus, anestrus, estrus, metestrus
    b. Anestrus, estrus, proestrus, metestrus
    c. Proestrus, estrus, metestrus, anestrus
    d. Anestrus, metestrus, estrus, proestrus

236. How often does estrus occur in normal, nonpregnant cows?
    a. Every 10 to 15 days
    b. Every 19 to 23 days
    c. Every 30 to 35 days
    d. Every 285 to 290 days

237. What is the normal average gestation period of guinea pigs?
    a. 75 days
    b. 63 days
    c. 21 days
    d. 10 days

238. How long do estrus and gestation normally last in mice?
    a. 4 to 5 days (estrus), 19 to 27 days (gestation)
    b. 16 days (estrus), 59 to 72 days (gestation)
    c. 21 days (estrus), 27 days (gestation)
    d. 32 days (estrus), 63 days (gestation)

239. Which is a response to estrogen?
    a. Inducing estrus via action on the brain
    b. Decreasing blood flow to the uterus
    c. Constricting the cervix
    d. Decreasing uterine contractions

240. Which is a response to progestins?
    a. Dilating the cervix
    b. Decreasing motility of the uterine muscles
    c. Increasing blood flow to the uterus
    d. Inducing estrus via action on the brain

241. What is the main hormonal influence during proestrus?
    a. FSH
    b. Luteinizing hormone (LH)
    c. Progestins
    d. Prostaglandin

242. Which term best describes the estrous cycle of cows, and how long is their estrous cycle?
    a. Seasonally polyestrous, 21 days
    b. Seasonally polyestrous, 6 months
    c. Polyestrous, 21 days
    d. Polyestrous, 6 months

243. The greatest amount of fetal growth occurs during the
    a. First trimester
    b. Second trimester
    c. Third trimester
    d. First week of gestation

244. The germinal layer in the early embryo that is responsible for most skin development is the
    a. Mesoderm
    b. Endoderm
    c. Keratoderm
    d. Ectoderm

245. Mammary glands are found in
    a. Males only
    b. Females only
    c. Males and females
    d. Sexually mature females only

246. How many mammae do horses have?
    a. 2
    b. 4
    c. 8
    d. 12

247. Which hormone is *not* a prerequisite for lactation?
    a. Estrogen
    b. Prolactin
    c. Testosterone
    d. Progesterone

248. Where are the ovaries located?
    a. Caudal to the urinary bladder
    b. Near the diaphragm
    c. Near the kidneys
    d. At the base of the brain

249. What is the literal definition of corpus luteum (CL)?
    a. Dead body
    b. Fluid-filled body
    c. Reproducing body
    d. Yellow body

250. The funnel-like structure of the oviduct adjacent to the ovary is the
    a. Infundibulum
    b. Corpus luteum
    c. Caruncle
    d. Cervix

251. When is puberty reached?
    a. Six months of age for all species
    b. When the reproductive organs first become functional
    c. After the first act of copulation
    d. One year of age for most species

252. During, or shortly after, which stage of the estrous cycle does ovulation occur?
    a. Metestrus
    b. Proestrus
    c. Anestrus
    d. Estrus

253. What is the relatively short period of quiescence (estrous inactivity) between estrous cycles in polyestrous animals?
    a. Diestrus
    b. Anestrus
    c. Triestrus
    d. Quadestrus

254. The luteal phase of the estrous cycle includes
    a. Estrus
    b. Proestrus
    c. Metestrus
    d. Estrus and proestrus

255. Metritis is inflammation of the
    a. Uterus
    b. Mammary gland
    c. Fallopian tube
    d. Vagina

256. What is dystocia?
    a. Quiet birth
    b. Difficult birth
    c. Early birth
    d. Overdue birth

257. What is the major male sex hormone?
    a. Endorphin
    b. Estrogen
    c. Testosterone
    d. Progesterone

258. Where do spermatozoa mature?
    a. Testes
    b. Vasa deferentia
    c. Scrotum
    d. Epididymis

259. What is the term for reflex emptying of the epididymis, urethra, and accessory sex glands?
    a. Erection
    b. Ejaculation
    c. Copulation
    d. Spermatogenesis

260. Hormones with masculinizing effects are known as
    a. Gonadotropins
    b. Estrogens
    c. Progestins
    d. Androgens

261. What action is *not* associated with testosterone?
    a. Promotes development of accessory sex glands
    b. Promotes development of secondary sex characteristics
    c. Decreases protein anabolism
    d. Increases libido

Correct answers are on pages 32–43.

262. Sperm can be fertile for up to how many hours in the reproductive tract of a ewe?
- a. 2
- b. 10
- c. 48
- d. 72

263. Which gland secretes gonadotropin-releasing hormone?
- a. Anterior pituitary
- b. Hypothalamus
- c. Posterior pituitary
- d. Thyroid

264. The release of prostaglandin F2-alpha from the uterus, as a result of nonpregnancy, causes
- a. A rise in estrogen levels
- b. Signs of estrus to begin immediately
- c. The animal to sweat
- d. Lysis of the corpus luteum

265. What is the major hormonal influence during metestrus?
- a. Estrogen
- b. Progesterone
- c. Oxytocin
- d. Gonadotropin-releasing hormone

266. During what part of the estrous cycle is the female most receptive to the male?
- a. Proestrus
- b. Estrus
- c. Metestrus
- d. Anestrus or diestrus

267. When is the usual breeding season for ewes?
- a. Summer
- b. Fall
- c. Winter
- d. Spring

268. Which hormone inhibits excessive uterine motility during gestation?
- a. Prostaglandin
- b. Oxytocin
- c. Estrogen
- d. Progesterone

269. What is the normal average length of gestation in sows?
- a. 21 days
- b. 114 days
- c. 150 days
- d. 285 days

270. What is the term for the time from fertilization of the ovum until birth of the fetus?
- a. Implantation
- b. Parturition
- c. Gestation
- d. Dystocia

271. What does the term *multiparous* mean?
- a. Having given birth to viable offspring in more than one gestation
- b. Having more than one period of estrus during the year
- c. Having more than two female offspring during one gestation
- d. Having offspring sired by more than one male during one gestation

272. In ruminants, the cotyledon of the placenta attaches to what structure on the uterus to form the placentome?
- a. Zonule
- b. Allantois
- c. Mesantois
- d. Caruncle

273. Which structure produces the ovum?
- a. Ovary
- b. Uterus
- c. Fallopian tube
- d. Fimbria

274. Rupture of a follicle releases
- a. Progesterone
- b. FSH
- c. An ovum
- d. Oxytocin

275. What is another name for *fallopian tubes*?
- a. Ureters
- b. Oviducts
- c. Uterine horns
- d. Broad ligaments

276. Which structure produces LH?
    a. Hypothalamus
    b. Posterior pituitary
    c. Thyroid gland
    d. Anterior pituitary

277. LH promotes growth of the
    a. Fetus
    b. Mammary glands
    c. Uterus
    d. Corpus luteum

278. What hormone is released from the corpus luteum?
    a. Progesterone
    b. Estrogen
    c. LH
    d. FSH

279. Nymphomania is caused by
    a. Too much progesterone
    b. Not enough estrogen
    c. Cystic ovaries
    d. Too much thyroid hormone

280. Which female is an induced or reflex ovulator?
    a. Cow
    b. Bitch
    c. Mare
    d. Queen

281. In the first stage of parturition, ACTH stimulates the fetal adrenal cortex to release
    a. Hydrocortisone
    b. Estrogen
    c. Progesterone
    d. FSH

282. Which hormone results in *strong* uterine contractions?
    a. Progesterone
    b. Estrogen
    c. Prostaglandin F2-alpha
    d. Oxytocin

283. What is the normal average length of gestation in goats?
    a. 21 days
    b. 114 days
    c. 150 days
    d. 285 days

284. What is the cutaneous sac containing the testes?
    a. Epididymis
    b. Labia
    c. Sheath
    d. Scrotum

285. In what two species is cryptorchidism most prevalent?
    a. Cats and dogs
    b. Cattle and goats
    c. Horses and pigs
    d. Sheep and dogs

286. The seminal plasma of all species contains
    a. Progesterone
    b. Fructose
    c. Urine
    d. Oxytocin

287. Enlargement of which structure is responsible for prolonged retention of the penis within the vagina during coitus in canines?
    a. Prostate gland
    b. Bulbourethral glands
    c. Vasa deferentia
    d. Bulbus glandis

288. What is a photoperiod?
    a. Length of daylight and darkness
    b. Time needed for a photic reaction
    c. Time it takes for light to move a specific distance
    d. Estrus induced by light

289. Which female has ovaries that resemble a cluster of grapes because of the large number of protruding follicles?
    a. Cow
    b. Ewe
    c. Sow
    d. Mare

290. The process by which ova are formed is termed
    a. Spermatogenesis
    b. Odontogenesis
    c. Oophorosis
    d. Oogenesis

Correct answers are on pages 32–43.

291. Which is *not* a layer of the fetal placenta?
    a. Caruncle
    b. Amnion
    c. Chorion
    d. Allantois

RESPIRATORY SYSTEM

292. Most *conditioning* of inspired air occurs in the
    a. Larynx
    b. Nares
    c. Nasal passages
    d. Pharynx

293. Which of the following is *not* a function of the respiratory system?
    a. Acid-base regulation
    b. Mastication
    c. Olfaction
    d. Phonation

294. The sites in the lung where gases are exchanged between the air and the blood are the
    a. Alveoli
    b. Bifurcations
    c. Bronchi
    d. Bronchioles

295. The short, irregular tubular structure in the neck region that acts as a valve to control air flow to the lungs is the
    a. Bronchus
    b. Larynx
    c. Pharynx
    d. Trachea

296. The transfer of oxygen and carbon dioxide between the air and blood in the lungs is accomplished by
    a. Blood pressure
    b. Diffusion
    c. Ion pumps
    d. Osmosis

297. The epithelium lining the alveoli is
    a. Pseudostratified columnar
    b. Simple cuboidal
    c. Simple squamous
    d. Stratified squamous

298. The main tubular structure in the neck region that carries air to and from the lungs is the
    a. Bronchus
    b. Larynx
    c. Pharynx
    d. Trachea

299. Which structure is *not* part of the upper respiratory tract?
    a. Bronchiole
    b. Larynx
    c. Pharynx
    d. Trachea

300. When the diaphragm contracts, it
    a. Compresses the lungs
    b. Creates positive pressure in the thoracic cavity
    c. Decreases the size of the thoracic cavity
    d. Increases the size of the thoracic cavity

301. Compared with blood entering the alveolar capillaries, air drawn into the alveoli of the lungs has
    a. Higher P_{CO_2} and higher P_{CO_2}
    b. Higher P_{CO_2} and lower P_{CO_2}
    c. Lower P_{CO_2} and higher P_{CO_2}
    d. Lower P_{CO_2} and lower P_{CO_2}

302. The epithelium lining the upper respiratory tract is
    a. Pseudostratified columnar
    b. Stratified squamous
    c. Simple squamous
    d. Transitional

303. External respiration takes place
    a. At the nares
    b. In the lungs
    c. In the upper respiratory tract
    d. Throughout the body tissues

304. Which of the following is a major function of the larynx?
    a. Filtering inspired air
    b. Olfaction
    c. Phonation
    d. Warming inspired air

305. Internal respiration takes place
    a. At the nares
    b. In the lungs
    c. In the upper respiratory tract
    d. Throughout the body tissues

306. The common passageway for the respiratory and digestive systems is the
    a. Larynx
    b. Nasal passage
    c. Pharynx
    d. Trachea

307. Proceeding caudally, the trachea bifurcates into two
    a. Mainstem bronchi
    b. Primary bronchioles
    c. Alveoli
    d. Secondary bronchioles

308. Which statement concerning the respiratory system is *least* accurate?
    a. Chemical control of breathing allows for correction of imbalances in various blood constituents.
    b. Mechanical control of breathing modulates rhythmic resting respiration.
    c. The apex of the lungs is in the caudal thorax.
    d. The lungs expand passively during inspiration.

309. Which of the following lists the respiratory structures in the order through which air passes during *exhalation*?
    a. Bronchi, trachea, larynx, pharynx, nasal passages
    b. Bronchi, trachea, pharynx, larynx, nasal passages
    c. Nasal passages, larynx, pharynx, trachea, bronchi
    d. Nasal passages, pharynx, larynx, trachea, bronchi

310. Exchange of oxygen and carbon dioxide between blood and the cells and tissues is termed
    a. External respiration
    b. Internal respiration
    c. Olfaction
    d. Phonation

SENSORY SYSTEM

311. Which cranial nerve mediates the sense of smell?
    a. Oculomotor
    b. Glossopharyngeal
    c. Olfactory
    d. Hypoglossal

312. What division of the nervous system contains the cranial nerves and paired spinal nerves?
    a. CNS (central)
    b. PNS (peripheral)
    c. ANS (autonomic)
    d. VNS (vagal)

313. Which cranial nerve innervates the throat area and the heart?
    a. Glossopharyngeal
    b. Spinal accessory
    c. Abducens
    d. Vagus

314. Which of the following is a response to increased sympathetic tone?
    a. Accelerated heart rate and amplitude
    b. Constricted bronchioles
    c. Dilated blood vessels in the intestinal tract
    d. Increased gastrointestinal secretions

315. Which structure acts as a light receptor?
    a. Uvea
    b. Sclera
    c. Cone
    d. Cochlea

Correct answers are on pages 32–43.

316. Which portion of the ear is essential for hearing and equilibrium?
    a. Inner
    b. Middle
    c. External
    d. Eardrum

317. Which cranial nerve carries impulses from the ear to the brain?
    a. Acoustic (VIII)
    b. Olfactory (I)
    c. Optic (II)
    d. Vagus (X)

318. Which cranial nerve provides parasympathetic innervation to the heart, lungs, stomach, and small intestine?
    a. Trochlear (IV)
    b. Vagus (X)
    c. Abducens (VI)
    d. Trigeminal (V)

319. Birds recognize feed primarily by
    a. Sight
    b. Odor
    c. Taste
    d. Touch

320. Which structure is *not* part of a nerve cell?
    a. Axon
    b. Dendrite
    c. Monocyte
    d. Axolemma

321. Which cranial nerve conducts motor impulses to the tongue?
    a. Oculomotor (III)
    b. Trigeminal (V)
    c. Vestibulocochlear (VIII)
    d. Hypoglossal (XII)

322. Which cranial nerve provides parasympathetic innervation to the cranial three-quarters of the body?
    a. Olfactory (I)
    b. Abducens (VI)
    c. Vagus (X)
    d. Spinal accessory (XI)

323. How many pairs of cranial nerves do dogs have?
    a. 6
    b. 8
    c. 10
    d. 12

324. Cerebrospinal fluid is found in the
    a. Kidney
    b. Central canal of the spinal cord
    c. Liver
    d. Anterior chamber of the eye

325. Outside the brain and spinal cord, nerve cells are usually found in clumps or aggregations called
    a. Receptors
    b. Ganglia
    c. Bundles
    d. Neuromas

326. The spinal cord is a communicating link between body tissues and the
    a. Brain
    b. Heart
    c. Liver
    d. Intestinal tract

327. Nerve fibers carrying information to the brain are termed
    a. Efferent
    b. Parasympathetic
    c. Motor
    d. Afferent

328. The presence of a myelin sheath on an axon tends to
    a. Accelerate all impulses
    b. Slow all impulses
    c. Accelerate only impulses to peripheral tissues
    d. Accelerate only impulses to the brain

329. What is the point at which the axon of one neuron meets the dendrite of another and over which nerve impulses can pass?
    a. Synapse
    b. Reflex arc
    c. Cyton
    d. Meninx

330. The eye converts light stimuli to nerve impulses via the
    a. Lens
    b. Pupil
    c. Retina
    d. Iris

331. The portion of the retina that is *not* sensitive to light stimuli is called the
    a. Blind spot
    b. Nonfunctional area
    c. Ciliary body
    d. Cornea

332. In what order does light pass through ocular structures on its way to the retina?
    a. Lens, cornea, pupil
    b. Cornea, lens, pupil
    c. Cornea, pupil, lens
    d. Pupil, cornea, lens

333. What is the pigmented sphincter-like structure of the eye that controls the amount of light entering the posterior eye?
    a. Sclera
    b. Iris
    c. Pupil
    d. Retina

334. An electrical charge moving along the membrane of a nerve fiber is called
    a. A stimulus
    b. An impulse
    c. A reflex
    d. A repolarization wave

335. Homeostasis or homeokinesis is the chief role of what part of the nervous system?
    a. Autonomic nervous system
    b. Central nervous system
    c. Cranial nerves
    d. Peripheral nervous system

336. What enzyme inactivates acetylcholine?
    a. Norepinephrine
    b. Cholinesterase
    c. Adrenolytic agent
    d. Acetylcholinesterase

337. What substance is a catecholamine?
    a. Acetylcholine
    b. Acetylcholinesterase
    c. Norepinephrine
    d. Nicotine

338. The scientific term for the *white of the eye* is
    a. Iris
    b. Retina
    c. Cornea
    d. Sclera

339. The central nervous system consists of the brain and the
    a. Sympathetic nerves
    b. Parasympathetic nerves
    c. Spinal cord
    d. Cranial nerves

340. Nerve fibers encased in a white sheath of fatty material are termed
    a. Parasympathetic
    b. Myelinated
    c. Sympathetic
    d. Golgi bodies

341. Which is *not* one of the three major subdivisions of the brain?
    a. Cerebrum
    b. Brainstem
    c. Cerebellum
    d. Occipital lobe

342. Which is *not* a layer of the meninges?
    a. Pons
    b. Dura mater
    c. Pia mater
    d. Arachnoidea

343. How many pairs of thoracic nerves does a dog have?
    a. 2
    b. 10
    c. 13
    d. 21

344. Spinal nerves are what type?
    a. Sensory (afferent)
    b. Motor (efferent)
    c. Autonomic
    d. Sensory and motor

Correct answers are on pages 32–43.

345. Branch-like structures that conduct impulses toward the nerve cell body are called
    a. Dendrites
    b. Axons
    c. Synapses
    d. Neurons

SKELETAL SYSTEM INCLUDING JOINTS

346. Articular cartilage consists of a thin layer of
    a. Periosteum
    b. Endosteum
    c. Epiphyseal cartilage
    d. Hyaline cartilage

347. The primary functions of long bones include all of the following *except*
    a. Mineral homeostasis
    b. Protection and support
    c. Protective cavity for the brain
    d. Blood formation

348. The study of skeletal systems with bones as the chief structures is called
    a. Angiology
    b. Osteology
    c. Esthesiology
    d. Arthrology

349. The axial skeleton includes all of the following *except* the
    a. Skull
    b. Sternum
    c. Appendages
    d. Vertebral column

350. Which joint type is found mainly in the skull?
    a. Suture
    b. Syndesmosis
    c. Gomphosis
    d. Synchondrosis

351. Most synovial joints are similar in structure and include all of the following *except*
    a. Articular cartilage
    b. Ligaments
    c. Joint capsule
    d. Tendons

352. Arthritis may lead to an increased production of
    a. Peritoneal fluid
    b. Synovial fluid
    c. Plasma
    d. Serum

353. A major function of osteoblasts is to
    a. Aid in bone growth and fracture repair
    b. Decrease bone resorption
    c. Increase bone calcification
    d. Aid in vitamin D synthesis

354. Which structure is a passage or a tube-like opening through bone?
    a. Fissure
    b. Fovea
    c. Fossa
    d. Meatus

355. Which of the following is a separate cranial bone of horses and cats but in other species is present only in the fetus and fuses with surrounding bones before birth?
    a. Temporal bone
    b. Interparietal bone
    c. Frontal bone
    d. Occipital bone

356. Which term describes movement of a part away from the median plane or a digit away from the axis of the limb?
    a. Flexion
    b. Extension
    c. Abduction
    d. Circumduction

357. Which joint type can, through simple sliding motion, move in one (uniaxial) direction only?
    a. Plane
    b. Hinge
    c. Pivot
    d. Condyloid

358. The os penis of the dog and cat and the ossa cordis found in the heart of ruminants are examples of
    a. Pneumatic bones
    b. Sesamoid bones
    c. Splanchnic bones
    d. Flat bones

359. Which of the following is an example of a saddle joint?
    a. Distal interphalangeal in a dog
    b. Scapulohumeral in a horse
    c. Atlantoaxial in a cow
    d. Metacarpophalangeal in an elephant

360. Which term describes implantation of a tooth into the alveolus of the mandible?
    a. Syndesmosis
    b. Gomphosis
    c. Diarthrosis
    d. Syschondrosis

361. Which enzyme is necessary for deposition of calcium salts in osteoid tissue to form true bone?
    a. Rennin
    b. Enterokinase
    c. Phosphatase
    d. Ribonuclease

362. Which areas of bone fuse early in life but cause bones to continue to increase in size as a result of the hereditary condition known as achondroplasia?
    a. Proximal epiphyses
    b. Distal epiphyses
    c. Diaphyses
    d. Metaphyses

363. Oversecretion by which gland causes demineralization of the skeleton called osteitis fibrosa or von Recklinghausen's disease?
    a. Parathyroid gland
    b. Endocrine gland
    c. Thymus gland
    d. Adrenal gland

364. Functions of long bones include all of the following *except*
    a. Providing support
    b. Absorbing concussion
    c. Aiding in locomotion
    d. Acting as levers

365. Functions of flat bones include all of the following *except*
    a. Protecting the brain
    b. Providing large areas for muscle attachment
    c. Shielding the heart and lungs
    d. Reducing friction

366. Nonarticular depressions or holes in bones include all of the following *except*
    a. Fossa
    b. Facet
    c. Fovea
    d. Foramen

367. Osteocytes are located in small cavities in bone called
    a. Centers of ossification
    b. Canaliculi
    c. Lacunae
    d. Haversian canals

368. Extracapsular (periarticular) ligaments are those outside the joint capsule and include all of the following *except*
    a. Collateral ligament
    b. Dorsal ligament
    c. Palmar ligament
    d. Proximal ligament

369. Which type of joint in the front limb has *no* connection with the bony thorax?
    a. Syndesmoid
    b. Sphenoid
    c. Ginglymoid
    d. Arthrodial

Correct answers are on pages 32–43.

370. Red marrow persists in which bone throughout life and is thus a convenient place for aspiration and examination?
    a. Scapula
    b. Maxilla
    c. Sternum
    d. Atlas

371. A vertebra consists of all of the following *except*
    a. Body
    b. Arch
    c. Processes
    d. Girdle

372. Which of the following gives bones rigidity and makes them more opaque on radiographs?
    a. Hemoglobin
    b. Granular white cells
    c. Inorganic salts
    d. Electrolytes

373. Within bone, blood vessels from the periosteum and endosteum communicate with those of the Haversian system via which canals?
    a. Volkmann's
    b. Alar
    c. Condyloid
    d. Syndesmoid

374. Articular, spinous, and transverse processes are all found on the
    a. Clavicle
    b. Vertebrae
    c. Ribs
    d. Pelvic girdle

375. Which of the following is an ellipsoid joint?
    a. Carpometacarpal
    b. Atlantoaxial
    c. Antebrachiocarpal
    d. Interphalangeal

376. The mandible forms synovial joints with the
    a. Frontal bone
    b. Parietal bone
    c. Occipital bone
    d. Temporal bone

377. The frontal and lacrimal sinuses have small openings into which meatus?
    a. Acoustic
    b. Ethmoidal
    c. Temporal
    d. Osseous

378. The ilium, ischium, and pubis have bodies that meet to form the
    a. Pelvic symphysis
    b. Tuber coxae
    c. Acetabulum
    d. Obturator foramen

Urinary System

379. What is the primary function of the urinary system?
    a. Removal of all liquid from the body
    b. Extraction of excess glucose from the blood
    c. Extraction of waste products from the blood
    d. Addition of glucose to the blood

380. The major force that affects filtration pressure through the kidneys is
    a. Hormone levels
    b. Blood pressure
    c. Osmotic pressure
    d. Oxygen levels

381. The urinary bladder is lined with what type of epithelium?
    a. Stratified squamous
    b. Cuboidal
    c. Transitional
    d. Stratified columnar

382. What is the *basic* functional unit of the kidney?
    a. Nephron
    b. Efferent tubule
    c. Afferent tubule
    d. Glomerulus

383. The hormone that regulates sodium resorption at the nephron is
    a. ADH
    b. Estrogen
    c. Progesterone
    d. Aldosterone

384. Which species has a lobulated kidney?
    a. Horses
    b. Sheep
    c. Goats
    d. Cattle

385. Most absorption in the kidney is
    a. Active
    b. Passive
    c. Constant
    d. By diapedesis

386. Where is the main filtration mechanism in the kidney?
    a. Collection ducts
    b. Glomerulus
    c. Henle's loop
    d. Pyramids

387. The vessel that carries blood to the nephron is the
    a. Pudendal artery
    b. Efferent arteriole
    c. Afferent arteriole
    d. Renal vein

388. Most domestic animals have kidneys that are shaped like a
    a. Tulip
    b. Pea
    c. Bean
    d. Heart

389. Which tubular structure conveys urine from the kidney to the bladder?
    a. Urethra
    b. Ureter
    c. Henle's loop
    d. Nephron

390. Increased excretion of urine is termed
    a. Diuresis
    b. Polyphagia
    c. Polydipsia
    d. Hypertrophy

391. What two hormones normally have the greatest influence on the kidneys?
    a. Progesterone and aldosterone
    b. Progesterone and ADH
    c. Oxytocin and ADH
    d. Aldosterone and ADH

392. What is the general term for inflammation of the kidney?
    a. Cystitis
    b. Nephritis
    c. Kidnitis
    d. Pancreatitis

393. What structure lies between the proximal and distal convoluted tubules?
    a. Bowman's capsule
    b. Malpighian corpuscle
    c. Henle's loop
    d. Glomerulus

394. What hormone is secreted by the kidneys?
    a. ADH
    b. Aldosterone
    c. Angiotensin
    d. Renin

395. What structure conveys urine from the bladder, to the exterior?
    a. Ureter
    b. Urethra
    c. Henle's loop
    d. Nephron

396. Urine cannot be expelled from the bladder without relaxation of the
    a. External sphincter
    b. Prostate
    c. Urethra
    d. Ureter

397. Angiotensin II promotes resorption of
    a. Calcium
    b. Phosphorus
    c. Sodium
    d. Nitrogen

Correct answers are on pages 32–43.

398. What hormone increases the permeability of renal tubular cells to water?
- **a.** LH
- **b.** ADH
- **c.** ACTH
- **d.** GnRH

399. What is the scientific term for emptying of the bladder?
- **a.** Defecation
- **b.** Polydipsia
- **c.** Polyphagia
- **d.** Micturition

400. The odor of urine is probably most influenced by an animal's
- **a.** Body temperature
- **b.** Body weight
- **c.** Diet
- **d.** Age

401. What is the scientific term for lack of urine production?
- **a.** Polyuria
- **b.** Oliguria
- **c.** Anuria
- **d.** Dysuria

402. What is normally the most plentiful chemical buffer in the body?
- **a.** Hemoglobin
- **b.** Nitrogen
- **c.** Amylase
- **d.** ADH

Answers

Cells and Tissues

1. **d** A red blood cell loses its nucleus as it matures.

2. **b** Three layers make up a cell membrane; a lipid layer is sandwiched between the two protein layers.

3. **d**

4. **b**

5. **a**

6. **c**

7. **d** Keratin is an insoluble protein, which makes stratified squamous epithelium very protective of underlying tissues.

8. **c**

9. **a** The wave-like motion of cilia helps move mucus and debris out of the respiratory system.

10. **c** Transitional epithelium is cuboidal when tissue is not in a contracted state, but it may become flattened when an organ is distended.

11. **c** Calcium is involved in the breakage and recoupling of cross linkages between myofilaments in a striated muscle fiber.

12. **d** a—skeletal muscle; b—smooth muscle; c—no such thing

13. **b** a—attachment between columnar epithelial cells; c—terminal area of the axon of a motor nerve fiber at the neuromuscular junction; d—site of impulse transmission between neurons

14. **c** a—skeletal muscle fibers may regenerate in this manner; b—mitotic division of smooth muscle fibers possible; d—possible means of smooth muscle regeneration

15. **d** The peritoneum, pleura, and pericardium all consist of flat expanded arrangements of loose connective tissue covered by mesothelium.

CIRCULATORY SYSTEM

16. **a**

17. **c** The right atrium receives carbon dioxide–rich blood from the systemic circulation.

18. **b** The mitral valve is the left atrioventricular valve.

19. **d** The right ventricle pumps blood to the pulmonary circulation.

20. **a** The aortic valve is the left ventricular outflow valve.

21. **a** The first heart sound is produced by closure of the two atrioventricular valves. The second heart sound is produced by closure of the two ventricular outflow valves.

22. **d** All the others carry oxygen-rich blood.

23. **d** Removal of the spleen is not life threatening. Removal of any of the other organs listed is fatal.

24. **d**

25. **c** The monocyte is an agranulocytic white blood cell.

26. **c** The monocyte is a macrophage and is important in the process of inflammation.

27. **c** Chordae tendineae are present on the atrioventricular valves.

28. **a**

29. **c** The pulmonary valve is the right ventricular outflow valve.

30. **a** All the other blood vessels carry carbon dioxide–rich blood.

31. **c**

32. **a**

33. **c**

34. **b** Simple squamous epithelium forms the very smooth endothelium that lines the entire circulatory system.

35. **d**

36. **d** The right ventricle pumps blood to the pulmonary circulation.

37. **a** Freshly oxygenated blood from the lungs flows back to the left atrium.

38. **b** The left ventricle pumps blood out to the systemic circulation.

39. **d** The tricuspid valve is the right atrioventricular valve.

40. **c** The pulmonary valve is the right ventricular outflow valve.

41. **d**

42. **a**

43. **a**

44. **a** The bundle of His conducts impulses from the atrioventricular node to the Purkinje fibers at the apex of the heart.

45. **a**

46. **d**

47. **d** The pulmonary valve is the right ventricular outflow valve.

48. **a** The mitral valve is the left atrioventricular valve.

49. **c** The aortic valve is the left ventricular outflow valve.

50. **b** The tricuspid valve is the right atrioventricular valve.

51. **d** The sinoatrial node is the pacemaker of the heart.

52. **a** The ductus arteriosus shunts blood from the pulmonary artery to the aorta of a fetus.

53. **a** The aortic valve is the left ventricular outflow valve.

54. **b** The Purkinje fibers conduct impulses from the bundle of His to the walls of the ventricles.

55. **d** Blood returning to the heart through the vena cava enters the right atrium and then passes through the right atrioventricular (tricuspid) valve.

56. **d** The vena cava returns blood to the heart from the systemic circulation.

57. **b**

58. **c** The pulmonary vein returns blood from the lungs to the left atrium.

59. **b** All the other choices are bony foramina.

60. **d**

61. **c**

62. **d** The mitral valve is the left atrioventricular valve.

63. **a** Blood from the pulmonary vein enters the left atrium.

64. **a** The general effect of the parasympathetic portion of the autonomic nervous system is to depress cardiac function.

65. **b** Pressure in the right atrium is higher than in the left atrium, resulting in right-to-left blood flow.

66. **b** Serum does not contain fibrinogen, which is essential for blood clotting.

67. **b**

68. **b**

69. **b** Blood flows from the heart through arteries, then through capillaries, then through veins, and back to the heart.

70. **d**

71. **a** Platelets and red blood cells do not normally have intact nuclei, and lymphocytes have single roundish nuclei.

Digestive System

72. **d**

73. **a** Herbivores rely on microbial fermentation to digest plant material.

74. **a**

75. **c**

76. **b**

77. **c**

78. **a**

79. **b** From proximal to distal, sections of the small intestine are the duodenum, jejunum, and ileum. The ilium is a bone of the pelvis.

80. **b**

81. **b**

82. **c**

83. **d**

84. **b**

85. **d** The rumen is where most of the microbial fermentation occurs in a ruminant.

86. **c**

87. **d**

88. **b**

89. **b** The duodenum is the first (most proximal) segment of the small intestine.

90. **d**

91. **a**

92. **a**

93. **b** The exocrine secretion of the pancreas consists primarily of various digestive enzymes.

94. **a**

95. **b**

96. **c**

97. **b** The anus and the esophagus are lined by stratified squamous epithelium. The pancreas is an accessory digestive organ.

98. **b** Chyme is the semi-fluid homogeneous material produced by the action of digestive enzymes and acid on the food in the stomach.

99. **b** Newborn ruminants are functionally simple-stomached animals. Until their forestomachs become active at weaning, the esophageal groove prevents milk from fermenting in the forestomach compartments.

100. **c** The ileum is the last segment of the small intestine.

101. **c** The villi of the small intestine increase the surface area of its lining, improving the efficiency of nutrient absorption.

102. **b** Blood cells are not normally formed in the liver of adult animals.

103. **b**

104. **c** Microbial fermentation is most important in digestion by herbivorous animals, (e.g., horses).

105. **a**

106. **a**

107. **c** The pharynx is the common passageway for both the respiratory and the digestive systems.

108. **c** Although saliva does contain some digestive enzymes, it contributes little to the digestive process.

109. **a** The esophagus merely conducts swallowed food from the pharynx to the stomach.

110. **a** The gas resulting from microbial fermentation in a ruminant must be periodically eliminated by eructation (burping) to prevent ruminal tympany (bloat).

111. **a**

ENDOCRINE SYSTEM

112. **c** The pituitary hormones function chiefly to regulate the activity of other endocrine glands.

113. **d** FSH is secreted by the anterior pituitary gland.

114. **b** Glucocorticoids are produced by the adrenal glands.

115. **c** Insulin is produced by the beta cells of the islets of Langerhans in the pancreas.

116. **d**

117. **d** Thyroxine (T_4) and calcitonin (Ca regulating hormone) are produced by the thyroid gland, insulin is produced by the pancreas, and parathormone is produced by the parathyroid gland.

118. **c** The release of oxytocin stimulates milk flow or letdown.

119. **b** a—pituitary gland location; c—adrenal gland location; d—pancreas location.

120. **a** The secretory products of exocrine glands are transported via ducts. Salivary and sweat glands are exocrine glands.

121. **b** Addison's disease results from insufficient adrenocortical hormones.

122. **d** Epinephrine and norepinephrine are secreted by the adrenal medulla; hence their name, adrenergics.

123. **c** Iodine is necessary for production of T_3 and T_4.

124. **a** Loss of weight is associated with hyperthyroidism; the others are related to hypothyroidism.

125. **b** Enlargement of the thyroid gland is termed a goiter.

126. **a** Potentiation (or synergism) is the term used to describe an increased effect.

127. **c**

128. **d** ADH helps control water loss by facilitating resorption of water from the distal portion of the nephron.

129. **a**

130. **c** The adrenal glands are located adjacent to the kidneys.

131. **d** A decrease in parathyroid hormone results in decreased blood calcium levels, and an increase in parathyroid hormone levels increases blood calcium levels.

132. **d** There are usually two, but the exact number and location vary among species.

133. **a** Diabetes mellitus is caused by lack of insulin or inability to use insulin.

134. **b** Glucagon is produced by the alpha cells. It has the opposite effect of insulin.

135. **c** Paracrine transmission uses interstitial fluid to diffuse hormones in the body; endocrine uses blood; neurocrine uses the synaptic clefts between neurons; and exocrine uses ducts to secrete to the exterior of the body.

136. **a** Pancreatic juices are not endocrine hormones.

INTEGUMENTARY SYSTEM

137. **c** Keratinized epithelium makes up the dry skin surface.

138. **d** Although long and coiled, the sweat glands are simple tubes.

139. **a** The cells that produce the hoof wall are located in the coronary band.

140. **d** The hoof wall has the lowest water content, and thus the firmest consistency.

141. **c** Sebaceous glands are simple sac-like (alveolar) structures.

142. **b** Salivary glands are part of the digestive system.

143. **a** The other three answers are true of the epidermis.

144. **c** The hair follicle is a "gland" of sorts whose product is the keratinized cylinder that we call a hair.

145. **a** The chestnut is a small vestigial mass of horn located in the vicinity of the carpus and tarsus.

146. **c** Vitamin E is not synthesized in the skin.

147. **c**

148. **d**

149. **a** Granules of melanin are deposited in the cortex of pigmented hairs by melanocytes in the hair follicles.

150. **a** Guard hairs are pulled into a more erect position by contraction of the arrector pili muscles. This creates more air spaces among the adjacent wool hairs, which are stretched up by the erect guard hairs.

151. **d**

152. **c**

153. **c** The dermis consists only of connective tissue.

154. **c**

155. **c**

156. **c**

MAMMARY GLANDS AND LACTATION

157. **a**

158. **b**

159. **d**

160. **c**

161. **a** In addition to providing a common origin for the gracilis and adductor muscles of each limb, the symphyseal tendon also gives rise to part of the suspensory apparatus.

162. **d**

163. **a**

164. **c** Secretion of colostrum takes place around the time of parturition, coinciding with an inordinately rapid drop in plasma levels of progesterone, and plasma estrogen increases to the highest levels observed during gestation.

165. **b**

166. **a** The levels of IgG-1 decrease in maternal plasma 2 to 3 weeks before calving; from this time until parturition, maximum concentrations of IgG-1 are present in lacteal secretions.

167. c

168. b

169. a Frequent milkings throughout episodes of acute mastitis can help remove inflammatory mediators that might be harmful if allowed to persist for extended periods.

170. c

171. d Tuberculosis is an even less common cause of enlarged mammary glands in horses.

Muscular System

172. a The intercostal muscles (between the ribs) enlarge the diameter of the chest when they contract, but the principal respiratory muscle is the diaphragm. This thin membranous sheet separates the thorax from the abdomen.

173. c Striated is striped or skeletal; smooth is unstriped or visceral; cardiac is found in the heart, and is also striated.

174. c Purkinje fibers are specialized cardiac muscle cells.

175. b

176. c Purkinje fibers carry the message from the sinoatrial node to the ventricles to contract.

177. c Fiber is the basic unit of structure and function in striated muscle and is made of normal sarcomeres.

178. b The triceps brachium is the main extensor of the elbow.

179. b The main action of the biceps brachium is to flex the elbow.

180. d Hip adductors are found on the medial side of the femur.

181. a The tibial tuberosity is the point of insertion for the quadriceps femoris on the tibia.

182. a The external oblique is the most superficial abdominal muscle.

183. b The maximum amount a muscle fiber can contract is one-half its resting length.

184. b The least movable attachment is called the origin, and the most movable is the insertion.

185. c Adductors are generally muscles that pull a limb toward the body axis.

186. a The gastrocnemius is the large muscle that flexes the stifle and extends the hock.

187. d Cutaneous muscles attach to the skin and are responsible for movement of the skin.

188. c Spasmodic muscle contractions used to maintain body temperature are called shivering.

189. a Sphincter muscles constrict a body opening as a result of their circular arrangement.

190. d Denervation atrophy results from loss of nerve supply to a muscle.

191. b The trapezius is the flat, triangular muscle found in the neck.

192. d The pectoral muscle (superficial and deep) is the main adductor of the shoulder.

193. a These muscles are known as hamstring muscles.

194. d Tendons are the connective tissue that attach muscles to bone.

195. b Flat sheets of tendons are known as fasciae; the other terms refer to joints.

Nervous System

196. a

197. d

198. d

199. a

200. a

201. c

202. a

203. d
204. c
205. a
206. a
207. c
208. a
209. a
210. a
211. a
212. a
213. b
214. c
215. c
216. b
217. a
218. c
219. a
220. b
221. b
222. a
223. b
224. d
225. d
226. d
227. c
228. a
229. d
230. b

REPRODUCTIVE SYSTEM

231. **d** a—bitch; b—ewe; c—cow.

232. **c** An ectopic pregnancy takes place outside of the uterus, such as in a fallopian tube.

233. **a** Oxytocin stimulates milk letdown; testosterone is the major male hormone.

234. **b** Sperm fertilizes the ovum in an oviduct.

235. **c**

236. **b** A cow's average estrous cycle is 19 to 23 days.

237. **b** The guinea pig's pregnancy lasts approximately 63 days.

238. **a**

239. **a** Estrogen works via the brain to cause estrual behavior (heat); estrogen would result in the opposite effects of b, c, d.

240. **b** Progestin maintains pregnancy by keeping the uterus quiescent; the other answers are responses to estrogen.

241. **a** FSH targets the ovary to bring about the growth and maturity of the follicles, which, in turn, secrete estrogen to stimulate the onset of estrus.

242. **c** Cows cycle throughout the year with approximately 21-day estrous cycles.

243. **c** The fetus grows the most during the third trimester.

244. **d** Ectoderm gives rise to many tissues and organs, including the skin.

245. **c** Males and females are both born with mammary glands, although these glands fully develop only in sexually mature females.

246. **a** Horses have two mammary glands.

247. **c** Testosterone plays no major role in lactation.

248. **c** The ovaries are located adjacent to the kidneys.

249. **d** The literal definition is yellow body.

250. **a** The infundibulum is the structure of the oviduct adjacent to the ovary.

251. **b** Puberty is reached when reproductive organs first become functional.

252. **d** During or shortly after estrus, ovulation occurs.

253. **a** Diestrus is the relatively short period of quiescence (rest) between estrous cycles in polyestrous animals; anestrus is a longer period of quiescence, as in seasonally polyestrous animals.

254. **c** Metestrus and diestrus make up the luteal phase of the estrous cycle.

255. **a** Because *metr-* refers to uterine tissue and *-itis* means inflammation, *metritis* is inflammation of the uterus.

256. **b** Because *dys-* means painful, bad, or difficult and *-tocia* relates to birth, *dystocia* is defined as a difficult birth.

257. **c** Testosterone is the major male sex hormone.

258. **d** The epididymes serve as a place for spermatozoa to mature before they are expelled by ejaculation.

259. **b** Ejaculation, the rhythmic contraction of the sex glands, results in expelling semen, which consists of sperm and secondary sex gland secretions.

260. **d** Androgens, such as testosterone, are hormones that have masculinizing effects.

261. **c** Testosterone promotes protein anabolism, resulting in increased male body size as compared with the female's body.

262. **c** Sperm may remain fertile in a ewe's reproductive tract for 30 to 48 hours.

263. **b** The hypothalamus releases GnRH in response to low levels of progesterone.

264. **d** This results in rapid regression or lysis of the corpus luteum.

265. **b** Progesterone is released from the corpus luteum, which is present during metestrus.

266. **b** Estrus is known as the period of heat.

267. **b** Most are polyestrous only in the fall, so they will give birth in the spring.

268. **d** Progesterone maintains a quiescent (quiet) uterus during gestation.

269. **b** Gestation in a sow lasts 114 days or 3 months, 3 weeks, 3 days.

270. **c** Gestation is the term used for the time an animal is pregnant.

271. **a** A multiparous female has given birth after more than one pregnancy.

272. **d** The cotyledon attaches to the caruncle to form the placentome.

273. **a** The ovaries produce and expel ova.

274. **c** Rupture of a follicle releases an ovum.

275. **b** Fallopian tubes are also known as oviducts or uterine tubes.

276. **d** The anterior pituitary gland releases LH.

277. **d** LH promotes the growth of the corpus luteum after the follicles rupture.

278. **a** The corpus luteum is the main source of progesterone during metestrus.

279. **c** Cystic ovaries may cause persistent estrual behavior as a result of continued estrogen release.

280. **d** Ovulation is stimulated by coitus in the cat.

281. **a** Fetal hydrocortisone crosses the placental barrier to stimulate uterine contractions that signal the onset of labor.

282. **d** Oxytocin brings about strong uterine contractions, which expel the fetus.

283. **c** The average length of gestation for goats is 150 days, the same as for sheep.

284. **d** The scrotum is the cutaneous sac containing the testes.

285. **c** Horses and pigs seem to have more cases of cryptorchidism or undescended testes than the other species listed.

286. **b** Fructose is a component of seminal plasma in all species.

287. **d** Enlargement of the bulbus glandis results in prolonged retention of the penis during coitus, or the tie.

288. **a** A photoperiod is the length of daylight, which regulates the heat cycles in some species.

289. **c** A sow has an ovary that resembles a cluster of grapes because the animal is litter bearing.

290. **d** Oogenesis is the process by which ova are formed.

291. **a** The caruncle is not a layer of the fetal placenta; it is a maternal structure.

RESPIRATORY SYSTEM

292. **c** The inhaled air is warmed, humidified, and filtered by the lining of the nasal passages.

293. **b** Mastication, the chewing of food, is a digestive system function.

294. **a** The alveoli are tiny grape-like clusters of air sacs, which are surrounded by capillary networks.

295. **b**

296. **b** The gases diffuse from areas of high concentration (pressure) to areas of low concentration (pressure).

297. **c**

298. **d** The trachea is commonly called the windpipe.

299. **a** Bronchioles are part of the lower respiratory system.

300. **d** Flattening of the diaphragm when it contracts increases the size (volume) of the thoracic cavity.

301. **c** Inhaled air contains more oxygen and less carbon dioxide than does blood entering the alveolar capillaries.

302. **a**

303. **b** External respiration is the exchange of oxygen and carbon dioxide between the blood and inspired air.

304. **c** None of the other choices is a significant function of the larynx.

305. **d** Internal respiration is the exchange of oxygen and carbon dioxide between the blood and the body's cells and tissues.

306. **c** The pharynx is a common passageway for both the respiratory and digestive systems.

307. **a**

308. **c** The lung apex is in the cranial part of the thorax.

309. **a** Exhaled air passes from the alveoli → bronchi → trachea → larynx → pharynx → nasal passages → outside world.

310. **b**

SENSORY SYSTEM

311. **c** The olfactory nerve mediates the sense of smell.

312. **b** The peripheral nervous system consists of 12 paired cranial nerves and paired spinal nerves that pass through the intervertebral foramina to supply the body and limbs.

313. **d** The vagus nerve (X) controls the pharynx, larynx, and heart.

314. **a** The sympathetic nervous system is used in emergency situations for rapid energy release to meet critical demands.

315. **c** Cones are the receptors for color and bright light.

86. When an endotracheal tube is being inserted in a horse, the animal should be placed
    a. In sternal recumbency with its head at a 90-degree angle to the neck
    b. In sternal recumbency with its head and neck extended
    c. In lateral recumbency with its head at a 90-degree angle to the neck
    d. In lateral recumbency with its head, neck, and back extended

87. Which of the following is *not* an advantage for endotracheal intubation?
    a. Ensures a patent airway
    b. Increases deadspace and allows for more efficient ventilation
    c. Prevents aspiration pneumonitis
    d. Improves oxygenation of arterial blood

88. Which animal is *most* likely to experience laryngospasm?
    a. Thoroughbred mare
    b. Hereford cow
    c. Persian cat
    d. Dalmatian dog

89. Which of the following is the *most* common complication with endotracheal intubation?
    a. Placement of the tube in the esophagus
    b. Physical damage to the teeth and oral mucous membranes
    c. Overinflated cuff injuring the trachea
    d. Underinflated cuff collapsing the trachea

90. The best method for determining the proper inflation of an endotracheal tube cuff is
    a. Use 1 ml of air for each millimeter of internal diameter of the tube
    b. Inject air while applying pressure from the reservoir bag until no air escapes around the tube
    c. Inject air until the bulb on the cuff tubing is too hard to collapse
    d. Use a 12 ml syringe and inject 12 ml of air into the cuff

91. The preferred method for treating a cat with laryngospasm is to
    a. Use a sharp stylet to wedge the endotracheal tube between the vocal cords
    b. Return the animal to its cage, and wait 20 minutes before trying again
    c. Place a drop of a topical anesthetic in the laryngeal area, wait a few minutes, and then intubate the animal
    d. Use a stiffer endotracheal tube that can force the vocal cords open

92. Which of the following is *not* an advantage of using an endotracheal tube?
    a. Prevents atelectasis of lung alveoli
    b. Encourages proper examination of the animal's mouth, pharynx, and larynx
    c. Provides a means for treating respiratory and cardiac arrest
    d. Increases the chances of airway obstruction

93. In a Siamese cat, the endotracheal tube should be removed
    a. As soon as the surgery or diagnostic technique is completed
    b. Only after the animal is fully conscious and able to maintain a free airway
    c. When the animal is taken off the anesthesia machine
    d. As soon as the animal begins to swallow and cough

94. In a Pug, the endotracheal tube should be removed
    a. As soon as the surgery or diagnostic technique is completed
    b. Only after the animal is fully conscious and able to maintain a free airway
    c. When the animal is taken off the anesthesia machine
    d. As soon as the animal begins to swallow and cough

Correct answers are on pages 62–69.

95. How should an endotracheal tube be secured to the animal?
    a. It is best *not* to secure the tube to the animal, so that it can move freely if the animal starts to wake up
    b. It should be secured by gauze strips around the head in cats and brachycephalic dogs, and caudal to the upper canines in other breeds of dogs
    c. It can be secured by several wraps of cloth and tape around the animal's nose and the tube
    d. A rubber band can be looped tightly around the tube and the animal's nose

MONITORING THE ANESTHETIZED PATIENT

96. Which statement concerning use of intravenous anesthesia in large animals is *least* accurate?
    a. It is routinely used for cast applications, castrations, and umbilical hernias.
    b. It works well on procedures that require complete immobilization of the patient.
    c. It should not be used on procedures that require more than 45 to 50 minutes to complete.
    d. It requires use of a preanesthetic for sedation and a barbiturate.

97. When monitoring the vital signs of an anesthetized patient, you must observe and record all of the following *except*
    a. Mucous membrane color and capillary refill time
    b. Heart rate and respiratory rate and depth
    c. Reflexes
    d. Pulse quality and strength

98. The responsibilities of the anesthetist during a surgical procedure include continuous monitoring of the patient's vital signs and recording observations at approximately
    a. 10-minute intervals
    b. 5-minute intervals
    c. 2-minute intervals
    d. 15-second intervals

99. Adequate oxygen may be evaluated subjectively during anesthesia by the
    a. Heart rate
    b. Respiratory rate
    c. Mucous membrane color and capillary refill time
    d. Pulse pressure

100. Hypoventilation that occurs in the anethetized patient is characterized by
    a. Decreased oxygen levels and increased carbon dioxide levels
    b. Decreased carbon dioxide levels and decreased oxygen levels
    c. Increased oxygen levels and decreased carbon dioxide levels
    d. Increased oxygen levels and increased carbon dioxide levels

101. In dogs recovering from anesthesia, the endotracheal tube should be removed
    a. When the palpebral reflex returns
    b. When the swallowing reflex returns
    c. When the pupils resume a central position
    d. When the animal shows voluntary movement of the limbs

102. Concerning physical stimulation of the recovering anesthetized patient, which statement is *least* accurate?
    a. Stimulation should not include rubbing the chest because it may interfere with respiration.
    b. Stimulation can include talking to the patient, moving the limbs, or pinching the toes.
    c. Stimulation increases the flow of information to the reticular activation center of the brain.
    d. A lack of stimulation may cause drowsiness in the conscious animal.

103. It is advisable to turn the anesthetized patient from side to side during the recovery period of anesthesia. Concerning this, which statement is *least* accurate?
    a. Turn the patient every 10 to 15 minutes until it regains conciousness.
    b. Turning the patient prevents pooling of blood in the dependent parts of the body.
    c. It is advisable to turn all animals dorsally rather than sternally to prevent gastric torsion.
    d. Turning the patient helps stimulate respiration and consciousness.

104. Once extubated, all animals should be placed in
    a. Right lateral recumbency with the neck extended
    b. Left lateral recumbency with the neck in a normal flexed position
    c. Sternal recumbency with the neck extended
    d. Whatever position is most comfortable for the patient

105. Following discontinuation of the anesthetic gas, periodic bagging of the patient with pure oxygen is advisable because it
    a. Helps reinflate collapsed alveoli
    b. Allows for a faster recovery
    c. Helps to flush anesthetic gas out of the hoses
    d. Allows expired waste gas to be evacuated by the scavenger system

106. In the anesthetized surgical patient, pale mucous membranes indicate all of the following *except*
    a. Inadequate oxygen levels
    b. Cyanosis
    c. Excessive blood loss
    d. Decreased tissue perfusion

107. In patients with which of the following characteristics is it recommended to wait a longer period before extubation because of the likelihood of vomiting or airway obstruction?
    a. Dolichocephalic
    b. Undershot mandible
    c. Brachycephalic
    d. Cleft palate

108. Providing good nursing care for the recovering anesthetized patient is the duty of the attending anesthetist. Which of the following is *not* advisable for a patient immediately following surgery?
    a. Providing ample bedding to prevent heat loss and increase comfort
    b. Providing fresh food and water following consciousness
    c. Providing a source of heat in hypothermia cases
    d. Administering postoperative analgesics as directed by the veterinarian

Correct answers are on pages 62–69.

109. The minimum acceptable heart rate (beats per minute) for the anesthetized canine patient is
    a. 60
    b. 70
    c. 85
    d. 100

110. It is cause for concern if an anesthetized cat's heart rate (beats per minute) falls below
    a. 160
    b. 120
    c. 100
    d. 140

111. An anesthetist should be aware of the effects of anesthetic agents on the patient. When used as preanesthetics, atropine and acepromazine can cause all of the following *except*
    a. Prolapse of the nictitating membrane
    b. Respiratory depression
    c. Reduced salivation and tear production
    d. Pupil dilatation in cats

112. Capillary refill time is noticeably prolonged (over 2 seconds) when the blood pressure drops below
    a. 100 to 120 mm Hg
    b. 140 to 160 mm Hg
    c. 70 to 80 mm Hg
    d. 50 to 70 mm Hg

113. Use of an indwelling catheter in an artery to monitor blood pressure is termed
    a. Direct monitoring
    b. Central venous pressure
    c. Indirect monitoring
    d. Peripheral venous pressure

114. When monitoring the mucous membrane color of an anesthetized patient with pigmented gingivae, you should include the following 2 alternative sites *except*
    a. Pinnae
    b. Tongue
    c. Buccal mucous membranes
    d. Membranes lining the prepuce or vulva

115. During the maintenance period of anesthesia, respiratory rates fewer than how many breaths/min may indicate excessive anesthetic depth and should be reported to the veterinarian?
    a. 5
    b. 8
    c. 10
    d. 12

116. Some anesthetists routinely *bag* their patient under inhalation anesthesia once every 5 minutes to help prevent
    a. Apnea
    b. Mydriasis
    c. Hypercapnia
    d. Atelectasis

117. The causes of true hyperventilation and tachypnea during anesthesia may include all of the following *except*
    a. Progression from light to moderate anesthesia
    b. Response to metabolic acidosis
    c. Response to a mild surgical stimulus
    d. Presence of pulmonary edema

118. If the rectum of a patient is covered by a surgical drape or is otherwise inaccessible to the anesthetist, a rough estimate of body temperature can be obtained by
    a. Touching the patient's nose or tail
    b. Touching the patient's feet or ears
    c. Touching the patient's tongue or mucous membranes
    d. Feeling the temperature of exhaled air

119. Throughout anesthesia, the animal's temperature should be maintained as close to normal as possible. Hypothermia can be prevented by all of the following measures *except*
    a. Warming the stainless-steel V trough before using it
    b. Administering warm intravenous fluids
    c. Use of a circulating warm-water heating pad
    d. Providing a comfortable air temperature in the surgery room

120. Malignant hyperthermia is a potentially fatal syndrome to the anesthetized patient. Which species is *most* prone to this condition?
    a. Cattle
    b. Pigs
    c. Dogs
    d. Goats

121. Use of succinylcholine in combination with general anesthetics may be advantageous to the surgeon during certain procedures, but it gives the anesthetist one less measure with which to monitor anesthetic depth. Which measure would be of no use in monitoring patients given succinylcholine?
    a. Eye position and pupil size
    b. Heart rate
    c. Jaw muscle tone
    d. Respiratory rate

122. Using ketamine as an anesthetic agent diminishes the value of which measure in assessing anesthetic depth?
    a. Pinna reflex
    b. Pedal reflex
    c. Jaw muscle tone
    d. Eye position

123. Which statement concerning eye position, pupil size, and responsiveness to light as indicators of anesthetic depth is *least* accurate?
    a. In stage III, plane 3, of anesthesia, the eyes are usually central to slightly eccentric, with normal pupils that are responsive to light.
    b. In stage III, plane 2, of anesthesia, the eyes are usually rotated ventrally with slightly dilated pupils.
    c. In stage II of anesthesia, the eyes are usually central, and the pupils may be dilated and responsive to light.
    d. In stage IV of anesthesia, the eyes are central with widely dilated pupils that are unresponsive to light.

124. The presence or absence of salivary and lacrimal secretions may give clues regarding anesthetic depth. In an animal that has *not* received an anticholinergic, which statement concerning observance of these secretions is most accurate?
    a. Production of tears and saliva increases with increasing anesthetic depth.
    b. Production of tears and saliva is totally absent in light anesthesia.
    c. Tear and saliva production diminishes as anesthetic depth is increased.
    d. Tear and saliva production increases in all stages of anesthesia in the absence of anticholinergics.

125. The anesthetized patient may respond to surgical stimulation if the anesthetic depth is inadequate. Response to a painful stimulus may be indicated by all of the following *except*
    a. A considerable increase in heart rate and an increase in blood pressure
    b. A decrease in lacrimation and salivation
    c. An increase in respiratory rate
    d. Sweating on the foot pads

Correct answers are on pages 62–69.

126. A 10-year-old dog has been anesthetized for removal of a skin tumor and is now maintained on 2% isoflurane. The anesthetist observes that its respirations are 8/min and shallow, its heart rate is 80 beats/min, its pupils are centrally positioned, its jaw tone is slack, and all its reflexes are absent. This animal is in what stage and plane of anesthesia?
    a. Stage III, plane 2
    b. Stage III, plane 3
    c. Stage III, plane 4
    d. Stage IV, plane 1

127. What should be your response or actions to the condition of this animal?
    a. It is adequately anesthetized; no adjustments are necessary
    b. You should try to stimulate the animal to lighten the plane of anesthesia
    c. You should notify the veterinarian of the dog's condition but not be alarmed
    d. You should reduce the vaporizer setting to 1.5% isoflurane and continue to monitor for signs of decreased depth

128. Which stage of anesthesia may be characterized by vocalization, struggling, and breath holding?
    a. Stage I
    b. Stage II
    c. Stage III, plane 1
    d. Stage III, plane 2

ANESTHETIC EMERGENCIES

129. A dog received the correct dose of xylazine intramuscularly. Second-degree heart block and bradycardia developed. Based on the *most* common cause of this adverse reaction, what would the best therapy be?
    a. No treatment is required
    b. Yohimbine
    c. Glycopyrrolate
    d. Doxapram

130. An abnormally elevated central venous pressure developing during anesthesia and surgery may indicate
    a. Intravenous fluid overload
    b. Increased cardiac output
    c. Dehydration
    d. Liver disease

131. A 1:10,000 dilution of epinephrine contains how much epinephrine per milliliter?
    a. 1.0 mg
    b. 0.01 mg
    c. 1 μg
    d. 0.1 mg

132. Cardiac arrhythmias that occur during anesthesia are commonly associated with all of the following *except*
    a. Normocapnia
    b. Excessive halothane concentration
    c. Hypoxemia
    d. Myocardial ischemia

133. Mean arterial blood pressure of the halothane-anesthetized horse
    a. Can be used as an indication of anesthetic depth
    b. Is not important
    c. Is not practical to monitor
    d. Is only important for long procedures

134. Surgical evaluation of a dog hit by a car revealed a PCV of 18% and plasma protein below 2.5 g/dl. All of the following are true *except*
    a. The patient is predisposed to pulmonary edema
    b. Fluid administration rates should be watched closely
    c. The patient should receive plasma or whole blood before surgery
    d. The patient should not receive fluid before surgery

135. The estimated blood volume in dogs is
    a. 40 ml/kg
    b. 60 ml/kg
    c. 70 ml/kg
    d. 80/ml/kg

136. The volume of blood administered to a patient is determined by all of the following *except*
    a. PCV of the donor
    b. PCV of the recipient
    c. Desired PCV
    d. Age of the recipient

137. While monitoring a horse during inhalation anesthesia, you note that the heart rate suddenly increases to 80 beats/min. Your *most* appropriate response is to
    a. Increase the delivered anesthetic concentration
    b. Administer 10 mg of butorphanol intravenously
    c. Evaluate the peripheral pulse, mucous membranes, and other vital organ function before responding
    d. Not be concerned because the horse is not moving

138. While monitoring a horse receiving oxygen at the rate of 8 L/min, halothane 1.5%, and fluids at the rate of 20 ml/kg/hr, you note that the blood pressure suddenly falls to 60 mm Hg and the peripheral pulse becomes weak. Your first response should be to
    a. Administer a vasoactive agent
    b. Lower the halothane concentration and increase fluid delivery rate
    c. Turn down the oxygen flow
    d. Not be concerned

139. For each milliliter of blood loss during surgery, the crystalloid fluid replacement volume should be
    a. 1 ml
    b. 3 ml
    c. 6 ml
    d. 10 ml

140. Whole blood should be administered in which of the following *presurgical* situations?
    a. PCV 30%
    b. PCV 14%
    c. Von Willebrand's positive
    d. Chronic anemia, PCV 25%

141. A 10-kg dog with a ventricular arrhythmia is treated with an IV lidocaine drip at 50 µg/min. How many drops per minute from a minidrip infusion set (60 drops/ml) are necessary if the concentration of lidocaine is 1 mg/ml?
    a. 3
    b. 5
    c. 30
    d. 50

142. The most common arrhythmia associated with use of thiobarbiturates in dogs during induction of anesthesia is
    a. Atrial fibrillation
    b. Ventricular tachycardia
    c. Bigeminy
    d. Second-degree atrioventricular block

Correct answers are on pages 62–69.

143. Tachycardia in an anesthetized patient may be an indication of any of the following *except*
    a. Hypotension
    b. Pain
    c. Light plane of anesthesia
    d. Xylazine overdose

144. A cardiac rhythm disturbance detected shortly after induction of anesthesia may be the result of any of the following *except*
    a. The induction agent
    b. Difficulty intubating
    c. Hypoxemia
    d. Breathing oxygen-enriched air

145. Hypothermia has become significant in a 4-kg anesthetized cat. The best way to restore body heat is
    a. With a warm-water blanket
    b. To submerge the animal in warm water
    c. With a heat lamp
    d. To warm the air in the breathing circuit by some method

146. In a cat that is too deeply anesthetized, all of the following may be present *except*
    a. Pale mucous membranes
    b. Tachycardia
    c. Bradycardia
    d. Voluntary movement

147. An isoflurane-anesthetized cat suddenly begins breathing 30 times a minute during a surgical procedure. Your first response should be to
    a. Turn down the oxygen flow rate
    b. Begin to bag the patient immediately
    c. Turn up the anesthetic concentration
    d. Evaluate vital organ function and endotracheal tube placement and make necessary adjustments

148. A 20-kg dog is resuscitated after cardiac arrest. The heart rate is now 160 beats/min with sinus rhythm, poor pulse quality, and pale mucous membranes. The most appropriate drug to administer is
    a. Epinephrine
    b. Doxapram
    c. Atropine
    d. Dobutamine

149. If a dog is too deeply anesthetized, all of the following may be seen *except*
    a. Tachycardia
    b. Bradycardia
    c. Pale mucous membrane
    d. Increased jaw muscle tone

150. A dog anesthetized with halothane in 99% oxygen develops ventricular tachycardia. What is the drug of choice for therapy?
    a. Propranolol
    b. Quinidine
    c. Lidocaine
    d. Atropine

151. Dobutamine is used in emergency anesthetic and clinical situations to
    a. Increase the respiratory rate
    b. Increase cardiac output
    c. Correct cardiac arrhythmias
    d. Decrease the heart rate

152. During cardiopulmonary cerebral resuscitation (CPCR) in a medium-sized dog, you should maintain a ventilation rate of how many breaths/min?
    a. 5
    b. 12
    c. 20
    d. 30

153. During CPCR, adequate cardiac massage is present when
    a. The electrocardiogram is normal
    b. The heart rate is 60 beats/min
    c. A peripheral pulse is present
    d. The mucous membranes are pink

154. The *only* accurate way to evaluate the effectiveness of respiration is by
    a. Observing abdominal and chest movements during respiration
    b. Counting the respiratory rate
    c. Feeling air move through the endotracheal tube or nostrils
    d. Measuring the arterial blood oxygen and carbon dioxide partial pressures

155. Dehydration greater than 10% is
    a. A seriously morbid state
    b. Nothing to worry about
    c. Not something that affects skin turgor
    d. Not associated with depression

156. Patients that have water withheld for long periods before surgery and general anesthesia may be prone to
    a. Vomiting during induction
    b. Dehydration and hypotension
    c. Nothing more than other patients
    d. Respiratory depression

157. When xylazine is used to induce vomiting before surgery,
    a. There is nothing to worry about
    b. Do *not* place an endotracheal tube
    c. Examine the airway for gastric contents before placing the endotracheal tube
    d. Do not administer atropine

158. Immediately after tracheal intubation in a 3-kg cat you notice extreme respiratory distress. The most likely cause is
    a. Light plane of anesthesia
    b. Hypoxemia
    c. Nothing; this is normal
    d. Bronchial intubation

159. After correctly placing, lubricating, and inflating the cuff of the endotracheal tube, you note a sudden decrease in heart rate. The most likely cause is
    a. Low oxygen flow
    b. Too deep a plane of anesthesia
    c. Cuff is underinflated
    d. Cuff may be overinflated, producing vagal-induced bradycardia

160. During CPCR, 2% lidocaine is used to treat ventricular arrhythmias. A complication that may occur after intravenous infusion of lidocaine is
    a. Bradycardia
    b. Coughing
    c. Tachycardia
    d. Vomiting

161. Indications of poor cardiac function include all of the following *except*
    a. Cyanosis in patients with a PCV of 45%
    b. Poor perfusion
    c. Cardiac arrhythmias
    d. Normal pulse

162. Sodium bicarbonate is used to
    a. Treat cardiac arrhythmias
    b. Produce positive inotropic effects
    c. Stimulate respiration
    d. Combat acidosis

163. Corticosteroids are used during CPCR for all of the following reasons *except* to
    a. Induce vasodilatation
    b. Aid in regulating fluid and electrolyte homeostasis
    c. Stimulate respiration
    d. Stabilize the cellular membranes

164. Doxapram may produce all of the following *except*
    a. CNS excitement
    b. Decreased venous return
    c. Respiratory alkalosis
    d. Hypoventilation

Correct answers are on pages 62–69.

Answers

Types of Anesthetics

1. **b**

2. **c**

3. **b**

4. **c** Diazepam is an ideal drug for use in the cardiovascular-compromised patient. In patients with impaired renal or hepatic function, recovery may be significantly prolonged as a result of the metabolic requirements.

5. **d**

6. **b**

7. **a** The combination of xylazine and butorphanol provides greater analgesia and muscle relaxation, with the effects of both drugs being enhanced. One benefit of this combination is that the dose of each drug is reduced, minimizing side effects and maximizing therapeutic effects.

8. **b** Detomidine is a much more potent sedative on a volume-per-volume basis.

9. **c** Acepromazine is an alpha blocker with significant potential to produce hypotension; however, this is rarely a problem in healthy, normovolemic patients.

10. **c**

11. **d** Although epidural anesthetics are used to provide analgesia, patient movement is still of concern and prevents their use in most surgical procedures.

12. **a** Isoflurane maintains better cardiac output and produces less sensitivity of the myocardium to catecholamines, thereby minimizing cardiac arrhythmias during anesthesia.

13. **d**

14. **d** Essentially all anesthetics except neuromuscular-blocking agents cross the placental barrier in significant amounts, depressing the fetus. Neuromuscular-blocking agents are highly ionized and have high molecular weights, minimizing placental transfer.

15. **d** Propofol is an alkylphenol, nonbarbiturate, highly lipid-soluble hypnotic agent used to produce short-term anesthesia.

16. **b** Glycopyrrolate, a quaternary ammonium drug with anticholinergic properties, has fewer side effects than atropine and does not cross the placental barrier.

17. **c** Low dosages of morphine (0.1 to 0.2 mg/kg) may be used in cats, but CNS excitement is often experienced.

18. **d** Atropine is often used to prevent bradycardia.

19. **b**

20. **b** Acepromazine has no analgesic effect.

21. **a** The anticholinergic effects of atropine on the intestinal tract of horses may include ileus, intestinal distention, and colic. Atropine use should be limited to treatment of bradycardia caused by increases in vagal tone.

22. **b** The phenothiazine tranquilizers all have the potential to produce paralysis of the penis in stallions.

23. **a**

24. **b** Percent weight in volume (w/v) expresses the number of grams of a constituent in 100 milliliters of solution. Percent solution × 10 = mg/ml (e.g., 10% × 10 = 100 mg/ml).

25. **b** The addition of depressant premedication to an anesthetic protocol may prolong the recovery time because of anesthetic drug enhancement.

26. **c**

27. **c**

28. **a** The adrenergic (sympathetic) effects of epinephrine increase heart rate.

29. **b** Nitrous oxide adds to the effect of other inhalation anesthetics; therefore, less of the more-potent agent is needed to produce anesthesia.

30. **a** The partial pressure of oxygen in arterial blood should be approximately five times the percent inspired oxygen. Breathing 100% oxygen would then yield a PaO_2 of 500 mm Hg. Oxygen 50% + N_2O 50% would yield a PaO_2 of 250 mm Hg. In some patients this might not be desirable.

31. **c** 2% × 10 = 20 mg/ml.

32. **b** 500 kg × 8 mg/kg = 4,000 mg total dose; 10% × 10 = 100 mg/ml; 4,000 mg/100 mg/ml = 40 ml.

33. **c** Apneustic respirations are characterized by an inspiratory hold and rapid expiration.

34. **d** Premedication agents are used to minimize undesirable autonomic effects.

35. **b** 5% × 10 = 50 mg/ml × 180 ml = 9,000 mg/150 kg = 60 mg/kg.

36. **c** Epidural lidocaine can be used to provide analgesia (preoperatively and postoperatively) for surgical procedures involving the rear limbs and anal area.

37. **d** Mask inductions in aggressive patients can be so stressful that they offset the benefit of avoiding premedication and induction agents.

38. **b** Elimination of and recovery from anesthesia using pentobarbital are partially dependent on the biotransformation that takes place in the liver. Prolonged recovery is to be expected in hepatic-impaired patients.

39. **b** Atropine decreases salivation.

40. **b** 0.1 mg/kg × 60 kg = 6 mg. The maximum dose is still 4 mg.

41. **d** All inhalation anesthetics are expected to decrease cardiac output at working concentrations.

42. **d** Phenylbutazone is a heavily protein-bound drug, as are barbiturates. The competition for protein sites allows more barbiturate to be free of protein and to produce its anesthetic effect.

43. **d** Subcutaneous thiobarbiturate causes severe tissue irritation and necrosis. It is not absorbed rapidly enough for adequate results.

44. **c** The more anesthetic agent administered, the greater the adverse effect.

45. **d** Increased heart rate, increased respiratory rate, and active palpebral reflex may be indications of light planes of anesthesia, but are not reliable. They may be signs of excessive anesthetic depth.

46. **d**

47. **a** Acepromazine lowers the seizure threshold and should not be used in animals with a history of seizures. Old dogs with adequate liver function tolerate acepromazine quite well in proper doses.

48. **d** Narcotics in the dog are commonly associated with respiratory depression, bradycardia, and analgesic activity. Excitement is rare.

49. **b** The MAC is the concentration in percent at 1 atmosphere that prevents gross purposeful skeletal muscle movement in response to a noxious stimulus in 50% of patients. It is an expression of the potency of the drug. Cardiopulmonary effects vary with the agent at 1 MAC.

50. **b**

51. **d**

52. **d** Methoxyflurane is highly soluble in tissue, and 50% of the drug must be metabolized for complete elimination from the body. This equates to longer recovery as compared with agents that are less soluble in tissue and require less metabolism.

53. **d**

54. **c** Ease of access and adequate size.

MACHINES AND EQUIPMENT

55. **d** Flows less than 1.5 times the minute ventilation allow rebreathing of carbon dioxide.

56. **c** The pressure in the cylinder begins to drop when all of the liquid nitrous oxide has been vaporized and the gas loses pressure. No change in full pressure (750 psi) takes place until that time.

57. **b** Adequate inflation of the normal lung requires approximately 20 cm H_2O.

58. **b**

59. **d** The absence of unidirectional valves allows rebreathing of carbon dioxide. Because the attachment of a nonrebreathing device to the fresh gas port bypasses the circuit, it can be used.

60. **a**

61. **b**

62. **a** Metabolic rate determines the minimum oxygen requirement.

63. **d**

64. **d** All vaporizers can be used with any breathing circuit.

65. **b**

66. **a**

67. **c**

68. **c**

69. **d** Normally soda lime should be changed on the basis of hours of use, depending on the size of the soda lime cannister.

70. **d**

71. **d**

72. **a**

73. **c**

74. **b**

75. **c**

76. **b**

77. **d**

78. **d**

79. **a**

80. **d**

81. **d**

INTUBATION

82. **d** The equine esophagus consists of entirely smooth muscle; therefore, the horse is not capable of regurgitation, except in severe cases of gastric torsion. In that case it is a reflux problem, not true regurgitation.

83. **c** Pigs, sheep, goats, llamas, and rabbits generally require a laryngoscope for intubation because of their oral and pharyngeal anatomy.

84. **b** If more than 5 ml are required to fill the cuff properly, a larger cuff should be used.

85. **a** To reduce deadspace and prevent endobronchial intubation, you should premeasure and mark the tip of the tube so it can be placed midway between the thoracic inlet and the larynx.

86. **d**

87. **b** The endotracheal tube, when properly fitted and placed, should decrease the deadspace.

88. **c** Cats and sheep are most likely to experience laryngospasm, and cats are more susceptible than sheep.

89. **a** All of the choices are complications involved in placing an endotracheal tube. However, misplacement of the tube into the esophagus occurs more frequently than the others.

90. **b** The ideal method for inflating a cuff is to compress the rebreathing bag (or an Ambu bag) while adding air to the cuff. This method should prevent over-inflation and tracheal necrosis.

91. **c** The safest way to treat laryngospasm is to apply 1 or 2 drops of lidocaine and wait a few minutes to allow the larynx to relax before proceeding.

92. **d** The endotracheal tube is specifically used to decrease the chances of having airway obstruction.

93. **d** In nonbrachycephalic animals, the endotracheal tube should be removed as soon as the animal is able to swallow and cough and at the first sign that it can chew on the tube. This must be done before the animal has had a chance to puncture the tube or injure itself on the tube.

94. **b** In brachycephalic breeds, the chances of respiratory complications are greater than in other animals. Therefore, the endotracheal tube should be left in place until the animal is conscious and able to maintain a patent airway.

95. **b** Although tape and rubber bands are used in some clinics, these are not recommended. The rubber bands may become tangled in the hair, and, if applied too tightly, can cause pressure necrosis. Tape will stick to the hair and may be difficult to remove in an emergency.

MONITORING THE ANESTHETIZED PATIENT

96. **b** Intravenous anesthesia (sedative plus a short-acting barbiturate) alone does not completely immobilize large animals and should not be used for procedures that require such control of movement.

97. **c** The term *vital sign* refers to measures that indicate the response of the animal's homeostatic mechanisms to anesthesia. These include heart rate, blood pressure, capillary refill time (CRT), central venous pressure, mucous membrane color, blood loss, respiratory rate, blood gases, and temperature. *Reflex* refers to an involuntary response to a stimulus.

98. **b** Continuous monitoring of the anesthetized patient may be impractical in many veterinary clinics. However, an attempt should be made to observe and evaluate an anesthetized animal at least once every 3 to 5 minutes.

99. **c** The color of mucous membranes and capillary refill time (CRT) are both used to evaluate oxygen levels in tissue. Pink mucous membranes suggest adequate oxygen levels, whereas bluish mucous membranes indicate cyanosis. A CRT of greater than 2 seconds indicates poor tissue perfusion with oxygenated blood.

100. **a** Every patient given an anesthetic drug is hypoventilating. During hypoventilation periods, oxygen levels decrease while carbon dioxide levels increase.

101. **b** Although some of the other reflexes may be present (e.g., palpebral, pedal), the appearance of the swallowing reflex is most often cited as the appropriate time to remove the endotracheal tube, as return of this reflex will help protect the animal from aspirating vomitus.

102. **a** Patient recovery may be hastened by gentle stimulation, which includes talking to the animal, gently pinching the toes, opening the mouth, gently moving the limbs, and rubbing the chest.

103. **c** It is advisable to turn all animals sternally (the feet are moved under the dog as it is turned rather than rolling the patient onto its back) to lessen the chance of gastric torsion, especially in deep-chested animals.

104. **c** Once extubated, all animals should be placed in sternal recumbency with the neck extended because this position helps maintain a patent airway.

105. **a** Periodic bagging with pure oxygen is advisable for as long as the recovering patient is connected to the anesthetic machine because it helps reinflate collapsed alveoli. Continued administration of a high flow rate of oxygen until extubation helps flush anesthetic gases out of the animal's system, and it also allows expired gas to be evacuated by the scavenger.

106. **b** Cyanosis is indicated by bluish coloring of the mucous membranes.

107. **c** Because of the structure of their nasal passages and palate, brachycephalic breeds are more prone to vomiting and possible airway obstruction after anesthesia.

108. **b** Food and water should not be offered immediately after consciousness is regained because many animals experience periods of nausea and vomiting after anesthesia.

109. **b**

110. **c**

111. **b** Phenothiazine drugs, such as acepromazine, do not cause respiratory depression and are considered to have a wide margin of safety.

112. **c**

113. **a** *Direct monitoring* refers to the measuring of arterial blood pressure through use of an indwelling catheter placed in the femoral or dorsal pedal artery. *Indirect monitoring* refers to use of external devices when recording blood pressure.

114. **a** Alternative sites for monitoring mucous membrane color include the tongue, buccal mucous membranes, conjunctivae of the lower eyelids, and lining of the prepuce or vulva.

115. **b**

116. **d** Atelectasis is a respiratory condition characterized by partially collapsed alveoli. It may be the result of shallow breathing, which causes a decrease in tidal volume. Bagging the patient helps prevent atelectasis by gently forcing air into the patient's breathing passages.

117. **a** Hyperventilation and tachypnea may be observed in animals progressing from moderate to light anesthesia.

118. **b** Feeling the temperature of the extremities, such as the paws and ears, can give an indication of the animal's body temperature.

119. **a** It is impractical and often impossible in many hospitals to *prewarm* the stainless-steel V trough before its use in surgery; the metal does not retain heat. Lining the trough with towels or newspapers would be a more practical way of keeping the animal away from the cold stainless steel.

120. **b** Although hyperthermia may occasionally be seen in dogs anesthetized with ketamine or halothane, pigs are more susceptible to this condition.

121. **c** Succinylcholine is a muscle-paralyzing agent that may be used to achieve pronounced muscle relaxation for certain procedures, but you will not have the degree of muscle relaxation as an indicator of anesthetic depth.

122. **d** Ketamine does not cause eye rotation, even at moderate depths of anesthesia.

123. **a** In stage III, plane 3, of anesthesia, the eye is usually central to slightly rotated and the pupils are moderately dilated and respond to light slowly or not at all.

124. **c** Production of tears and saliva diminishes with increasing depth of anesthesia and is totally absent in deep surgical anesthesia. Ophthalmic solutions and ointments are used to prevent corneal drying.

125. **b** A light plane of anesthesia may be indicated by increasing lacrimation and salivation.

126. **b** Stage III, plane 3, is the indicated depth of anesthesia with the signs listed.

127. **d** The anesthetic plane is probably too deep for the given procedure. The age of the animal is also a risk factor. You should try to lighten the plane of anesthesia by adjusting the vaporizer setting to 1.5% and watch for signs of lightening, such as increased heart rate and respiratory rate, lacrimation, sweat on the foot pads, and movement. Maintain anesthesia on a setting that will permit the surgery without pain.

128. **b** Stage II is characterized as the "excitement stage" with the signs listed. This stage should be avoided by giving a bolus of anesthetic to take the animal past this phase of excitement.

ANESTHETIC EMERGENCIES

129. **c** The anticholinergic effects of glycopyrrolate block the vagal-induced bradycardia and second-degree heart block commonly associated with xylazine.

130. **a**

131. **d** $1/10,000 = 0.0001 \times 100 = 0.01\% \times 10 = 0.1$ mg/ml.

132. **a** Normal carbon dioxide levels do not induce arrhythmias.

133. **a**

134. **d**

135. **d**

136. **d**

137. **c**

138. **b**

139. **b**

140. **b**

141. **c** 10 kg $\times 50$ µg/kg/min $= 500$ µg/min; 500 µg $= 0.5$ mg $= 0.5$ ml $= 30$ drops/min.

142. **c**

143. **d**

144. **d**

145. **d** It is difficult to warm the patient by surface application of warm objects.

146. **d**

147. **d**

148. **d**

149. **d**

150. **c**

151. b   158. d
152. b   159. d
153. c   160. a
154. d   161. d
155. a   162. d
156. b   163. c
157. c   164. d

Notes

Section 3

Animal Care

Patricia Creamer, CAHT *Sarah McLaughlin, DVM*
Kay Knox, RVT, LAT *Mary Lou Shea, CAHT*
Teresa Sonsthagen, RVT

Recommended Reading

Allen MD: Carbohydrate nutrition, *Vet Clin North Am Food Anim Pract* 7:327-340, 1991.

Burkholder WJ, Thatcher CD: Enteral nutritional support of sick horses. In Smith BP, editor: *Large animal internal medicine*, St Louis, 1990, Mosby.

Corbin JE: Nutritional requirements of dogs. In Kronfield DS, editor: *Canine nutrition: a collection of papers*, Philadelphia, 1973, University of Pennsylvania School of Veterinary Medicine.

Crane SW, Grosdidier SR: Clinical nutrition. In McCurnin DM: *Clinical textbook for veterinary technicians*, ed 3, Philadelphia, 1994, WB Saunders.

Haylor JM: Nutritional management in disease. In Smith BP, editor: *Large animal internal medicine*, St Louis, 1990, Mosby.

Johnson LW: Nutrition, *Vet Clin North Am* 5:37-54, 1989.

Knox KE: Swine behavior and restraint techniques, *Vet Tech* 15:256-261, 1994.

Koterba AM, Drummond WH, Kosch PC: *Equine clinical neonatology*, Philadelphia, 1990, Lea & Febiger.

Leman AD, Straw BE, Mengeling WL, et al: *Diseases of swine*, ed 7, Ames, 1992, Iowa State University Press.

Morris ML: Nutrition. In Catcott EJ, editor: *Canine medicine*, Santa Barbara Calif, 1971 American Veterinary Publications.

Mylrea PJ: Digestion in young calves fed whole mik ad-lib and its relationship to calf scours, *Res Vet Sci* 7:407-416, 1966.

National Research Council: *Nutrient requirements of swine*, ed 9, Washington DC, 1988, National Academy Press.

Pork industry handbook, West Lafayette Ind, 1994, Cooperative Extension Service, Purdue University.

Ralston SL: Diagnosis of common mineral imbalances. In Smith BP, editor: *Large animal internal medicine*, St Louis, 1990, Mosby.

Roy JHB: *The calf*, ed 4, London, 1980, Butterworth.

Smith BP, editor: *Large animal internal medicine*, St Louis, 1990, Mosby.

Smith MC, Sherman DM: *Goat medicine*, Philadelphia, 1994, Lea & Febiger.

Wilkinson JM: Nutrition. In Andrews AH, Blowey RW, Boyd H, Eddy RG, editors: *Bovine medicine: diseases and husbandry of cattle*, Oxford, 1992, Blackwell Scientific Publications.

Practice answer sheet is on page 319.

Questions

HOUSING

General

1. Which of the following housing conditions is *most* likely to lead to heaves in horses?
   a. Low temperature in the stable
   b. Hay stored in the loft
   c. Screen partitions between stalls
   d. Fresh wood shavings for bedding

2. Which species is *least* likely to require frequent cage cleaning?
   a. Rats
   b. Mice
   c. Gerbils
   d. Hamsters

3. Preventive measures against kennel cough in shelters include ensuring that the number of air changes per hour is *not* fewer than
   a. 2 to 5
   b. 7 to 10
   c. 12 to 15
   d. 17 to 20

4. Low environmental humidity puts neonatal puppies and kittens at risk for
   a. Chilling
   b. Dehydration
   c. Diarrhea
   d. Retardation

5. The minimum relative humidity in a neonatal puppy housing unit should be
   a. 30%
   b. 50%
   c. 70%
   d. 90%

6. During the first week of life, orphan puppies and kittens should be reared in an environmental temperature of
   a. 32.2° C (90° F)
   b. 26.7° C (80° F)
   c. 21.1° C (70° F)
   d. 15.6° C (60° F)

7. To keep animals germ free inside a barrier unit, the air pressure inside compared with that outside must be
   a. Higher
   b. Lower
   c. Equal
   d. Much lower

8. In an isolation unit where sick animals are housed, the air pressure in the unit compared with that in the quarters housing healthy animals must be
   a. Higher
   b. Lower
   c. Equal
   d. Much higher

9. Very low humidity in a colony of rats may precipitate a problem known as
   a. Stud tail
   b. Wet tail
   c. Fan tail
   d. Ring tail

10. A roll-bar in a farrowing crate keeps the sow from contacting the pen wall as she lies down; the function of the roll-bar is to prevent
    a. Injuring the teats
    b. Upsetting the food
    c. Crushing the young
    d. Breaking the pen wall

11. The squeeze-back is a desirable feature in a cage housing for
    a. Cats
    b. Rats
    c. Dogs
    d. Monkeys

12. Adult males of which species should *not* be group-housed?
    a. Rats
    b. Mice
    c. Guinea pigs
    d. Gerbils

13. For good sanitation, outdoor runs should have bottoms constructed of
    a. Dirt
    b. Grass
    c. Gravel
    d. Wood

14. Shoebox caging is required for housing rodents that are being
    a. Bred
    b. Culled
    c. Weaned
    d. Born

15. Ducks and geese that eat moldy feed frequently succumb to
    a. Dermatophytosis
    b. Aspergillosis
    c. Pediculosis
    d. Actinobacillosis

16. Filter caps on rodent shoebox cages reduce the
    a. Ammonia levels
    b. Horizontal transmission of pathogens
    c. Cage temperatures
    d. Litter sizes of pregnant females

17. The most common health problem encountered when shipping animals is
    a. Heat prostration
    b Dehydration
    c. Suffocation
    d. Starvation

18. A well-built doghouse has all of the following properties *except*
    a. Windproof against drafts
    b. Raised off the ground
    c. Insulated against cold
    d. Spacious and roomy inside

19. In extreme hot weather, dairy cattle should be fed
    a. Early in the day
    b. Close to midday
    c. Early in the evening
    d. Close to midnight

20. The best type of feeding bowl for dogs is one made of
    a. Plastic
    b. Steel
    c. Enamel
    d. Ceramic

21. Although there is good serologic evidence that animals in shelters are exposed to many of the same pathogens, not all shelters experience a disease problem. The difference can best be explained by variance in the
    a. Degrees of pathogenic virulence
    b. Standards of management practice
    c. Types of climatic conditions
    d. Genetic make-up of the animals

22. An *inappropriate* use of a puppy crate is for
    a. Housebreaking
    b. Traveling
    c. Punishing
    d. Sleeping

23. When livestock are exposed constantly to rain, what epidemics often occur?
    a. Coccidioidomycosis
    b. Dermatophilosis
    c. Tuberculosis
    d. Mitosis

24. In a barn housing cows, steers, and calves in separate pens, the incoming air should flow over the pens in which order?
    a. Cows, steers, calves
    b. Steers, calves, cows
    c. Calves, cows, steers
    d. Calves, steers, cows

25. Puppies that are isolated from normal environmental stimuli during their critical socialization period develop a condition known as
    a. Neurosis
    b. Psychosis
    c. Hypnosis
    d. Kennelosis

Correct answers are on pages 90–96.

26. Spikes, loose nails, and barbed wire must be removed from equine quarters to decrease the danger of
    a. Rabies
    b. Colibacillosis
    c. Tetanus
    d. Strangles

SWINE

27. The height of a nipple watering device must be adjusted according to the size of the pigs in the pen. It should be set at a level that is
    a. Even with the elbow of the pigs
    b. Just above the shoulder of the pigs
    c. Halfway between the shoulder and the elbow of the pigs
    d. At eye level of the pigs

28. The number of nipple watering devices in group pens varies according to the size and number of animals involved. A pen of 20 pigs should have a *minimum* of
    a. 1 nipple per pen
    b. 2 nipples per pen
    c. 3 nipples per pen
    d. 4 nipples per pen

29. What is a newborn piglet's lower critical temperature?
    a. 70° to 75°F
    b. 65° to 70°F
    c. 110° to 115°F
    d. 90° to 95°F

30. At what temperature is a lactating sow *most* comfortable?
    a. 90° to 95°F
    b. 70° to 75°F
    c. 50° to 60°F
    d. 75° to 80°F

31. The environmental temperature should be monitored routinely in a farrowing unit. Where should thermometers be placed?
    a. At the herdsman's eye level
    b. At the herdsman's waist
    c. Near the entrance to the room
    d. Near the floor at the pigs' level

32. What can a producer do to provide an acceptable environment for a lactating sow and her offspring?
    a. Keep the sow comfortable and let the piglets huddle against her for warmth
    b. Heat the entire farrowing area to a comfortable level for the piglets and let the sow cool herself through perspiration
    c. Keep the overall area comfortable for the sow and provide zone heat for the piglets
    d. Set the room temperature at a level halfway between the two extremes

33. Fences and dividers between groups of pigs should be constructed so that
    a. The slats are positioned horizontally
    b. The slats are positioned vertically
    c. The top of the fence is no higher than the largest pig's back
    d. The bottom of the fence is at least 8 inches above the floor of the pen

34. As you walk through the nursery section of a swine production unit, you notice that most of the pigs in the room are lying piled against the front of the pens. What does this behavior tell you about the environment?
    a. The pigs are comfortable
    b. The pigs are cold
    c. The humidity level is too low
    d. The humidity level is too high

35. The humidity level in a swine barn should be maintained between
    a. 30% and 40%
    b. 50% and 60%
    c. 70% and 80%
    d. 10% and 20%

36. Where is the dunging area most likely to be located in a pen that has adequate space for hogs?
    a. Near the front
    b. All over
    c. In the center
    d. At the rear

37. What common vice might become apparent if pigs are crowded into a pen with insufficient space for the number of animals?
    a. Tail biting
    b. Hyperactivity
    c. Self-mutilation
    d. Bar biting

38. Excessive carbon monoxide levels in a swine barn are usually associated with
    a. Too many animals in a building or room
    b. Overheating of the animals in a building or room
    c. Incomplete combustion of fuel in a heater
    d. Excessive waste buildup in the pits

39. Chutes used for moving swine should be constructed so that the sides
    a. Have no openings
    b. Have vertical bars
    c. Have horizontal bars
    d. Are wider at the bottom than at the top

40. Feeders in finishing hog pens should have
    a. One feeder space per pig
    b. Wide openings so that two pigs can eat per hole
    c. One feeder space per 6 to 10 pigs
    d. Shallow feeder spaces

41. In finishing buildings with pits, exhaust fans should pull air out of the building from the
    a. Pit area
    b. Ceiling
    c. Sides of the building
    d. Ends of the building

NUTRITION

General

42. Energy-producing nutrients include all of the following *except*
    a. Sugars
    b. Amino acids
    c. Minerals
    d. Fatty acids

43. Fiber serves as a major energy source for
    a. Monogastric mammals
    b. Herbivorous animals
    c. Carnivorous animals
    d. Snakes

44. Adenosine triphosphate (ATP) is a high-energy storage molecule used directly or indirectly to drive other cellular processes that require energy. These processes include all of the following *except*
    a. Transport of molecules and ions across cell membranes against concentration gradients that maintain the internal environment of the cell
    b. Synthesis of chemical compounds
    c. Contraction of muscle fibers and other fibers producing motion of the cells
    d. Synthesis of other low-energy compounds

45. Of the following, which takes priority in increasing the amino acid requirements of an animal?
    a. Growth and lactation
    b. Maintenance
    c. Exertional work
    d. Exercise

46. The most important ingested nutrient is
    a. Minerals
    b. Fats
    c. Vitamins
    d. Water

47. Which of the following is an example of a dietary macromineral?
    a. Iron
    b. Calcium
    c. Zinc
    d. Copper

Correct answers are on pages 90–96.

48. The definition of nutrients is
    a. Materials used to manufacture a finished feed
    b. Quantitative distribution of the individual nutrients within the finished formula
    c. A nourishing substance, food, or component of food, including minerals, vitamins, fats, protein, carbohydrates, and water
    d. Portions and select ingredients

49. A normal growth rate for puppies (per kilogram of anticipated adult weight) is
    a. 2 to 4 g/day
    b. 4 to 5 g/day
    c. 1 to 2 g/day
    d. 3 to 6 g/day

50. Vitamins that are classified as fat-soluble include all of the following *except*
    a. A
    b. D
    c. E
    d. B

51. All of the following are causes for obesity in companion animals *except*
    a. Overfeeding when young
    b. Genetic predisposition
    c. Diet high in protein
    d. Surgical neutering of males and females (which deregulates satiety and increases the desire to eat)

52. Which would provide the best information on the mineral status of a horse?
    a. Feed analysis
    b. Muscle analysis
    c. Blood and urine analyses
    d. Hair analysis

53. Sudden ration changes can result in any of the following *except*
    a. Cachexia
    b. Laminitis
    c. Diarrhea
    d. Colic

54. Enteral feeding is indicated in a horse with
    a. Rabies
    b. Dementia
    c. Ileus
    d. Dysphagia

55. Prolonged undernutrition in adult horses adversely affects all of the following *except*
    a. Wound healing
    b. Immune system
    c. Skeletal structures
    d. Gastrointestinal tract

56. A horse with cardiac disease may *not* require a major dietary change. The *only* change may be to restrict intake of
    a. Hay
    b. Grain
    c. Salt
    d. Water

57. Horses with active laminitis should be fed
    a. Grain only
    b. Alfalfa hay and grain
    c. Alfalfa hay only
    d. Average-quality hay and no grain

58. Horses prone to esophageal obstruction should *not* be fed
    a. Pellets
    b. Grain
    c. Hay
    d. Salt

59. All of the following are nutrients required for normal horn and hoof formation *except*
    a. Lipids
    b. Vitamin K
    c. Amino acids
    d. Protein

60. A first line of attack to improving voluntary feed intake in a hospitalized patient is to
    a. Initiate vitamin supplementation
    b. Improve palatability of feeds
    c. Feed stimulants
    d. Give drugs to treat the primary condition

61. During pregnancy, goats require extra dietary energy during the last
    a. 4 months
    b. 3 months
    c. 2 months
    d. 1 week

62. Urea toxicity in small ruminants typically occurs within 1 hour after ingestion. Signs include all of the following *except*
    a. Low packed cell volume (PCV)
    b. Frequent urination and defecation
    c. Incoordination
    d. Muscle and chin tremors

63. In goats, night blindness, poor appetite, weight loss, unthrifty appearance with a poor haircoat, and a thick nasal discharge have resulted from a lack of vitamin
    a. B
    b. K
    c. D
    d. A

64. Lack of which vitamin in goats can cause nutritional muscular dystrophy (white muscle disease)?
    a. E
    b. B
    c. D
    d. A

65. Lack of which nutrients can cause retarded growth and rickets in goat kids?
    a. Vitamin B and magnesium
    b. Vitamins E and C
    c. Vitamin C and calcium
    d. Vitamins A and B

66. Goats spend more time eating each day than sheep. Goats ruminate approximately how many hours a day?
    a. 10
    b. 8
    c. 6
    d. 4

67. Goats are most at risk for developing the metabolic condition termed *ketosis* during
    a. Middle of gestation
    b. Late lactation
    c. Early gestation
    d. Late gestation

68. Goats that consume excessive concentrates may be predisposed to
    a. Ketosis
    b. Rumen acidosis
    c. Rumen alkalosis
    d. Parturient paresis

69. Sudden changes in a goat's diet (consumption of unaccustomed quantities of grain or of lush pasture when first turned out in the spring) can lead to incomplete digestion in the rumen. The ingesta that passes to the small intestine then favors overgrowth of clostridia and production of epsilon toxin. This produces a syndrome called
    a. Parturient paresis
    b. Urolithiasis
    c. Posthitis
    d. Enterotoxemia

70. A llama's stomach is functionally similar to, but anatomically different from, a true ruminant stomach. How many compartments does a llama's stomach have?
    a. 2
    b. 3
    c. 4
    d. 5

Correct answers are on pages 90–96.

71. Llamas, like true ruminants, can break down which feed constituent into short-chained fatty acids with the assistance of bacteria and protozoa?
    a. Cellulose
    b. Water
    c. Calcium
    d. Phosphorus

72. Which statement concerning feeding of llamas is most accurate?
    a. They must be fed once daily.
    b. They must be fed twice daily.
    c. They must be fed free choice.
    d. They should be fed on a regular schedule.

73. A *predominant* deficiency of which nutrient causes angular limb deformities, given current North American feeding practices of llamas?
    a. Phosphorus
    b. Calcium
    c. Vitamin A
    d. Vitamin D

74. Which nutrient represents the greatest fraction of dairy cattle diets after weaning and is essential to optimizing milk production?
    a. Minerals
    b. Vitamins
    c. Carbohydrates
    d. Protein

75. When formulating cattle rations, which part of the bovine digestive tract warrants most consideration?
    a. Rumen
    b. Omasum
    c. Abomasum
    d. Reticulum

76. Cattle add large quantities of saliva to their feed during chewing and also regurgitate during rumination. The most important effect of this is to
    a. Add more moisture to forage materials
    b. Buffer the acids produced in the rumen
    c. Aid chewing and swallowing
    d. Keep the tongue moist

77. Which of the following comprises the major gaseous energy loss as a result of fermentation in the rumen?
    a. Oxygen
    b. Ethane
    c. Carbon dioxide
    d. Methane

78. Neonates unable to tolerate gastrointestinal feeding are often administered TPN. What do the letters TPN stand for?
    a. Thiamin/protein/nitrogen mix
    b. Total parenteral nutrition
    c. Typical program for neonates
    d. Triglyceride potassium nutrients

79. To supply adequate nutrition via the intravenous route, solutions used must be
    a. Hypertonic
    b. Hypotonic
    c. Isotonic
    d. Catatonic

80. Which foal has the greatest nutritional requirement?
    a. Healthy active foal
    b. Foal with an umbilical infection
    c. Newborn foal
    d. Premature foal with septicemia

81. Hyperlipidemia is usually caused by intolerance of lipids and is characterized by cloudy serum and
    a. Hypoglycemia
    b. Hyperactivity
    c. Increased serum triglycerides
    d. Acidosis

82. Which of the following is *not* recommended for a weak foal?
    a. Bucket feeding
    b. Bottle feeding
    c. Nasogastric intubation
    d. Intravenous nutrition

83. Weight loss is most commonly associated with any of the following circumstances *except*
    a. Anorexia
    b. Increased nutrient demands
    c. Protein calorie malnutrition
    d. Aflatoxicosis

84. To avoid abomasal bloat in calves, the amount of milk fed at one time should *not* exceed
    a. 500 ml
    b. 4 L
    c. 2 L
    d. 20% of body weight

85. Healthy calves can handle what percent of their body weight of milk per day without developing diarrhea?
    a. 1% to 5%
    b. 10% to 15%
    c. 16% to 20%
    d. 25%

86. When a calf suckles and ingests warm milk, the reticular groove is stimulated to close so that milk and saliva pass directly into the
    a. Abomasum
    b. Rumen
    c. Reticulum
    d. Duodenum

87. When the newborn lamb is nursing but receives no nutrition at all in cold environmental conditions, fat reserves last only about
    a. 4 hours
    b. 1 to 2 days
    c. 5 days
    d. 1 week

88. The neonatal calf is a preruminant and does not become a full ruminant until 3 to 4 months of age, depending on
    a. Its sex
    b. The season
    c. Its breed
    d. Its diet

89. Most problems associated with use of milk replacers for raising neonatal calves, foals, kids, and lambs can be traced to three main management practices *except*
    a. Use of improper milk replacer formula
    b. Feeding an inadequate amount per day
    c. Use of contaminated milk replacer powder
    d. Suboptimum environment and management, such as competition for feed

90. Lack of which vitamin can cause deafness, tissue malfunction, and large coarse skin lesions in dogs?
    a. A
    b. K
    c. B_1
    d. B_{12}

For questions 91 through 94, select the correct answer from the four choices below.

    a. Vitamin E
    b. Vitamin K
    c. Vitamin B_1
    d. Vitamin B_{12}

91. Synthesized in the intestinal tract of dogs and other animals under normal conditions

92. Needed by dogs in heavy training to facilitate development of erythrocytes to carry oxygen from the lungs to the muscles

Correct answers are on pages 90–96.

93. Very important in reproduction; usually called the antisterility vitamin, it is a biologic antioxidant and is considered necessary for several bodily functions

94. Another name for thiamine; it is necessary in carbohydrate utilization; deficiency can lead to loss of appetite, weight loss, and even convulsions

95. The major consideration in evaluating a dog's diet is
    a. Maintenance requirements
    b. Reproduction and lactation
    c. Carbohydrate content
    d. Digestibility

96. Which term refers to the quantities of nutrients necessary to maintain a constant body weight in mature dogs at rest?
    a. Maintenance requirements
    b. Reproduction and lactation
    c. Palatability
    d. Digestibility

97. Which condition is most likely to increase a dog's nutritional requirements?
    a. Sedentary lifestyle
    b. Pregnancy and lactation
    c. Old age
    d. Obesity

98. The most important factor in a dog's diet is
    a. Availability of water
    b. Sufficient protein
    c. Sufficient carbohydrates
    d. Digestibility and utilization of nutrients

99. Which nutrient comprises the greatest part of most dog rations, supplying energy and the bulk needed for proper intestinal function?
    a. Protein
    b. Fat
    c. Carbohydrates
    d. Vitamins and minerals

100. During lactation, the feed intake of queens typically:
    a. Stays the same
    b. Increases about 1.5 times
    c. Increases about 2-3 times
    d. Increases about 50%

101. In home-cooked diets for dogs and cats, what are the most common nutritional deficits?
    a. Protein and fat
    b. Water and magnesium
    c. Vitamin A and copper
    d. Salt and protein

102. Because of their high fiber content and bulky nature, dry dog food should *not* be fed to dogs with
    a. Diarrhea
    b. Ascites
    c. Anemia
    d. Pancreatitis

103. Which clinical condition is often mistaken for obesity and may conceal malnutrition?
    a. Diarrhea
    b. Ascites
    c. Anemia
    d. Pancreatitis

104. With which clinical condition are severe abdominal pain, cardiovascular shock, vomiting, and diarrhea commonly associated in older dogs, but only rarely seen in horses and pigs?
    a. Diarrhea
    b. Ascites
    c. Anemia
    d. Pancreatitis

105. In which condition should dietary ash be reduced and 5 g of NaCl per pound of food be added to stimulate water intake and thus achieve moderate diuresis?
    a. Diarrhea
    b. Ascites
    c. Pancreatitis
    d. Urolithiasis

SWINE

106. Newborn piglets raised in confinement must be supplemented with
    a. Zinc
    b. Iron
    c. Copper
    d. Manganese

107. Why do piglets need this supplement?
    a. The calcium obtained from nursing binds the mineral and makes it useless
    b. They are born without any and must have it to survive
    c. They are born with low levels in their tissue and do not have an adequate dietary source while nursing
    d. It is depleted during digestion

108. Swine must have access to drinking water at all times. If deprived of water for an extended period, they
    a. Develop sodium chloride toxicity
    b. Become hyperactive
    c. Begin to bite the tail of other pigs in the same pen
    d. Develop potassium deficiency

109. Goosestepping (excessive lifing of the rear legs during walking) is most likely to be caused by a deficiency of
    a. Copper
    b. Vitamin D
    c. Zinc
    d. Pantothenic acid

110. Soybean meal is often a basic component of swine diets. What does this ingredient provide?
    a. Fat
    b. Protein
    c. Mineral
    d. Vitamin

111. A nursery pig is presented for necropsy. The history states that it was healthy yesterday afternoon and was found dead this morning. Necropsy reveals "mulberry heart disease." What dietary deficiency is the *most* likely cause of this pig's sudden demise?
    a. Vitamin E
    b. Vitamin C
    c. Vitamin K
    d. Vitamin B_2

112. Creep feed should be given to piglets a few days after birth. How much protein should be available in the ration?
    a. 10% to 12%
    b. 18% to 20%
    c. 7% to 9%
    d. 2% to 3%

113. What is the protein requirement in an adult breeding sow?
    a. 20% to 25%
    b. 3% to 4%
    c. 10% to 12%
    d. 15% to 17%

114. Sows often develop constipation during late gestation and early lactation. What should the producer do to minimize this problem and keep them at optimum performance?
    a. Increase the daily ration
    b. Add fiber to the ration
    c. Confine the animals to prevent exercise
    d. Decrease the daily ration

115. Finely ground hog feed (particle size 600 to 800 μ) can increase the incidence of
    a. Gastric ulcers
    b. Reproductive problems
    c. Respiratory infections
    d. Lameness

Correct answers are on pages 90–96.

116. Antibacterials are routinely added to hog feed to increase performance and feed efficiency. What group of animals benefits the most from this practice?
    a. Breeding boars
    b. Breeding sows
    c. Finishing hogs
    d. Nursery and grower pigs

117. What ingredient can be added to the diet of hogs to provide increased energy and reduce dust in the feed?
    a. Fat
    b. Water
    c. Soybean meal
    d. Silage

118. During what season should sows and boars be fed additional energy to optimize breeding efficiency?
    a. Spring
    b. Summer
    c. Fall
    d. Winter

119. Hogs fed a diet deficient in zinc develop
    a. Cataracts
    b. Ear necrosis
    c. Ulcers
    d. Hyperkeratosis

120. What is a consequence of feeding swine from the floor for prolonged periods?
    a. Formation of trichobezoars (hairballs)
    b. Lacerations on the tongue and in the mouth
    c. None; pigs will not eat from the floor
    d. Floor damage

PHYSICAL RESTRAINT

General

121. If used improperly, which restraint instrument is most likely to cause broken bones, strangulation, and death?
    a. Cat bag
    b. Nose lead
    c. Restraint gloves
    d. Capture pole

122. Because of their bellows-like breathing, which species should be held loosely if grasped around the thorax?
    a. Birds
    b. Ferrets
    c. Cats
    d. Hamsters

123. If a bird is presented to you in a cage containing toys, perches, and water and food dishes, what is the best procedure for capturing the bird?
    a. Throw a towel over the bird and grasp it
    b. Turn the lights down and reach in behind the bird
    c. Talk gently and coax the bird to stand on your finger
    d. Remove all the paraphernalia from the cage and then reach in behind the bird

124. To collect blood from the cephalic vein of a dog or cat, you should place the animal in
    a. A sitting position and lift the head to expose the ventral aspect of the neck
    b. Lateral recumbency and steady the uppermost back leg
    c. A sitting position and steady a front leg
    d. Lateral recumbency and lift the uppermost rear leg out of the way to expose the medial surface of the other rear leg

125. For oral administration of liquid medication to a dog or cat, you should
  a. Tilt the head up slightly and roll the lips over the canine teeth to open the mouth
  b. Leave the head in a horizontal position and administer the liquid between the lips and cheek
  c. Tilt the head straight up and open the mouth using the index finger of your other hand
  d. Tilt the head straight up, administer the liquid between the lips, and stroke the throat

126. Of the following steps to place a cat in a cat bag, which should be first?
  a. Close the zipper
  b. Place the bag on the table
  c. Hook the bag around the cat's neck
  d. Place the cat in the center of the bag

127. In prolonged attempts to capture a sheep or pig in a paddock or pen, it is extremely easy to cause
  a. An abortion
  b. Hyperthermia
  c. A limb fracture
  d. Death from shock

128. When applying a chain twitch to a horse, you should
  a. Place it on the upper lip and tighten with intermittent pressure
  b. Place it on the upper lip and tighten as much as possible
  c. Place it on the ear and tighten with intermittent pressure
  d. Place it on the lower lip and tighten as much as possible

129. Which piece of restraint equipment is most commonly used on horses?
  a. Twitch
  b. Hobbles
  c. Cradle
  d. Halter

130. When disturbed by attempts at physical restraint, a horse's initial response usually is to
  a. Kick
  b. Bite
  c. Run
  d. Rear

131. When restraining a foal for treatment or diagnostic procedures, you should
  a. Lead the mare out of sight of the foal
  b. Keep the mare nearby, within sight of the foal
  c. Leave the mare with the foal, but heavily sedate the mare
  d. Pick the foal up off the ground so it cannot run away

132. Which piece of restraint equipment usually remains permanently attached to bulls used for breeding?
  a. Halter
  b. Nose lead
  c. Bull staff
  d. Nose ring

133. Which animals have the strongest instinct to remain in a group when threatened?
  a. Sheep
  b. Goats
  c. Pigs
  d. Chickens

134. The knot or hitch used to tie together two ropes of different sizes is a
  a. Bowline
  b. Sheet bend
  c. Halter tie
  d. Clove hitch

135. The knot or hitch that can be used for breeding hobbles is a
  a. Bowline on a bight
  b. Clove hitch
  c. Halter tie
  d. Reefer

Correct answers are on pages 90–96.

136. The knot or hitch used to secure a lead rope to a stationary object is a
    a. Square
    b. Clove hitch
    c. Bowline
    d. Halter tie

137. The knot or hitch used to secure a rope to a vertical bar without slippage is the
    a. Clove hitch
    b. Halter tie
    c. Half hitch
    d. Bowline

138. A nonslip knot or hitch that is safe to place around an animal's neck is the
    a. Bowline
    b. Halter tie
    c. Clove hitch
    d. Sheet bend

139. When "tail jacking" a cow, grasp the tail
    a. By the end and pull it to one side as far as possible
    b. At the base and elevate it dorsally and to the right
    c. By the end and elevate it dorsally and to the left
    d. At the base and elevate it dorsally and directly in the midline

140. When carrying a rabbit, it is important to support its hindquarters so the animal does *not*
    a. Scratch you with its hind feet
    b. Struggle and possibly fracture its spine
    c. Injure its ear
    d. Defecate and urinate

141. After securing a mouse by its tail, the head and body can be restrained by
    a. Twirling the mouse until it is dizzy and then quickly grasping the scruff of its neck
    b. Placing the mouse on a smooth surface, pulling caudally on its tail, and then quickly grasping the scruff of its neck
    c. Grasping the loose skin along its back
    d. Placing the mouse on a grate, pulling back on its tail, and then quickly grasping the scruff of its neck

142. The apparatus usually used to restrain beef cattle is the
    a. V-trough
    b. Stock
    c. Squeeze chute
    d. Stanchion

143. The apparatus used to restrain horses is the
    a. Stock
    b. Squeeze chute
    c. Stanchion
    d. Tilt table

144. The apparatus used to restrain pigs weighing up to 80 lb is the
    a. Stock
    b. Squeeze chute
    c. V-trough
    d. Tilt table

145. The apparatus ideal for restraining a bull to facilitate hoof trimming is the
    a. Stock
    b. Squeeze chute
    c. Tilt table
    d. Alley way

146. Which procedure is *not* a distraction technique?
    a. Taping the legs together
    b. Firm petting
    c. Twitching
    d. Blowing on the face

147. What is the best time of day to restrain sheep in the summer?
    a. Midafternoon
    b. Afternoon
    c. Early morning
    d. Midmorning

148. To judge whether a dog is being aggressive, observe its body language. An aggressive dog
    a. Looks from side to side
    b. Holds its head low between the shoulders
    c. Wags its tail
    d. Has eyes darting from one thing to another

149. To judge whether a dog is nervous, observe its body language. A nervous dog
    a. Holds its head low between the shoulders
    b. Stares straight at you
    c. Has raised shoulder hair
    d. Has eyes darting from one thing to another

150. To protect yourself if attacked by a dog, you should
    a. Run
    b. Kick or hit at it
    c. Roll yourself into a ball and protect your neck and face with your arms
    d. Stand still and call for help

151. When confronted by a dog inside a kennel that is snarling, growling, and lunging at the bars, which restraint instrument is safest for you and the dog?
    a. Restraint gloves
    b. Capture pole
    c. Blanket
    d. Rope leash

152. A cat that was quiet and manageable before going into a cage has turned into a snarling mass of fangs and claws. What is the most likely cause of this behavior change?
    a. Someone hit it or beat it
    b. It has been frightened
    c. It is defending its territory
    d. It is lonely

153. The cardinal rule when working with cats is to
    a. Make sure doors and windows are firmly locked
    b. Always wear restraint gloves
    c. Put them in a cat bag for easier handling
    d. Always cover their head with a blanket or towel

154. Normal behavior for a cat in a new place is to
    a. Cower in a corner
    b. Lose bladder and bowel control
    c. Sit in one spot
    d. Look around and investigate

155. Which of these is *not* a warning sign of an angry cat?
    a. Hissing and spitting
    b. Rubbing up against the cage bars
    c. Ears lowered
    d. Crouching low with tail lashing

156. When restraining a rooster, be most careful of the
    a. Beak
    b. Spurs
    c. Wings
    d. Feet

157. When restraining a large parrot, be most careful of its
    a. Beak
    b. Wings
    c. Talons
    d. Spurs

Correct answers are on pages 90–96.

158. Of domestic fowl, which poses the *least* threat to a handler?
- **a.** Ducks
- **b.** Geese
- **c.** Turkeys
- **d.** Chickens

159. Of the caged birds listed below, which one has the *least* tolerance for handling?
- **a.** Cockatiels
- **b.** Canaries
- **c.** Parrots
- **d.** Conures

160. Which behavior trait can you use to advantage when trying to restrain a pig?
- **a.** Strong herding instinct
- **b.** Easily trained
- **c.** Their love of rooting in the ground
- **d.** A strong stubborn streak

161. Which restraint equipment is most useful when moving pigs from one place to another?
- **a.** A bucket
- **b.** Small fences
- **c.** A hurdle or portable barrier
- **d.** A dog

162. It is acceptable and humane to lift a newborn pig by the
- **a.** Tail
- **b.** Ear
- **c.** Front leg
- **d.** Back leg

163. Of the cattle listed below, which is most likely to be docile?
- **a.** Dairy bull
- **b.** Beef bull
- **c.** Dairy cow
- **d.** Beef cow

164. When handling cattle with horns, stand
- **a.** Directly in front of the animal
- **b.** To the left of the animal
- **c.** To the left and front of the animal
- **d.** To one side, directly behind the horns

165. If you need to tie a cow's tail out of the way, it is best to tie it to:
- **a.** The cow's own body
- **b.** A fence rail no higher than its hock
- **c.** A nail directly overhead
- **d.** The front of the chute or stanchion

166. To lift a full-grown rabbit out of its cage, you should grasp it by the
- **a.** Ears
- **b.** Lumbar vertebrae
- **c.** Shoulders
- **d.** Scruff of the neck

167. Rats can be safely and humanely picked up by
- **a.** The scruff of the neck
- **b.** Grasping them over the shoulders
- **c.** Grasping the tail
- **d.** Grasping a back leg

168. Which species can have a seizure if handled too harshly?
- **a.** Gerbils
- **b.** Guinea pigs
- **c.** Mice
- **d.** Rats

169. To restrain a snake, you should
- **a.** Grasp it behind the head and let the rest of the body hang down
- **b.** Grasp it behind the head and support the rest of the body with your other hand
- **c.** Grasp it with one hand at midupper body and the other at midlower body
- **d.** Grasp it by the tail and let the rest of the body hang down

170. A horse standing with its ears erect and moving and its head erect is most likely
- **a.** Depressed
- **b.** Nervous
- **c.** Alert
- **d.** Angry

208. Hazardous components of a cleaner or disinfectant are stated in the manufacturer's
   a. SOPS
   b. GLPS
   c. VFAS
   d. MSDS

209. Alcohol's optimum disinfecting ability occurs at a dilution factor of
   a. 50%
   b. 70%
   c. 90%
   d. 100%

210. When hypochlorite solution comes in contact with formaldehyde, the gas produced is a very
   a. Effective disinfectant
   b. Dangerous carcinogen
   c. Pleasant deodorant
   d. Weak antiseptic

211. When disinfecting using two products, the rule is to
   a. Use one disinfectant at a time
   b. Mix the disinfectants together
   c. Dilute each disinfectant by half
   d. Select one bactericial and one bacteriostatic disinfectant

212. Selection of a disinfectant ideally depends on the
   a. Result required
   b. Purchase price
   c. Ease of application
   d. Product stability

213. Ultrasonic cleaners are used to
   a. Sanitize instruments
   b. Disinfect instruments
   c. Sterilize instruments
   d. Lubricate instruments

214. Ultrasonic cleaners work through creating
   a. Steam under pressure
   b. High-frequency sound waves
   c. Mechanical scrubbing
   d. Radiation

215. In hand-cleaning equipment after surgery, the degree of cleanliness is most influenced by the
   a. Contact time with the cleaner
   b. Degree of mechanical friction
   c. Thoroughness of subsequent rinsing
   d. Temperature of the wash water

216. Floors are cleaned best using a
   a. Wet vacuum
   b. Dry vacuum
   c. Wet mop
   d. Dry mop

217. During busy days in surgery, the area in the suite most likely to need decontamination is the
   a. Doorway to the operating room
   b. Cabinets holding surgical packs
   c. Scrub sink floor and walls
   d. Air conditioning and heating duct grills

218. When washing hands, it is important to remember that the highest density of bacteria occurs
   a. Under the nails
   b. Over the knuckles
   c. Between the digits
   d. On the palm

219. Nursing mares and foals should *not* be put into pastures that were grazed the previous year by
   a. Stallions
   b. Mares
   c. Foals
   d. Yearlings

220. Pastures should be free of
   a. Rocks
   b. Ponds
   c. Trees
   d. Fences

221. If stabling horses on clay floors, once a year you should
   a. Apply a sealant to the clay floor
   b. Soak the floor with disinfectant
   c. Replace the clay surface
   d. Culture the clay for microbes

Correct answers are on pages 90–96.

222. For effective sanitation, lights in the surgical suite should be
    a. Recessed into the ceiling
    b. Close to the air inlet
    c. Fitted with fluorescent bulbs
    d. Activated by entry of personnel

223. Soap for hand washing is most likely to harbor microbes if it is in
    a. A pressurized dispensing pump
    b. Solid bar form
    c. An aerosol cannister
    d. A sponge-brush combination

224. Before it is taken into the surgery room, portable equipment should be
    a. Wiped with a dry sterile cloth
    b. Fumigated with formaldehyde gas
    c. Damp dusted with a disinfectant
    d. Scrubbed with a sanitizer

225. Colonization of coliform bacteria on the hands may be promoted by using hand cleaners that contain
    a. An iodophor
    b. Chlorhexidine
    c. Hexachlorophene
    d. Alcohol

Answers

HOUSING

General

1. b
2. c
3. c
4. b
5. b
6. a
7. a
8. b
9. d
10. c
11. d
12. b
13. c
14. d
15. b
16. b
17. a
18. d
19. a
20. b
21. b
22. c
23. b
24. d
25. d
26. c

SWINE

27. **b** The pig should have to reach up slightly to drink from a nipple watering device to minimize waste. In addition, the pigs are less likely to come into contact with the nipple, causing damage to themselves or the device.

28. **b** Providing two nipples in a pen of 20 pigs allows all of the animals access to water. Generally, swine producers are encouraged to install a minimum of two watering devices per pen.

29. **d** Newborn piglets do not have the ability to regulate their body temperature, and supplemental heat must be provided.

30. **b** Sows have a thick layer of body fat and are more comfortable at lower temperatures than newborn piglets.

31. **d** The environmental temperature can fluctuate in the room. Thermometers should be placed at the pigs' level to ensure that the pigs are comfortable.

32. **c** If a sow is too warm, milk production decreases, resulting in smaller pigs. In addition, an uncomfortable sow changes position often and could crush her pigs. Keeping her comfortable is, therefore, to the advantage of the piglets. They should be provided with a source of heat well away from the sow.

33. **b** Vertical slats prevents the pigs from climbing the fence.

34. **b** Comfortable pigs spread out in the sleeping area of the pen. When they are cold, the pigs pile up to conserve body heat.

35. **b** Humidity levels between 50% to 60% tend to minimize growth of bacteria. In addition, levels below 60% keep other contaminants (gases, respirable dust) low.

36. **d** Pigs tend to defecate in a far corner of the pen, as they are in a vulnerable position at this time.

37. **a** Tail biting is commonly seen when pigs are overcrowded. Producers often remove the tails from newborn piglets to alleviate this vice as the animals grow older.

38. **c**

39. **a** If pigs see obstructions or movement in front of them, they stop moving.

40. **c** One feeder space per 6 to 10 pigs allows the animals ample access to the food supply and is economical for the producer to provide.

41. **a** Animal wastes that collect in the pits produce noxious gases that should not be pulled back into the building. Exhaust fans must be set up so that they move the air from the pit area out of the building.

NUTRITION

General

42. **c** Minerals

43. **b** Grazing animals. Mammals lack fiber-degrading enzyme systems, so fiber is not digested in a monogastric mammal.

44. **d** Should be "synthesis of other *high-energy* components."

45. **a**

46. **d** Dehydration is a common clinical problem in sick patients unwilling or unable to eat and drink.

47. **b** Calcium, iron, zinc, and copper are examples of microminerals.

48. **c** a—the definition of ingredients; b—the definition of nutrient profile; d—the definition of formula.

49. **a** 2 to 4g/day/kg of anticipated adult weight. Puppies should be weighed when there is concern about lactation.

50. **d** Vitamin B is water soluble.

51. **c**

52. **a**

53. **a** Cachexia is a profound and marked state of constitutional disorder, general ill health, and malnutrition.

54. **d** Dysphagia. Difficulty in swallowing may be exactly the time to initiate enteral feeding.

55. **c**

56. **c**

57. **d**

58. **a**

59. b

60. d

61. c

62. a Actually, an elevated PCV is seen with small ruminants with urea toxicity.

63. d

64. a

65. c

66. b

67. d The disease is also termed *pregnancy toxemia*.

68. b

69. d *Overeating* disease.

70. b

71. a

72. d Owners may have a lifestyle whereby they feed twice a day or free choice. The most important point is that they should feed regularly.

73. a.

74. c

75. a

76. b

77. d

78. b

79. a

80. d

81. c

82. b Bottle feeding may cause aspiration pneumonia in a weak foal.

83. d Aflatoxicosis is caused by toxic metabolites of certain molds and usually produces liver damage with possibly some weight loss; it is not a common cause.

84. c

85. c

86. a

87. b

88. d

89. c

90. a

91. b

92. d

93. a

94. c

95. d

96. a

97. b

98. a

99. c

100. c

101. c

102. a

103. b

104. d

105. d

SWINE

106. b Piglets are born with very low iron reserves and do not obtain much iron while nursing the sow. Piglets raised outdoors obtain iron from the dirt lots.

107. c

108. a With water deprivation, sodium accumulation can lead to convulsions and death. Affected pigs should be rehydrated slowly over a period of several hours.

109. d A deficiency of pantothenic acid in the diet leads to deterioration of the sciatic nerve. Affected pigs exhibit an abnormal gait.

110. b Soybean meal provides a readily available source of protein (44% to 48.5%) and satisfies the amino acid requirements of pigs.

111. **a** Mulberry heart disease is a classic finding in pigs suffering from vitamin E deficiency; it is characterized by degeneration of cardiac muscle.

112. **b** Protein requirements vary with the age and growth period of the pig's life. Increased amounts of amino acids are necessary for muscle development in the young animal.

113. **c** Breeding sows have reached their growth potential and do not need high levels of protein for muscle development. Protein is the most expensive ingredient in a ration, and excessive amounts are used by the sow as energy, which is not economical.

114. **b** Sows are limit-fed to prevent obesity. More fiber adds bulk to the diet without increasing calories.

115. **a** Studies show that the production of digestive acids increases when the pig ingests finely ground particles of feed.

116. **d** Young pigs grow rapidly, and addition of antibacterials to the diet increases feed efficiency and the rate of gain during this period of the pig's life.

117. **a** Fats or oils provide a readily available source of energy to the diet, with the added benefit of reducing the level of dustiness of the feed.

118. **b** Sows tend to decrease their feed intake during hot weather, and reproductive performance decreases as a result of an energy deficit. Additional energy in the ration maintains optimal breeding performance.

119. **d** Zinc is a key element in the metabolism of protein, carbohydrates, and lipids. A deficiency of the mineral results in hyperkeratosis.

120. **a** Hogs that are floor fed for extended periods ingest hair that is constantly shed. Accumulation of hair in the stomach leads to development of a large hairball (trichobezoar), which can obstruct the digestive tract.

PHYSICAL RESTRAINT

General

121. **c** Restraint gloves decrease your tactile perception to the extent that you could cause strangulation, broken bones, and ultimately death.

122. **a** The lungs of birds cannot inflate if the thorax is grasped tightly.

123. **d** Removing all paraphernalia reduces the chance that the bird will injure itself in attempts to escape.

124. **c** The cephalic vein is on the cranial (dorsal) surface of the front leg.

125. **b** The head should remain horizontal and the mouth closed. Stroking the throat induces swallowing.

126. **b** Place the open bag on the table.

127. **b** The insulation of a sheep's heavy wool coat and a pig's layer of body fat can lead to overheating if the animal is chased excessively.

128. **a** The twitch is placed on the upper lip, with pressure applied intermittently to keep the horse's attention on the twitch and at the same time preserve circulation to the lip.

129. **d** The halter is the main tool of restraint for horses.

130. **c** Running is a horse's first instinct when threatened. If it cannot run away, it will fight.

131. **b** The foal and mare should remain within eyesight of each other. If not, both will fret and struggle to be reunited.

132. **d** Nose rings are permanently inserted through the nasal septum of bulls.

133. **a**

134. **b**

135. **a** When this knot is tied in the middle of a long rope, it forms a nonslip noose that can go around the animal's neck. The long ends can be wrapped around the rear legs and secured so the mare cannot kick.

136. **d** This quick-release knot should be the only knot used to tie a lead rope to a stationary object.

137. **a** A clove hitch will not slip, even when one end is pulled.

138. **a**

139. **d** The tail should be grasped at the base and elevated straight up. Moving the tail toward one side or holding the tail by the end can damage the tail.

140. **b** Rabbits carried without support of the rear legs can struggle to the extent that they fracture their spine.

141. **d** A mouse will instinctively grasp a grate with its forefeet. You can then quickly grasp it by the scruff of the neck.

142. **c** A squeeze chute is usually used to restrain beef cattle. Dairy cattle usually are restrained in stanchions.

143. **a** Stocks are used to protect the veterinarian or technician while working on a horse.

144. **c** Pigs weighing up to 80 pounds can be placed on their back in a V trough.

145. **c** A tilt table is ideal for trimming cattle hooves. The animal is led to the side of the tabletop, which is in a vertical position. After the animal is strapped to it, the table is moved to a horizontal position so that the animal is in lateral recumbency.

146. **a** Taping the legs is considered a restraint technique.

147. **c** Early morning is the coolest time and allows the owner to observe the flock for signs of distress throughout the rest of the day.

148. **b** Head held low between the shoulders is a classic stance of an aggressive dog.

149. **d**

150. **c**

151. **b** The capture pole allows you to remain a safe distance from the dog, and the noose will not cause the animal to choke if used properly.

152. **c** Cats are territorial and establish territory quickly.

153. **a** Cats can squeeze through very small spaces. To prevent escape from a cage, examination room, or hospital, all doors should remain latched or locked securely.

154. **d** The cat's natural instinct is to investigate a new territory.

155. **b**

156. **b**

157. **a**

158. **a** A duck's bill is blunt and can pinch but not break the skin. Also, ducks are small; consequently their wings do not cause painful bruises.

159. **b** The canary is typically the most affected by handling, although the other birds can also have an adverse reaction to rough treatment.

160. **d** Pigs are notorious for being stubborn. This trait can be used to advantage and is the reason the hog snare works so effectively.

161. **c** A hurdle or barrier made of a solid piece of plastic or fiberglass placed in the path of a pig will turn it in the desired direction.

162. **d** Lifting by any of the other body parts may cause injuries.

163. **c** Dairy cows are usually accustomed to handling and do not react as the other three may.

164. **c** This the safest area as long as you stand well beyond the reach of the animal's head.

165. **a** Never tie a tail to anything but the animal's body. If you forget to untie the tail and the cow bolts, the tail may be pulled off.

166. **d** Anywhere else, and the rabbit or handler may be injured.

167. **b** Anywhere else, and the rat may be injured.

168. **a**

169. **b** A snake's body must be supported in the middle so that the vertebrae are not damaged.

170. **c**

171. **b**

172. **a** Most horses are trained to respond to *whoa* or *hold still* and a few other commands.

173. **d** Anything lower or longer and the animal can get tangled in the rope.

174. **b** Horses are very adept at reading body language, and quickly detect signs of nervousness, no matter how subtle.

175. **d** Placing it anywhere else will cause extreme discomfort to the horse, and it may act up even more strongly.

176. **d** Pulling on the wool of sheep can damage subcutaneous tissues and the fleece, and may cause hemorrhages.

177. **c** Using a crook anywhere else can harm the animal.

178. **b** Save steps and aggravation by learning which goat is the lead goat. A dog will only cause them to scatter more.

179. **b**

180. **a** All fences and paddocks must be at least 6 feet high because a goat can easily jump anything lower.

SWINE

Restraint and Behavior

181. **c** The snare must control the pig's head. When the pig feels the pressure of the snare, it will pull backward.

182. **d** The sow's vision will be effectively blocked, causing her to back up. The other items mentioned might work, but the handler's hand and arms would be at risk from the bars of the crate.

183. **b**

184. **b** Although catching by the tail is acceptable when piglets are only a few days old, a 7- to 10-day-old pig weighs too much for the animal to be lifted from the ground by the tail alone.

185. **d** The rope snare can be placed around the sow's snout, and the end can be secured to the bars of the farrowing crate. A large sow can swing a regular hog snare against the bars of the crate and severely injure the handler's arms and hands.

186. **a** Pigs cannot dissipate heat because they do not have functional sweat glands. It is always wise to schedule such activities early in the day to avoid overheating the animals.

187. **d** It is always easier to catch pigs when they are confined in a small area. Bringing them into the area just before the arrival of the veterinarian can avoid problems associated with water deprivation.

188. **c** Hog tongs facilitate snaring. One handler applies the tongs to the back of the neck, which causes the animal to squeal. As soon as a second person places the snare, the tongs are released. This procedure is usually less stressful than chasing the gilt around the pen.

189. **a** The gilt is exhibiting a porcine stress syndrome reaction. If the restraint is continued, the reaction may progress and the gilt will die.

190. **c** The size of the pig often dictates the best restraint technique, and the number of animals involved affects the choice because of the time involved in applying a technique. Techniques that are effective with a single 10-kg pig may be too difficult or time consuming to apply to 25- to 100-kg hogs.

191. **a** Pigs are territorial and establish a dominance order when new animals are introduced. It is important to pen together pigs of similar size to minimize fighting. The aggression is normally short lived as the pigs determine the dominance order.

192. **b** Swine have a tendency to move as a group but will not hesitate to separate when stressed.

193. **c** Pigs are reluctant to move into a dimly lit area. Lighting the passageway of the barn encourages them to enter the building. However, it is important that the light not shine directly into the eyes of the pigs.

194. **d** The herding panel would be most effective because it can be used to block the pigs' vision if they attempt to run to the back of the trailer.

195. **b** The handler should easily be able to manipulate the herding panel, which is used to block the pig's vision. A pig will not attempt to walk through a solid panel.

SANITATION

196. a
197. b
198. d
199. c
200. d
201. c
202. b
203. c
204. b
205. b
206. b
207. c
208. d
209. b
210. c
211. a
212. a
213. a
214. b
215. b
216. a
217. c
218. a
219. c
220. b
221. c
222. a
223. b
224. c
225. c

Dentistry

Marsha E. Madsen, RVT, MS   Terri Raffel, CVT

Recommended Reading

Burger WL: The role of the technician in small animal dentistry. I, *Vet Tech* 14:491–495, 1993; II, *Vet Tech* 14:649-653, 1993.

Frost P: *Canine dentistry*, ed 4, Vero Beach Fla, 1993, JH Day Communications.

Hawkins J: Applied dentistry for veterinary technicians, *Vet Tech* 12:75–96, 1991.

Hawkins J: *Waltham applied dentistry*, Vernon Calif, 1993, Waltham USA.

Holstrom SE, Frost P, Gammon RL: *Veterinary dental techniques for the small animal practitioner*, Philadelphia, 1992, WB Saunders.

McCurnin DM, editor: *Clinical textbook for veterinary technicians*, ed 3, Philadelphia, 1994, WB Saunders.

Questions

1. The root length of an upper canine is how long compared with the length of the exposed portion of that tooth?
   a. $\frac{1}{2}$ the length
   b. Same length
   c. 3 times the length
   d. $1\frac{1}{2}$ times the length

2. The upper fourth premolar communicates with which sinus?
   a. Mandibular
   b. Occipital
   c. Maxillary
   d. Orbital

3. The crown of a tooth is defined as
   a. That portion above the gum line and covered by enamel
   b. The most terminal portion of the root
   c. That portion below the gum line
   d. The layer of bony tissue that attaches to the alveolar bone

4. The range for acceptable gingival sulcal measurements in cats is
   a. 1 to 3 mm
   b. 0.5 to 1 mm
   c. 1.5 to 4.5 mm
   d. 0.005 to 0.007 mm

Practice answer sheet is on page 321.

Correct answers are on pages 102–103.

5. When performing dental prophylaxis, you should be sure to wear
   a. Cap, mask, gloves
   b. Gown, gloves, mask
   c. Cap, eye protection, gloves
   d. Mask, eye protection, gloves

6. In which grade of periodontal disease does early pocket formation occur without initial bone loss?
   a. Grade I
   b. Grade II
   c. Grade III
   d. Grade IV

7. A curet
   a. Is used strictly as a supragingival instrument
   b. Can be used either supragingivally or subgingivally
   c. Is the most important dental instrument
   d. Is used to irrigate the teeth with air or water

8. What drug should *not* be given to pregnant dogs because it may cause discoloration of the puppies' teeth?
   a. Amoxicillin
   b. Tetracycline
   c. Chloramphenicol
   d. Penicillin

9. The occlusal surface of a caudal tooth is defined as the
   a. Surface facing the hard palate
   b. Surface nearer the cheek
   c. Chewing surface of the tooth
   d. Surface nearer the tongue

10. The normal adult canine mouth has how many permanent teeth?
    a. 40
    b. 42
    c. 48
    d. 52

11. The instrument used to measure pocket depth is a periodontal
    a. Explorer
    b. Scaler
    c. Curet
    d. Probe

12. A complication that may develop if subgingival plaque is improperly removed is
    a. Etched tooth enamel
    b. Torn epithelial attachment
    c. Overheated tooth
    d. Bitten technician

13. Which tooth has three roots?
    a. Upper canine
    b. Lower first premolar
    c. Lower first molar
    d. Upper fourth premolar

14. Which statement concerning the polishing aspect of dental prophylaxis is *least* accurate?
    a. A slow speed should be used.
    b. Adequate prophy paste is needed for lubrication and polishing.
    c. The polisher should remain on the tooth for as long as is needed to polish the tooth.
    d. If teeth are not polished, the rough enamel will promote bacterial plaque formation.

MATCHING

For questions 15 through 18, choose the answer that identifies the situation described in the question.

   a. Plaque
   b. Attrition
   c. Calculus
   d. Erosion

15. The wearing away of teeth by tooth-against-tooth contact during mastication.

16. The hard mineralized substance on the tooth surface.

17. The loss of tooth structure by chemical means.

18. The thin film covering a tooth that comprises bacteria, saliva, and food particles.

19. What is the *minimum* age for a cat to have all of its permanent teeth?
    a. 6 months
    b. 8 months
    c. 10 months
    d. 1 year

20. Generally speaking, most dental instruments should be held as you would a
    a. Knife
    b. Pencil
    c. Hammer
    d. Toothbrush

21. Of cats and dogs aged 6 years and older, approximately what percentage have periodontal disease?
    a. 20%
    b. 35%
    c. 50%
    d. 85%

22. Removal of calculus and necrotic cementum from the tooth roots is called
    a. Curettage
    b. Splinting
    c. Root planing
    d. Scaling

23. Prevention of periodontal disease involves all of the following *except*
    a. Daily teeth brushing or mouth rinsing
    b. Regular exercise
    c. Routine professional scaling and polishing
    d. Proper diet

24. To prevent the pulp tissue from thermal damage during ultrasonic scaling, which of the following should be done?
    a. Use constant irrigation
    b. Change tips frequently
    c. Use slow rotational speed
    d. Use appropriate amounts of paste

25. Ideally, the cutting edge of the scaler should be held at what angle to the tooth surface?
    a. 5 to 10 degrees
    b. 35 to 45 degrees
    c. 15 to 30 degrees
    d. 45 to 90 degrees

26. The purpose of fluoride treatment is to
    a. Prevent thermal damage and lubrication
    b. Strengthen enamel and help desensitize teeth
    c. Remove plaque and strengthen the enamel
    d. Irrigate and lubricate

27. Mrs. Walker comes to pick up her dog after dental prophylaxis has been performed. Which of the following topics would *not* need to be discussed as a part of the discharge instructions?
    a. Chewing exercises
    b. Home care
    c. How to give injections
    d. Dietary concerns

28. Once plaque has formed on a tooth, how long does it take to mineralize into calculus?
    a. About 7 days
    b. 2 weeks
    c. 4 weeks
    d. 2 months

29. The most common dental procedure performed on horses is
    a. Quidding
    b. Floating
    c. Repelling
    d. Scaling

30. Which tissue is *not* part of the periodontium?
    a. Periodontal ligament
    b. Alveolar bone
    c. Root
    d. Gingiva

Correct answers are on pages 102–103.

31. The correct dental formula for an adult dog is
    a. 2(I 3/3 C 1/1 P 3/4 M 3/3) = 42
    b. 2(I 3/3 C 1/1 P 4/4 M 3/2) = 42
    c. 2(I 3/3 C 1/1 P 4/4 M 2/3) = 42
    d. 2(I 4/4 C 1/1 P 3/4 M 3/3) = 46

32. The correct dental formula for an adult cat is
    a. 2(I 3/3 C 1/1 P 3/2 M 1/1) = 30
    b. 2(I 4/4 C 1/1 P 2/3 M 1/1) = 34
    c. 2(I 3/3 C 1/1 P 2/3 M 1/1) = 30
    d. 2(I 3/3 C 1/1 P 3/2 M 2/1) = 32

Questions 33 to 36

    a. Apical
    b. Rostral
    c. Furcation
    d. Buccal

33. The space between the roots of the same tooth.

34. The tooth surface facing the cheeks or lips.

35. The directional term for toward the root.

36. The directional term for toward the front of the head.

37. Chlorhexidine contributes to dental prophylaxis by
    a. Slowly dissolving calculus
    b. Bonding to the cell membrane and inhibiting bacterial growth
    c. Bleaching stained teeth
    d. Decreasing tooth sensitivity

38. In normal occlusion, the bite is termed
    a. Scissor bite
    b. Straight bite
    c. Occlusal bite
    d. Razor bite

39. What is the proper dilution of chlorhexidine solution for use in the mouth?
    a. 20%
    b. 2.0%
    c. 0.2%
    d. 10%

40. Topical fluoride
    a. Will stain remaining calculus red
    b. Helps to desensitize teeth and slows the rate of plaque formation
    c. Should never be used on feline teeth
    d. Enhances osteoclastic activity and helps desensitize teeth

41. The depth of a normal gingival sulcus is
    a. 1 to 1.5 mm
    b. 1 to 3 mm
    c. 2 to 4 mm
    d. 2 to 5 mm

Questions 42 through 45

    a. Periodontal probe
    b. Explorer
    c. Scaler
    d. Curet

42. Instrument used for root planing.

43. Instrument used to detect subgingival calculus.

44. Instrument to measure the depth of the gingival sulcus.

45. Instrument used for removal of supragingival calculus.

46. An elongation of one side of the animal's head results in
    a. Anterior crossbite
    b. Wry mouth
    c. Brachygnathism
    d. Prognathism

47. The bulk of a tooth is composed of
    a. Enamel
    b. Pulp
    c. Dentin
    d. Cementum

48. The most common mistake made in treating periodontal disease is
    a. Inadequate removal of supragingival calculus
    b. Inadequate root planing
    c. Insufficient polishing
    d. Iatrogenic trauma to subgingival tissues

49. As a dentifrice for use in small animals, baking soda
    a. Is an excellent choice
    b. Should be mixed with salt and water to form a paste
    c. Should be mixed with fluoride gel to form a paste
    d. Should not be used as a dentifrice for animals

50. After polishing with a prophylactic paste containing fluoride, a rinse with diluted chlorhexidine
    a. Is less effective because the fluoride interferes with bonding of chlorhexidine to tissues
    b. Results in temporary blue staining of the teeth
    c. Enhances the activity of both fluoride and chlorhexidine
    d. May be toxic to the patient

51. If the lower incisors seem to be excessively loose in a brachycephalic or miniature-breed dog,
    a. The teeth should be extracted
    b. The depth of the gingival sulcus should be tested
    c. The dog is calcium deficient
    d. The dog has advanced periodontal disease

52. Fractured deciduous teeth
    a. Should be left in place until they are normally shed
    b. Should be repaired
    c. Are insignificant
    d. Should be extracted

53. The first dental examination should occur when
    a. The animal is 2 to 3 years old
    b. The owner requests it
    c. A problem such as drooling or bad breath is noticed
    d. The animal is 6 to 8 weeks old

54. The deciduous incisors
    a. Erupt at $3\frac{1}{2}$ to 4 weeks of age
    b. Have roots that are proportionately longer than the roots of permanent incisors
    c. Are the most frequently retained teeth
    d. Are not usually replaced with permanent incisors until the dog is 6 months old

55. Nerves and blood vessels enter the tooth through the
    a. Apical delta
    b. Crown
    c. Pulp
    d. Sulcus

56. When one or more of the upper incisors rest caudal to the lower incisors and the rest of the occlusion is normal, this is called
    a. Level bite
    b. Wry mouth
    c. Anterior crossbite
    d. Anodontia

57. The term *polyodontia* refers to
    a. Retained deciduous teeth
    b. Supernumerary teeth
    c. Both supernumerary teeth and retained deciduous teeth
    d. Tooth loss as a result of periodontal disease

Correct answers are on pages 102–103.

Answers

1. **d** None of the other lengths is appropriate.

2. **c** The upper fourth premolar communicates directly with the maxillary sinus.

3. **a** The other answers describe other portions of a tooth.

4. **b** The other answers are inappropriate ranges.

5. **d**

6. **c** Early bone loss in the late stage of grade III can be verified by radiographic examination.

7. **b**

8. **b** None of the other drugs has this effect on neonatal dentition.

9. **c** The other answers describe other surfaces of a tooth.

10. **b**

11. **d** This is the only instrument that can be used for measurement.

12. **b** Excessive force may degrade epithelial attachment.

13. **d** The other teeth listed have 1 or 2 roots.

14. **c** Prolonged application creates overheating and damage to the tooth.

15. **b**

16. **c**

17. **d**

18. **a**

19. **a** Complete eruption of permanent dentition can occur as early as 6 months.

20. **b** A modified pen grip is the preferred method of holding dental instruments.

21. **d**

22. **c** This best describes the action.

23. **b** Exercise does not contribute to the prevention of periodontal disease.

24. **a** Constant irrigation helps prevent temperatures from rising too high.

25. **d** This is the most effective angle.

26. **b**

27. **c** Injections are generally not necessary after dental prophylaxis.

28. **a** Mineralization of plaque occurs fairly rapidly.

29. **b** Floating is the process of filing sharp edges off cheek teeth.

30. **c**

31. **c**

32. **a**

33. **c**

34. **d**

35. **a**

36. **b**

37. **b** Chlorhexidine bonds to the cell membrane and inhibits bacterial growth for up to 24 hours. The other choices do not describe actions of chlorhexidine. Fluoride decreases tooth sensitivity.

38. **a**

39. **c** All other choices are too concentrated.

40. **b** Fluoride does not stain the remaining calculus red, it is beneficial to feline teeth, and it inhibits (not enhances) osteoclastic activity.

41. **b**

42. **d**

43. **b**

44. **a**

45. **c**

46. **b** Brachygnathism refers to elongation of the maxilla (on both sides of the dog's head); prognathism refers to elongation of the mandible (on both sides of the head); anterior crossbite refers to malocclusion of the incisors.

47. **c**

48. **b** Both *a* and *c* refer to surfaces above the gingival sulcus, and it is in the sulcus that most of the damage from periodontal disease occurs. Proper removal of all calculus from the subgingival tooth surfaces is essential to proper treatment of periodontal disease. Although iatrogenic trauma to subgingival tissues may be a problem, it would not be considered the most common mistake in treatment of periodontal disease.

49. **d** Baking soda contains large amounts of sodium that can be absorbed into the pet's system. Remember, dogs and cats swallow their "toothpaste." Because many pets that require frequent brushing may also have heart disease, this extra sodium could be life threatening.

50. **a** If chlorhexidine is used, the prophylactic paste should not contain fluoride. After the teeth are polished, the teeth and subgingival surfaces can be flushed with dilute chlorhexidine, and then fluoride gel can be applied to the teeth.

51. **b** In many of these types of dogs, the incisor teeth may not be in individual bony sockets but suspended in connective tissue, which allows them to be quite mobile. These may be healthy teeth.

52. **d** The permanent tooth bud lies very close to the deciduous tooth and could become infected if the deciduous tooth is fractured and left in place.

53. **d** The animal should have its first dental examination when it comes in for its first vaccinations and should have a dental examination on every visit after that. Waiting for problems, such as drooling or bad breath, to occur allows dental disease to progress to a point where it may be more difficult to treat successfully.

54. **b**

55. **a**

56. **c**

57. **b**

Notes

Emergency Care

Robin Duntze, DVM   *Paula Voglewede, RVT*

Recommended Reading

Bonagura J, Crisp M, editors: *The Kal Kan Waltham symposium: Emergency medicine and critical care,* Vernon Calif, 1991, Kal Kan Foods.

Kirby R, Stamp L, editors: Critical care, *Vet Clin North Am Small Anim Pract,* vol 19, no 6, 1989.

Kirk R, Bonagura J, editors: *Current veterinary therapy XI,* Philadelphia, 1990, WB Saunders.

Kirk RW, Bistner SI, Ford RB: *Handbook of veterinary procedures and emergency treatment,* ed 5, Philadelphia, 1990, WB Saunders.

McCurnin DM: *Clinical textbook for veterinary technicians,* ed 3, Philadelphia, 1993, WB Saunders.

Pratt PW: *Medical, surgical, and anesthetic nursing for veterinary technicians,* ed 2, St Louis, 1994, Mosby.

Questions

EMERGENCY ASSESSMENT

1. Which would be considered the *least* important physical measure evaluated during triage of a patient?
    a. Heart rate
    b. Respiratory rate
    c. Capillary refill time
    d. Weight

2. Patients in shock have
    a. An initial decrease in heart rate that then increases as the patient nears death
    b. A decreased heart rate
    c. An initial increase in heart rate that then decreases as the patient nears death
    d. An increased heart rate

3. The mucous membranes of patients in hemorrhagic shock are
    a. Cyanotic
    b. Pale or white
    c. Brick red
    d. Unusually warm

4. The mucous membranes of patients with severe anemia and respiratory distress are
    a. White
    b. Purple or blue
    c. Brick red
    d. Pink

Practice answer sheet is on page 323.

Correct answers are on pages 115–118.

5. Normal urine output in cats and dogs is
   a. 1 to 2 ml/kg/hr
   b. 3 to 4 ml/kg/hr
   c. 0.5 ml/kg/hr
   d. 10 ml/kg/hr

6. According to the principles of triage, which patient should first be seen by the veterinarian?
   a. Cat with a closed fracture
   b. Dog in respiratory distress
   c. Dog with otitis externa
   d. Cat with a small laceration on a paw pad

7. Rapid shallow breathing usually indicates
   a. Pleural space disease
   b. Lung tissue disease
   c. Upper airway obstruction
   d. Asthma

8. Petechial hemorrhages on the mucous membranes can indicate
   a. Trauma
   b. Methemoglobinemia
   c. Anemia
   d. Thrombocytopenia

9. Which is *not* a characteristic of traumatic shock?
   a. White mucous membranes
   b. Cool extremities
   c. Capillary refill time under one second
   d. Weak femoral pulses

10. According to the principles of triage, which patient should first be seen by a veterinarian?
    a. Dog with a small laceration on a pinna
    b. Dog with acute gastric dilatation–volvulus
    c. Cat with dystocia, not in shock, no kitten in birth canal
    d. Cat with possible linear foreign body in the bowel

11. Which sign is *not* an indication of dystocia?
    a. Green or black vulvar discharge
    b. Profuse vulvar hemorrhage
    c. Pup or kitten in the birth canal for 5 minutes
    d. More than 1 hour of vigorous contractions with no pup or kitten produced

12. Which is *not* usually a sign of acute gastric dilatation–volvulus?
    a. Unproductive attempts to vomit
    b. Hypersalivation
    c. Abdominal distention
    d. Profuse diarrhea

13. Crackles on thoracic auscultation indicate
    a. Asthma
    b. Upper airway obstruction
    c. Fluid in the lungs
    d. Pleural space disease

14. An owner describes his male cat as lethargic and constipated; he has observed the cat straining in the litter box. You suspect that the cat is actually suffering from
    a. Peritonitis
    b. Urethral obstruction
    c. Intestinal obstruction
    d. An upper respiratory viral infection

15. If the hindquarters are elevated in a dog with a severe diaphragmatic hernia, what effect does this have on respiration?
    a. No change in respiratory rate or depth
    b. Respiratory rate decreases and respiration becomes less labored
    c. Respiration becomes more labored
    d. A cough is induced

16. You are assessing a cat with spinal injury. When you pinch its toe, a positive response to deep pain is indicated by
    a. No response
    b. Withdrawal of the foot without meowing
    c. Vomiting
    d. Withdrawal of the foot and meowing

17. Signs of impending cardiopulmonary arrest include all of the following *except*
    a. Alertness
    b. Dilated pupils
    c. Agonal breathing
    d. No femoral pulse

18. A patient with multiple pelvic fractures has *not* urinated in over 24 hours. You suspect the patient may also have
    a. A ruptured bladder
    b. A diaphragmatic hernia
    c. Renal failure
    d. Urethral calculi

19. A free-roaming dog is brought to your clinic for listlessness and dyspnea. When performing venipuncture, you notice that the animal seems to have a prolonged clotting time. You suspect that the patient may have ingested
    a. Anticoagulant rodent poison
    b. Ethylene glycol
    c. Strychnine
    d. Organophosphate insecticide

20. Which statement concerning status epilepticus is most accurate?
    a. It occurs only in geriatric animals.
    b. It is a life-threatening medical emergency.
    c. It is treated by administering acepromazine.
    d. It will resolve spontaneously.

21. Signs of organophosphate toxicity include all of the following *except*
    a. Salivation
    b. Lacrimation
    c. Dyspnea
    d. Dilated pupils

22. Normal capillary refill time in dogs is
    a. Under one second
    b. 1 to 2 seconds
    c. 2 to 4 seconds
    d. 4 to 6 seconds

FIRST AID

23. An owner calls your clinic and tells you that his cat has just been hit by a car. You recommend that he
    a. Immediately bring the cat in to be examined by a veterinarian
    b. Observe the cat at home for an hour, and call back if problems occur
    c. Bring the cat for examination by a veterinarian the following day
    d. Bring the cat to you for initial examination, so you can determine if the animal needs to be seen by a veterinarian

24. A dog has been hit by a car and the owner calls your clinic. The owner says the dog has a dangling leg. You recommend to the owner that he
    a. Start cardiopulmonary resuscitation immediately, then bring the pet to the clinic
    b. Observe the pet at home for an hour, and bring it to the clinic if there is no improvement
    c. Observe the pet at home for 24 hours, and bring it to the clinic if there is no improvement
    d. Splint the leg, if possible, and bring the pet to the clinic immediately

Correct answers are on pages 115–118.

25. An owner calls your clinic and tells you that his puppy has just eaten rat poison that you know contains an anticoagulant. What should you recommend?
    a. Do not induce emesis, and immediately bring the pet to the clinic for examination and treatment
    b. Induce emesis, then immediately bring the pet to the clinic for examination and treatment
    c. Induce emesis; no further treatment required
    d. Induce emesis, then bring the pet to the clinic only if it shows signs of toxicity

26. An owner calls your clinic and tells you that his cat has just ingested antifreeze (ethylene glycol). What should you recommend?
    a. Do not induce emesis, and immediately bring the pet to the clinic for examination and treatment
    b. Induce emesis, then immediately bring the pet to the clinic for examination and treatment
    c. Induce emesis; no further treatment required
    d. Induce emesis, then bring the pet to the clinic only if it shows signs of toxicity

27. An owner of a diabetic cat calls your clinic and says that her cat has just had a seizure and collapsed. She gave the cat its usual dose of insulin that morning. You recommend that she give
    a. Another dose of insulin, then bring the cat to the clinic for medical attention
    b. Some corn syrup or sugar solution, then observe the cat at home
    c. Some corn syrup or sugar solution, then bring the cat to the clinic for medical attention
    d. Another dose of insulin, then observe the cat at home

28. An owner has just treated his 5-week-old kitten with a flea dip containing lindane. The cat is acting slightly lethargic, and the owner now notices that the label on the dip says *for dogs only*. The owner calls your clinic. You should advise him to
    a. Observe the kitten at home
    b. Rinse the kitten with mild dish soap, then bring the animal to the clinic for examination
    c. Rinse the kitten with mild dish soap, then administer acetaminophen for discomfort
    d. Induce emesis, then observe the kitten at home

29. An owner calls your clinic because he has noticed that his cat has a string protruding from under the tongue. You should advise him to
    a. Attempt to gently pull out the string
    b. Induce emesis
    c. Cut the string and administer laxatives at home
    d. Bring the cat to the clinic for examination

30. An owner calls your clinic because she has noticed a fishhook embedded in her dog's lower lip. You should advise her to
    a. Attempt to gently pull out the fishhook
    b. Observe the dog at home; most fishhooks fall out spontaneously within 24 hours
    c. Attempt to gently push the fishhook through the skin, then cut and remove it; if this is not successful, seek prompt medical attention
    d. Administer aspirin for discomfort and see the veterinarian within 48 hours for treatment

31. The first measure used to control active bleeding is
    a. Direct digital pressure
    b. A tourniquet
    c. A pressure bandage
    d. Electrocautery

32. A dog has a lacerated paw pad. The owner has placed a small bandage over the wound, but blood is soaking through. Appropriate treatment is to
   a. Remove the bandage and apply digital pressure to the wound
   b. Apply a pressure bandage over the owner's original bandage
   c. Remove the bandage and apply a tourniquet to the limb
   d. Do nothing; no further treatment is required if the bleeding is not excessive

33. An owner calls the clinic and tells you that her small poodle has stopped breathing. What should you recommend?
   a. Attempt no treatment; immediately transport the pet to the hospital
   b. Attempt mouth-to-mouth resuscitation and chest compressions; immediately transport the pet to the hospital
   c. Close the dog's mouth and attempt mouth-to-nose resuscitation and chest compressions; immediately transport the pet to the hospital
   d. Attempt resuscitation; transport the pet to the hospital if attempts at resuscitation are unsuccessful

34. A patient with a head or neck injury should be transported to the hospital in which position?
   a. Head elevated, neck neutral
   b. Head elevated, neck flexed
   c. Head lowered, neck neutral
   d. Head lowered, neck flexed

35. A patient with a possible herniated intervertebral disc should be
   a. Allowed to move freely; if no improvement is evident in 24 hours, see the veterinarian
   b. Allowed to move freely; see the veterinarian immediately
   c. Kept strictly quiet and confined; if no improvement is evident in 24 hours, see the veterinarian
   d. Kept strictly quiet and confined; see the veterinarian immediately

36. Which item would be *least* likely to be found on a crash cart used for emergency situations?
   a. Laryngoscope
   b. Intravenous catheter
   c. Otoscope
   d. Ambu bag

37. A patient comes to your clinic apneic and cyanotic. A quick oral examination reveals a hard ball lodged in the glottal opening. You should
   a. Place the patient in an oxygen cage
   b. Attempt to pass a nasal oxygen catheter
   c. Attempt to pass an endotracheal tube
   d. Perform the Heimlich maneuver; if unsuccessful, prepare the patient for tracheotomy

38. A 16-year-old, 3-kg poodle comes to your clinic cyanotic with agonal respirations and frothy fluid coming from the nose and mouth. You should
   a. Administer intravenous fluids at 90 ml/kg/hr
   b. Administer furosemide intramuscularly, then place the patient in an oxygen cage
   c. Swing the patient to remove as much fluid as possible from the airway, then initiate cardiopulmonary resuscitation
   d. Prepare the patient for immediate tracheostomy

Correct answers are on pages 115–118.

39. The veterinarian for whom you work has authorized you to start infusing intravenous fluids in a 0.25-kg Yorkshire Terrier pup who is critically ill. You are unable to insert a catheter into a jugular or cephalic vein. An alternate site for catheter placement is the
    a. Intraosseous canal of the femur
    b. Carotid artery
    c. Lingual vein
    d. Ear vein

40. The veterinarian for whom you work has directed you to give a whole blood transfusion to a 0.3-kg kitten with severe anemia from flea infestation. You are unable to insert a catheter into a vein. An alternate route for the transfusion is
    a. Subcutaneous injection
    b. Intramuscular injection
    c. Intraperitoneal injection
    d. Per os

41. You are instructing an owner to apply an emergency muzzle to his injured dog. Which is the *least* appropriate material for the muzzle?
    a. Rope
    b. Metal chain dog leash
    c. Pantyhose
    d. Necktie

42. Which of the following is *least* likely to be available for at-home induction of emesis?
    a. Apomorphine
    b. Syrup of ipecac
    c. Hydrogen peroxide
    d. Mustard and water solution

43. All of the following should be included in the first aid procedure for acute gastric dilatation–volvulus *except*
    a. Induce emesis
    b. Treat for shock
    c. Attempt to pass a stomach tube
    d. Trocarize the stomach

44. All of the following should be included in the first aid procedure for epistaxis *except*
    a. Elevate the nose
    b. Apply warm compresses to the nose
    c. Apply an ice pack to the nose
    d. Keep the patient quiet

45. Which statement concerning administration of activated charcoal via stomach tube is *least* accurate?
    a. Check tube placement by administering a small amount of water; listen for coughing or gagging
    b. Measure the tube from the tip of the nose to the 9th through 13th rib
    c. Measure the tube from the tip of the nose to the thoracic inlet
    d. Use a roll of tape as a speculum to keep the mouth open and prevent the animal from biting the tube

46. Oxygen can be administered to a patient via any of the following routes *except*
    a. Endotracheal tube
    b. Tracheotomy tube
    c. Chest tube
    d. Nasal oxygen catheter

47. The initial first aid procedure for a patient with heat stroke is
    a. Intravenous fluid administration
    b. Cool-water enema
    c. Oxygen administration
    d. Cool-water bath

48. First aid for a dog with paraphimosis includes all of the following *except*
    a. Lubricate the penis
    b. Apply ice packs to the penis
    c. Apply hypertonic solutions to the penis
    d. Apply a warm compress to the penis

49. Initial first aid treatment for a dog with an open fracture includes all of the following *except*
    a. Copiously clean and flush the wound
    b. Cover the wound
    c. Apply a temporary splint to the limb
    d. Make radiographs of the fracture

50. Which statement concerning first aid for seizure is most accurate?
    a. Grasp the animal's tongue and pull it forward to prevent airway obstruction.
    b. Administer oral anticonvulsants.
    c. Keep the animal quiet, and prevent it from injuring itself.
    d. Immediately start infusion of intravenous fluids.

51. An owner calls your hospital and says that his Pekingese has suffered a proptosis. Your advice to the owner should include all of the following *except*
    a. Apply pressure to the globe to replace it in the socket
    b. Protect the globe from further trauma
    c. Keep the globe moist
    d. Bring the dog to the veterinarian immediately

52. An owner calls and says that his Rottweiler has been shot in the abdomen but appears perfectly fine. What should you recommend?
    a. Observe the animal at home for vomiting or abdominal pain
    b. See the veterinarian immediately
    c. See the veterinarian at your earliest convenience
    d. Observe the animal for hemorrhage

53. First aid treatment for a cat with an open pneumothorax may include all of the following *except*
    a. Thoracentesis
    b. Oxygen administration
    c. Covering the wound
    d. Radiographic examination

54. Which statement concerning emergency treatment of cats with urethral obstruction is *least* accurate?
    a. Cats must always be sedated to have a urinary catheter passed
    b. Sometimes the obstruction can be relieved by massaging the tip of the penis
    c. Cats with a slow, irregular heart rate probably have a high serum potassium level
    d. If the obstruction is not relieved, the cat will die

55. Which procedure is *not* routinely performed to resuscitate neonates following cesarean section?
    a. Clean the nose and mouth of secretions
    b. Rub them with a towel to stimulate breathing
    c. Administer a drop of oxytocin under the tongue
    d. Ligate the umbilical cord

56. Inducing emesis after ingestion of a solid toxin is probably no longer of value after how much time has elapsed since ingestion?
    a. 10 minutes
    b. 30 minutes
    c. 1 to 4 hours
    d. 24 hours

57. Which is *not* an immediate consideration in cardiopulmonary resuscitation?
    a. Airway
    b. Circulation
    c. Bleeding
    d. Breathing

CRITICAL CARE

58. During cardiopulmonary arrest, which route is the *least* effective for drug administration?
    a. Intraosseous
    b. Intratracheal
    c. Intramuscular
    d. Intravenous

Correct answers are on pages 115–118.

59. At what rate should cardiac compressions be administered to a dog in cardiopulmonary arrest?
    a. 80 to 120/min
    b. 60 to 80/min
    c. 110 to 140/min
    d. 25 to 30/min

60. What should the ventilation rate be during cardiopulmonary arrest in a cat?
    a. 40 to 45/min
    b. 15 to 20/min
    c. 25 to 30/min
    d. 35 to 40/min

61. At what rate should fluids be infused intravenously in a dog in shock?
    a. 90 ml/kg/hr
    b. 50 ml/kg/hr
    c. 40 ml/kg/hr
    d. 20 ml/kg/hr

62. What is the minimal mean arterial blood pressure at which adequate perfusion is maintained to the brain and heart?
    a. 40 mm Hg
    b. 60 mm Hg
    c. 80 mm Hg
    d. 100 mm Hg

63. What is the most common vessel used to assess the pulse in a dog?
    a. Dorsal pedal artery
    b. Aorta
    c. Sublingual vein
    d. Femoral artery

64. All of the following are signs of shock *except*
    a. Weak and thready pulse
    b. Vasodilatation
    c. Prolonged capillary refill time
    d. Tachycardia

65. Central venous pressure is used in monitoring
    a. Pulse quality
    b. Temperature
    c. Hydration status
    d. Heart rate

66. All of the following can be used to check mucous membrane color *except* the
    a. Sclera
    b. Gingiva
    c. Vulva
    d. Prepuce

67. Dehydration is assessed by all of the following *except*
    a. Moistness of mucous membranes
    b. Skin turgor
    c. Packed cell volume and total protein
    d. Nasal discharge

Questions 68 and 69.

A 20-kg Springer Spaniel is brought to the clinic because of anorexia and lethargy. Dehydration is estimated at 8%. The maintenance requirement of fluids is 66 ml/kg/day.

68. To correct this dog's dehydration, how much fluid should it receive over 24 hours?
    a. 2920 ml
    b. 1600 ml
    c. 1320 ml
    d. 1336 ml

69. What is the hourly rate of fluid infusion to provide two times daily maintenance requirements?
    a. 55 ml
    b. 110 ml
    c. 235 ml
    d. 1320 ml

70. Placement of a jugular catheter is *contraindicated* in which situation?
    a. Vomiting
    b. Pancreatitis
    c. Thrombocytopenia
    d. Renal failure

71. What is the *first* consideration in cardiac arrest?
    a. Ventilate the animal
    b. Apply cardiac compressions
    c. Be sure the airway is patent
    d. Intravenous catheter placement

72. Tissue perfusion can be assessed by all of the following *except*
    a. Capillary refill time
    b. Blood pressure
    c. Mucous membrane color
    d. Temperature

73. During triage, which patient should be attended to *first*?
    a. Dog with a penetrating wound of the abdomen
    b. Cat in respiratory arrest
    c. Cat with an intestinal foreign body
    d. Dog with gastric dilatation–volvulus

74. Signs seen during cardiopulmonary arrest include all of the following *except*
    a. Absence of pulse
    b. No breathing
    c. Loss of consciousness
    d. Tachycardia

75. Hyperthermic patients should be treated immediately with
    a. A cool-water bath
    b. Ice packs
    c. Corticosteroid injection
    d. An alcohol bath

76. What is the recommended dosage for intratracheal drug administration during cardiac arrest?
    a. 1.5 times the intravenous dosage
    b. Same as the intravenous dosage
    c. Double the intravenous dosage
    d. Half the intravenous dosage

77. At what rate should fluids be infused intravenously in a cat in shock?
    a. 20 ml/kg/hr
    b. 40 ml/kg/hr
    c. 60 ml/kg/hr
    d. 80 ml/kg/hr

78. A client calls you on the telephone and is worried about her Irish Wolfhound. The dog ran loose in the neighborhood, and it is now retching and pacing the floor. The abdomen looks a little distended. What should you do?
    a. Record the client's phone number and tell her the doctor will call her back
    b. Tell the owner to immediately bring the dog in for examination
    c. Advise the owner to give 3% hydrogen peroxide to induce vomiting
    d. Tell the owner that the dog may have eaten garbage and to call the hospital in the morning if the animal is not feeling better

79. A 6-year-old mongrel is brought to your hospital with anisocoria, loss of consciousness, and involuntary urination. What is the most likely cause of these signs?
    a. Urethral obstruction
    b. Warfarin poisoning
    c. Seizure
    d. Organophosphate poisoning

80. A 3-year-old female cat is brought to your hospital with petechiae on her abdomen, bleeding gums, and lethargy. What is the most likely cause of these signs?
    a. Head trauma
    b. Heatstroke
    c. Seizure
    d. Rat poison exposure

81. When advising an owner to move an injured animal, all of the following are appropriate *except*
    a. If a back injury is suspected, place the animal on a board to move it
    b. Muzzle the injured animal because it may bite when being moved
    c. Call the veterinary hospital to notify it of your expected arrival time
    d. Give a baby aspirin before moving the animal to reduce pain

Correct answers are on pages 115–118.

82. Intraosseous infusion can be used in all of the following cases *except*
    a. Young and debilitated animals
    b. Epinephrine and atropine administration in an arrest
    c. Animals with septicemia
    d. Rapid access to the circulatory system in hypovolemic animals

83. What is the preferred route of fluid administration in a critically ill animal?
    a. Intravenous
    b. Subcutaneous
    c. Oral
    d. Intramuscular

84. Which of the following is a colloid?
    a. Hypertonic saline
    b. Lactated Ringer's solution
    c. Hetastarch
    d. Dextrose

85. Whole blood is indicated over packed red blood cells in which case?
    a. Acute blood loss during surgery
    b. Disseminated intravascular coagulation
    c. Autoimmune hemolytic anemia
    d. Acute blood loss caused by trauma

86. Nutritional support can be given in several ways. What is the preferred method?
    a. Per os
    b. Partial parenteral nutrition
    c. Total parenteral nutrition
    d. Per rectum

87. The normal body temperature for a dog is
    a. 37.5° C to 38.9°C (100° F to 102° F)
    b. 36.9° C to 38.3°C (98.6° F to 101° F)
    c. 35.6° C to 37.2°C (96° F to 99° F)
    d. 38.3° C to 40° C (101° F to 104° F)

88. A dog is considered tachycardic if the heart rate is
    a. Greater than 180
    b. Lower than 180
    c. Greater than 100
    d. Lower than 100

89. What is normal urinary output for a dog?
    a. 30 ml/kg/day
    b. 2 ml/kg/hr
    c. 1 ml/kg/hr
    d. 40 ml/kg/day

90. Which of the following is *not* a sign of a blood transfusion reaction?
    a. Fever
    b. Vomiting
    c. Tachycardia
    d. Seizure

91. The normal blood pH for a dog is
    a. 6.4
    b. 7.0
    c. 7.4
    d. 8.0

92. Which electrolyte imbalance is most likely to be found in a cat with total urethral obstruction?
    a. Hyperkalemia
    b. Hypokalemia
    c. Hyponatremia
    d. Hypercalcemia

93. All of the following are ways to monitor the heart rate in an unanesthetized animal *except*
    a. Stethoscope
    b. Electrocardiographic monitor
    c. Pulse rate
    d. Esophageal stethoscope

94. All of the following are noninvasive ways of monitoring a critically ill patient *except*
    a. Blood pressure measurement using a Doppler unit
    b. Temperature measurement using a tympanic thermometer
    c. Blood pressure measurement using an arterial catheter hooked to a transducer
    d. Blood pressure measurement using a Dinamap

95. What is the *last* priority in preparing for an emergency?
    a. Oxygen source
    b. Endotracheal tubes
    c. Heating pad
    d. Intravenous catheters

96. Closed-chest cardiopulmonary resuscitation is most effective in dogs weighing up to
    a. 10 kg
    b. 20 kg
    c. 30 kg
    d. 35 kg

Answers

EMERGENCY ASSESSMENT

1. **a** The patient's weight does not reveal the seriousness of its condition.

2. **c** Compensatory mechanisms initially cause an increase in heart rate; as the patient nears death these mechanisms fail and the heart rate drops.

3. **b** Blood loss causes pale mucous membranes as a result of diminished peripheral vascular perfusion.

4. **a** Patients must have adequate amounts of hemoglobin before cyanosis is demonstrated.

5. **a**

6. **b** Of the listed conditions, respiratory distress is the most critical.

7. **a** Fluid or masses in the pleural space restrict lung expansion, and the patient compensates with rapid shallow respiration.

8. **d** Abnormally low platelet counts interfere with blood clotting. One sign of thrombocytopenia may be petechial hemorrhages on mucous membranes.

9. **c** Traumatic shock is characterized by capillary refill times over 2 seconds.

10. **b** Of the conditions listed, acute gastric dilatation–volvulus is the most critical.

11. **c** Pups and kittens normally take longer than 5 minutes to traverse the birth canal.

12. **d** Diarrhea is not associated with gastric dilatation–volvulus.

13. **c** Crackles are produced as air is forced through fluid-filled airways.

14. **b** One should suspect urethral obstruction in male cats that are straining on the litter box until that problem is ruled out.

15. **c** Entry of abdominal organs into the chest cavity causes labored breathing.

16. **d** The patient must indicate with vocalization that it feels deep pain. Withdrawal is a spinal reflex.

17. **a** The patient's mental status is not a reliable indicator of impending arrest.

18. **a** Trauma sufficient to cause multiple pelvic fractures may also cause a ruptured bladder.

19. **a** Ingestion of anticoagulant rodenticides causes prolonged clotting times.

20. **b** Status epilepticus is a life-threatening medical emergency; without prompt treatment, brain damage or death may result.

21. **d** Organophosphate toxicity causes miosis.

22. **b**

FIRST AID

23. **a** Because of the potential for serious injury, all animals hit by a car should be immediately examined by a veterinarian.

24. **d** All animals hit by a car should be evaluated immediately. The fractured leg should be splinted, if possible, to prevent further injury during transport.

25. **b** Emesis should be induced because this is a noncorrosive toxin. The pet should be brought for antidotal treatment before signs of toxicity occur.

26. **b** Emesis should be induced because this is a noncorrosive toxin. The pet should be brought in for antidotal treatment before signs of toxicity occur.

27. **c** Because the cat had a morning dose of insulin, hypoglycemia may have caused the seizure.

28. **b** All cutaneous toxins should be removed via thorough washing.

29. **d** All of the other choices are potentially harmful to the cat.

30. **c** Most fishhooks are barbed and must be pushed through the skin for removal.

31. **a**

32. **b** Removing the bandage would remove any clot that had started to form. For most lacerated extremities, a pressure bandage is applied; tourniquets are used only when bandages cannot effect hemostasis.

33. **c** Mouth-to-nose resuscitation is more successful in pets and should be initiated during transport to the hospital.

34. **a** Elevating the head reduces intracranial pressure; a neutral neck minimizes cord compression or fracture displacement.

35. **d** A patient with a possible herniated disc should be strictly confined to minimize further cord damage. It should be immediately examined by a veterinarian to assess the extent of injury and start appropriate therapy.

36. **c** All the other equipment is used for cardiopulmonary resuscitation and life support.

37. **d** The Heimlich maneuver is used to relieve upper airway obstruction; if unsuccessful, a tracheotomy will be necessary.

38. **c** This patient has cardiopulmonary arrest. The airway should be cleared of secretions before instituting other resuscitation measures.

39. **a** The medullary cavity of the femur can accept large volumes of fluid.

40. **c.** Although this route is not ideal, red blood cells will be absorbed from the peritoneal cavity.

41. **b** Metal chain may injure the animal and is difficult to apply.

42. **a** Apomorphine is a controlled drug and unlikely to be found in a home.

43. **a** Inducing emesis is contraindicated in gastric dilatation–volvulus. Vomitus cannot be passed if the stomach is twisted.

44. **b** Warm compresses may increase circulation and worsen the epistaxis.

45. **c** The tube will not be placed in the stomach.

46. **c** Administration of oxygen via a chest tube would result in pneumothorax.

47. **d** Initial first aid can be performed by pet owner at home.

48. **d** A warm compress may increase circulation and worsen the paraphimosis.

49. Radiographic films are not a first aid measure and should be made only when wounds are cleaned and the patient's condition is stable.

50. **c** Other measures may be contraindicated or unnecessary.

51. **a** Pressure may cause further injury to the globe.

52. **b** Because of the high risk of peritonitis, most emergency clinicians recommend exploratory surgery as soon as possible after penetrating abdominal injuries.

53. **d** A radiographic examination should not be performed until the patient's condition is stabilized.

54. **a** Cats with prolonged uretheral obstruction may be comatose and often require no sedation for urinary catheterization.

55. **c** Doxapram is usually administered under the tongue; oxytocin is not given to neonates.

56. **c** After this time, the toxin has been absorbed into the system.

57. **c** The others are all principles of cardiopulmonary resuscitation.

CRITICAL CARE

58. **c** Drugs administered by the intramuscular route in patients with cardiac arrest are not absorbed quickly because of decreased perfusion of muscles.

59. **a**

60. **c**

61. **a**

62. **b**

63. **d** The femoral artery is the largest vessel to palpate the pulse and is usually easy to feel.

64. **b** Vasoconstriction occurs in shock.

65. **c**

66. **a** The conjunctiva, not the sclera, is used.

67. **d**

68. **a** $0.08 \times 20 \times 1,000 = 1,600$ ml; $20 \times 66 = 1,320$ ml; ($1,600$ ml + $1,320$ ml = $2,920$ ml)

69. **b** $20 \times 132 = 2,640 \div 24 = 110$ ml/hr

70. **c** Low platelet count causes more chance of bleeding; the jugular vein should not be used for fear of causing a large hematoma near the trachea.

71. **c**

72. **d**

73. **b** Respiratory function is an immediate concern.

74. **d** Bradycardia is seen during cardiopulmonary arrest.

75. **a** Ice packs may shock the system; alcohol may cause toxicity.

76. **c**

77. **b**

78. **b** Time is important and gastric dilatation–volvulus is life threatening.

79. **c**

80. **d**

81. **d** Medication should not be given without the doctor's consent.

82. **c** Intraosseous infusion may cause osteomyelitis in animals with septicemia.

83. **a** The intravenous route provides direct access to the intravascular space.

84. **c**

85. **b** Platelets are needed in disseminated intravascular coagulation; platelets are not present in packed red blood cells.

86. **a**

87. **a**

88. **a**

89. **c**

90. **d**

91. **c**

92. **a** Because potassium cannot be excreted properly, the cat becomes hyperkalemic.

93. **d** An animal must be anesthetized to insert an esophageal stethoscope.

94. **c** An arterial catheter is invasive.

95. **c** A heating pad is secondary to respiratory function.

96. **b** Effective pulses are hard to detect in dogs weighing more than 20 kg; it would be necessary to open the chest in these large dogs.

Notes

Hospital Management

Randal M. Shirbroun, DVM   *George W. Younger, DVM*

Recommended Reading

Accreditation policies and procedures of the AVMA Committee on Veterinary Technician Education and Activities, Schaumburg Ill, 1993, AVMA.

Becklin KJ, Sunnarborg EM: *Medical office procedures*, ed 3, Lake Forest Ill, 1992, Glencoe–Macmillan/McGraw–Hill.

Furumoto HH: Practice management, *Vet Clin North Am Small Anim Practice*, vol 13, no 4, 1983.

Hannah H: *Legal briefs for the Journal of the American Veterinary Medical Association*, Schaumburg Ill, 1986, AVMA.

McCurnin, DM, editor: *Clinical textbook for veterinary technicians*, ed 3, Philadelphia, 1994, WB Saunders.

National Association of State Public Health Veterinarians: Compendium of animal rabies control, *JAVMA* 206:14–18, 1995.

Professional Liability: quarterly report of the AVMA Professional Liability Insurance Trust, Schaumburg Ill, 1995, AVMA.

Smith BR, Computers in veterinary practice, *Vet Clin North Am Small Anim Pract*, vol 16, no 4, 1986.

Tannenbaum, J: *Veterinary ethics*, ed 2, St Louis, 1995, Mosby.

Veterinary accreditation—a reference guide for practitioners, Washington DC, 1994, APHIS/USDA.

Waltham veterinary hospital manual, Vernon Calif, 1993, Waltham U.S.A.

Practice answer sheet is on page 325.

Correct answers are on pages 127–129.

Questions

Record Keeping

1. In accepting checks as payment for veterinary services, you should record or verify certain items. Which of the following is *not* considered essential?
   a. Client's name and current address
   b. His or her driver's license number
   c. The initials of the employee who accepted the check
   d. Home or work telephone number or place of employment

2. Which of the following is *not* considered a legal reason for maintaining medical records?
   a. Hospital-employed accountants and attorneys require them
   b. They are essential in the defense of legal actions for malpractice or incompetence
   c. They are used to establish that a legal contract existed for the care of a patient and collection of a fee
   d. Many states and some professional associations require them

3. Of the five schedules used to identify controlled substances, this schedule has the *least* potential for abuse, and the drugs are primarily antitussive and antidiarrheal, containing limited quantities of certain narcotic and stimulant drugs.
   a. Schedule I
   b. Schedule III
   c. Schedule IV
   d. Schedule V

4. Upon the loss of a controlled substance, the veterinarian or veterinary technician must
   a. Notify the local police department
   b. Alert the FBI in your area
   c. Notify the DEA field office
   d. Both a and c are required

5. The duties of the veterinary technician, as related to controlled substances, typically includes all of the following *except*
   a. Ordering
   b. Dispensing
   c. Record keeping
   d. Storage procedures

6. Extremely popular during the past few years, what may be the greatest cost-saving feature ever developed for filing and retrieval of records?
   a. Digital phasing
   b. Color coding
   c. Chronologic filing
   d. Geographic filing

7. What filing system operates generally by state or country and then alphabetically or numerically by account name or number?
   a. Geographic filing
   b. Subject filing
   c. Numeric filing
   d. Open filing

8. Which system's greatest benefit is speed of filing and finding? Although this system requires a cross index, it can increase efficiency 40% to 50%.
   a. Alphabetic system
   b. Numeric filing
   c. Subject filing
   d. Chronologic filing

9. A patient's medical record is the accumulation of all data pertaining to the patient and typically includes all of the above *except*
   a. History and physical examination
   b. Laboratory and radiology reports
   c. Special procedure reports
   d. Photographs of the client

10. The most immediate and tangible increase in income from hospital computer use may result from the *reminder and recall* system. Evidence has shown a return rate increase of what percentage range with followup contact with clients via reminder cards or calls?
    a. 10% to 20%
    b. 80% to 90%
    c. 1% to 5%
    d. 40% to 50%

11. Basic considerations in planning the physical arrangement of a veterinary hospital include all of the following *except*
    a. Efficient flow of traffic
    b. Economy of time
    c. Economy of energy
    d. Avant garde design

12. If an incorrect entry is made in a medical record, the accepted procedure is to
    a. Erase the entire entry and start again
    b. Draw an ink line through the incorrect entry, initial it, and insert the date of the change in the margin; the correct entry is then made on the following line
    c. Begin a new medical record, copying all previous entries
    d. Erase only the incorrect entry; initial and follow with the correct entry on the following line

13. The original medical record, along with x-ray films and laboratory reports or electrodiagnostic tests, is the property of the
    a. Owner of the patient
    b. The veterinary hospital
    c. The owner of the practice
    d. Both b and c

14. A comprehensive medical record should contain all of the following *except*
    a. Clinical signs
    b. Patient's pedigree history
    c. Vaccination status
    d. Discharge summary

15. Which of the following medical record formats takes more time to compile? Because it makes available more historical data and other information, this format supports case planning and provides protection in the event of litigation.
    a. Problem-oriented medical records
    b. Conventional method
    c. Situation method
    d. Master problem list

16. Each practice or clinic sets its own rules for purging active records. How long are records generally kept in a practice?
    a. 3 years
    b. 5 years
    c. 1 years
    d. 10 years

17. In which form of color coding is one color assigned to each digit from 0 to 9, and the colors vary on the record according to the number? This system prevents chart misfiles.
    a. Alphabetic
    b. Sequential
    c. Numeric
    d. Microlegal

18. A signed authorization form from the animal's owner should be obtained before any information in the medical record can be released to
    a. The owner
    b. Another veterinarian
    c. An insurance company
    d. A release is needed for a, b, and c

Correct answers are on pages 127–129.

19. Which separate financial record consists of a chronologic listing of every daily transaction? This includes client and patient identification, service rendered, fee charged, and amount paid.
    a. Daybook
    b. Ledger card
    c. Business record form
    d. Charge or fee slip

20. Which of the following is *not* an ingredient of the inventory control system?
    a. Supply ledger or card file
    b. Want sheet
    c. Actual count of items in the hospital
    d. Ledger sheet

21. Arriving with supplies, which form usually includes a list of items in the package? It is checked against the contents to ensure everything is enclosed.
    a. Bill
    b. Packing slip
    c. Invoice
    d. Inventory record

22. In the routine of processing shipments of veterinary products, what is the usual sequence of document handling?
    a. Packing slip, bill, invoice, and inventory record
    b. Invoice, bill, packing slip, and inventory record
    c. Packing slip, invoice, inventory record, and bill
    d. Inventory record, packing slip, invoice, and bill

23. The bill usually lists all of the following *except*
    a. Invoice numbers
    b. Total amount of each invoice
    c. Total amount of purchases made during the month
    d. Packing slip numbers and dates shipped

24. A veterinarian who dispenses or regularly administers controlled substances must take an inventory of all substances on hand on the same date every
    a. 1 year
    b. 5 years
    c. 2 years
    d. 3 years

25. Records for what schedule of drugs must be kept separate from all other controlled substance records?
    a. Schedule II
    b. Schedule I
    c. Schedule III
    d. Schedule IV

ETHICS AND JURISPRUDENCE

26. In which of the following situations might a veterinary technician's error result in the veterinarian's being found guilty of malpractice?
    a. When the error endangers an animal or a client
    b. When the veterinarian is aware of the error
    c. When the veterinarian is present when the error is made
    d. A veterinary technician's error would never result in the veterinarian's liability

27. If an owner insists on restraining his or her animal and is then injured, are there grounds for a malpractice suit against the veterinary clinic?
    a. Yes; the veterinary clinic has an obligation to always protect clients from injury
    b. Yes, but only if the animal was not previously known to be vicious
    c. Yes, but only if the injury occurs as a direct result of the animal's being frightened by examination or treatment
    d. No; there is no potential liability in such a case

28. In which of the following situations would the veterinarian definitely *not* be held liable for damages?
    a. During rectal palpation, a mare becomes excited and fractious and her rectum is torn, resulting in peritonitis and death
    b. A dog escapes from a clinic's outdoor run and is never seen again
    c. A 2-year-old child opens a zip-lock bag containing medication for a dog, eats several tablets, and is poisoned
    d. An animal dies as a result of the owner's not following written directions relating to treatment

29. Prescriptions
    a. Need not be signed
    b. Are not considered legal documents
    c. Should be recorded, and records should be maintained
    d. Are not necessary for extra-label drug dispensing

30. Which of the following is appropriate when a disgruntled client alleges malpractice that may precipitate a law suit?
    a. Apologize and state that the mistake can be corrected
    b. Respond angrily and indignantly to the client; these types of people understand only forceful language
    c. Offer to waive (skip) the charges for the procedure and care in question
    d. Show concern for the client

31. Medical records
    a. Are the undisputed property of the client and must be sent to any client moving from the area
    b. Do not include radiographic films and laboratory reports
    c. Should be retained even if the client moves away
    d. Can be shared with anyone requesting copies

32. The recommended procedure for an unvaccinated dog with a known exposure to a rabid animal is
    a. Quarantine for 10 days
    b. Quarantine for 30 days
    c. Immediate vaccination, then quarantine for 10 days
    d. Euthanasia

33. Which of the following label statements indicates a prescription product?
    a. Sold only to graduate veterinarians
    b. Caution: federal law restricts this drug for use by or on the order of a licensed veterinarian
    c. For veterinary use only
    d. Caution: use only as directed

34. According to a recent clarification from the federal government, who may sign health certificates and other official veterinary documents?
    a. Only the veterinarian
    b. The veterinarian, or a veterinary technician on the advice of the veterinarian
    c. Any employee of the clinic, as long as the employee has power of attorney and the signature is initialed by the employee
    d. Any employee of the clinic may apply the veterinarian's signature stamp

35. To issue an interstate health certificate, a veterinarian must be accredited and
    a. Have seen the animal(s) within the last 7 days
    b. Have seen the animal(s) within the last 30 days
    c. Have seen the animal(s) on the day the certificate is signed
    d. Familiar with the herd of origin, even though the specific animal(s) in question have not been seen

Correct answers are on pages 127–129.

36. To be moved across most state lines or into Canada, dogs must be vaccinated against
    a. Parvovirus infection
    b. Rabies
    c. Canine distemper
    d. Lyme disease

37. Which of the following does *not* require a valid veterinarian-client-patient relationship for dispensing?
    a. Dimethylsulfoxide (DMSO)
    b. Prostaglandins
    c. Canine parvovirus vaccine
    d. Oxytocin

38. Brucellosis vaccination tags are what color and are applied to which ear of cattle?
    a. Silver, right
    b. Green, left
    c. Silver, left
    d. Orange, right

39. If an entire cattle herd is tested on _____ occasions _____ months apart for brucellosis, it may qualify as a(n) _____ herd.
    a. 2, 10 to 14, validated free
    b. 3, 12, accredited free
    c. 2, 10 to 14, certified free
    d. 2, 6 to 8, qualified negative

40. Which federal government agency is responsible for monitoring and enforcing regulations on the interstate shipment of livestock?
    a. Department of the Interior
    b. Animal and Plant Health Inspection Service
    c. Drug Enforcement Administration
    d. Food and Drug Administration

41. Cattle are tested for tuberculosis by injection with tuberculin in what site and reexamined how long after the injection?
    a. Neck, 24 hours
    b. Caudal fold, 24 hours
    c. Ear, 48 hours
    d. Caudal fold, 72 hours

42. Which statement concerning rabies vaccination is most accurate?
    a. Rabies vaccine may be dispensed to clients.
    b. Some rabies vaccines provide protection to dogs and cats for 3 years and are licensed as such.
    c. There is no rabies vaccine approved for horses.
    d. There are no rabies vaccines labeled for subcutaneous use.

43. Rabies vaccines licensed to be administered only intramuscularly are to be injected
    a. In the thigh
    b. In the gluteals
    c. In the pectorals
    d. Over the crest of the shoulders

44. When may a rabies tag be issued without completing a rabies certificate?
    a. If the tag replaces a lost tag
    b. If the owner does not want or need a certificate
    c. If the owner is simply using the tag for identification
    d. It should never be issued without completing a rabies certificate, even in the case of a lost tag

45. The recommended procedure for a dog that has just bitten a person is
    a. Quarantine and observation for 10 days
    b. Quarantine and observation for 30 days
    c. Advise the owner to closely observe the dog for a few days
    d. Shoot the dog in the head

46. Chloramphenicol is
    a. Legal for use in calves and baby pigs less than 2 weeks old
    b. Legal for use in food animals when the requirements of extra-label drug use are met
    c. Illegal for use in any food animals
    d. Illegal for use in all animals

47. The FDA checks and licenses drugs and biologics before they can be sold. Which aspects are evaluated by the FDA?
    a. Cost effectiveness and probable demand
    b. Safety and efficacy
    c. Profit margin (markup) and packaging
    d. Market niche

48. Who can purchase an over-the-counter (OTC) drug?
    a. Anyone
    b. Only veterinarians
    c. Only veterinarians and registered feed mills
    d. Only physicians

49. If a drug has been identified as a carcinogen, what would you expect the residue tolerance to be?
    a. One part per million
    b. One part per billion
    c. One part per trillion
    d. Residues detected at any level would not be tolerated

50. After being cited for a first-time residue violation, a feedlot must
    a. Pay a fine not to exceed $10,000
    b. Send five head of cattle to be slaughtered and tested for residues before sending the next load of cattle to slaughter
    c. Eliminate use of all drugs at the feedlot
    d. Do nothing; there is no required action after a *first-time* violation

51. Extra-label use of feed medications is
    a. Permitted by veterinary prescription
    b. Strictly illegal
    c. Permitted if a Form 1900 is secured
    d. Permitted under the guidelines of Form FD 2656

52. Controlled substances with no accepted medical use are classified as
    a. Schedule I
    b. Schedule II
    c. Schedule III
    d. Schedule IV

53. How long must controlled substance records be maintained?
    a. 90 days
    b. 1 year
    c. 2 years
    d. 5 years

54. Which species may be legally vaccinated against rabies using an injectable rabies vaccine?
    a. Ferret
    b. Skunk
    c. Wolf
    d. Raccoon

55. Which bovine brucellosis ear tattoo is *incorrect*?
    a. 3V8
    b. 5V2
    c. 4V1
    d. 1V0

56. A written consent form
    a. Is not considered part of a patient's medical record
    b. Is not necessary for surgery when verbal consent has been given
    c. Should be used when a client requests that a child-proof container not be used for dispensed medication
    d. Is not necessary for euthanasia when the owner is a recognized client

Correct answers are on pages 127–129.

57. Which of the following would be considered ethical and appropriate on the part of a veterinary technician?
    a. Telling a client that Mrs. J, another client, owns an animal that has a contagious disease
    b. Confiding to a client that Dr. A has had recent mishaps in surgery and suggesting that Dr. B perform the requested surgical procedure
    c. Explaining that the reason our fees are higher than those of the clinic down the street is because they do not do things as well as we do
    d. Refusing to reduce the charges for professional services without the approval of the veterinarian

58. Which of the following may be legally performed by a veterinary technician?
    a. Castrating a cat
    b. Diagnosing feline panleukopenia
    c. Administering an intravenous anesthetic
    d. Prescribing ampicillin for treatment of a respiratory infection in a pup

59. The accrediting body for veterinary technology education programs in the United States is the
    a. North American Veterinary Technician Association (NAVTA)
    b. AVMA Committee on Veterinary Technician Education and Activities (CVTEA)
    c. United States Department of Agriculture (USDA)
    d. Association of Veterinary Technician Educators (AVTE)

60. A client takes a Rottweiler to a two-veterinarian clinic for castration. The client indicates to the receptionist that the dog has a bad disposition and the receptionist records this information on the patient's medical record. Dr. X castrates the dog without incident. When the client returns the next day to pick up the dog, Dr. Y asks the veterinary technician to take the dog to the reception area, which is crowded with other clients. As the dog's leash is handed to the client, the dog jerks away and attacks another client's dog. Who is *least* liable for damages claimed by the second client?
    a. The owner of the Rottweiler
    b. The veterinary technician
    c. Dr. X
    d. Dr. Y

61. If a veterinarian and employer commits acts that a veterinary technician considers to be unethical, the technician should
    a. Do or say nothing at all
    b. Warn clients
    c. Discuss the concerns with the veterinarian
    d. Immediately report the veterinarian to the State Board of Examiners

62. A client takes a dog for vaccination against parvovirus. The only canine parvovirus vaccine in the clinic has an expiration date that indicates it expired 2 months earlier. What should be done?
    a. The vaccine should be used at the recommended dose
    b. The vaccine should be used at twice the recommended dose
    c. Feline panleukopenia vaccine should be used
    d. A new appointment should be made for a date after a shipment of new vaccine has arrived

63. Ethically speaking, veterinary technicians involved in animal research should
   a. Avoid unnecessary suffering and pain in their subjects
   b. Avoid any use of live animals
   c. Become active in militant animal rights organizations and sabotage any research techniques with which he or she disagrees
   d. Use only invertebrates and amphibians in research

64. Which statement concerning ethics is most accurate?
   a. Because declawing cats is excessively painful and considered unethical, euthanasia should be performed when cats cannot be discouraged from causing damage with their front claws.
   b. Clients should not be allowed to be present when their pet is euthanized.
   c. From an ethical standpoint, a client's request for euthanasia of a terminally ill pet should always be denied; euthanasia is never ethical.
   d. It is appropriate to send a sympathy card to the client following the death of a pet.

Answers

Record Keeping

1. c
2. a
3. d
4. d
5. b
6. b
7. a
8. b
9. d
10. a
11. d
12. b
13. d
14. b
15. a
16. a
17. c
18. d
19. a
20. d
21. b
22. c
23. d
24. c
25. a

ETHICS AND JURISPRUDENCE

26. **a** The veterinary technician is an agent of the veterinarian.

27. a

28. **d** By issuing written directions, the clinic fulfills its obligation. The client has an obligation to follow those written directions. The veterinarian could reasonably be found liable for damages in the other three situations: injury to a patient, disappearance of a patient in his or her custody, and failure to dispense medication in child-proof packaging.

29. **c** Prescriptions are legal documents and must be signed, and records of prescriptions should be maintained. Drugs dispensed for "extra-label use" must be handled on a prescription basis.

30. **d** The AVMA Professional Liability Insurance Trust recommends that potential fault not be acknowledged. It is appropriate to empathize with the client in an unfortunate situation.

31. **c** Medical records are the property of the clinic and are strictly confidential.

32. **d**

33. **b**

34. **a**

35. **a**

36. **b**

37. **c** DMSO, prostaglandins, and oxytocin are prescription products and, as such, require a valid veterinary-client-patient relationship to dispense.

38. **d**

39. **c**

40. **b**

41. **d**

42. **b** Rabies vaccine may not be dispensed. It may only be used by a veterinarian or, in some states, under the direct supervision of a veterinarian.

43. **a**

44. **d** If a client has lost a rabies tag, a new one may be issued; however, a new certificate should be issued (including the original vaccination information) with the new tag number.

45. **a**

46. **c** Chloramphenicol is specifically forbidden for use in food animals by the FDA because of the potential of fatal aplastic anemia in some people consuming tissues of treated animals.

47. **b**

48. **a**

49. **d**

50. **b**

51. **b** Label dosage regimens and indications of feed additives must be strictly observed in all cases by all individuals, including veterinarians.

52. **a**

53. **c**

54. **a**

55. **b** The first digit indicates the quarter of the year of brucellosis vaccination. The digit following the *V* shield indicates the year of vaccination. For example, a heifer vaccinated in November of 1995 would have a tattoo of 4V5.

56. **c** A written consent form should be used for surgery, euthanasia, and other risky or expensive procedures. A completed and signed written consent form is considered part of the medical record from a legal standpoint.

57. **d** Confidentiality should be maintained at all times. It is not ethical to criticize professional colleagues. It is not appropriate for a veterinary technician to reduce fees without the veterinarian's approval.

58. **c** According to the AVMA Model Practice Act, veterinary technicians may not perform surgery, make diagnoses, or prescribe treatments.

59. **b**

60. **a** The veterinary hospital is usually considered responsible for the safety of clients and patients on the premises and should take appropriate steps to minimize any possible risk. The owner of the dog has met his obligation under the law by informing the hospital of the dog's disposition.

61. **c** Ethical concerns should first be discussed with the person involved. It would be inappropriate to voice the concerns to clients.

62. **d** Outdated products should never be used. Panleukopenia vaccine is not a satisfactory substitute for canine parvovirus vaccine.

63. **a**

64. **d** Euthanasia is a viable, ethical option in a number of situations. Declawing cats is considered by many veterinarians to be an ethical alternative to needless euthanasia. It is appropriate for the client to be present when a pet is euthanized, if requested.

Notes

Notes

Section 7

Laboratory Animals

Beth Harries, MEd, LVT   *Karen Hrapkiewicz, DVM*

Recommended Reading

American Association for Laboratory Animal Science: *Training manual series* (Vol 1, *Assistant laboratory animal technician*; Vol 2, *Laboratory animal technician*), Cordova Tenn, 1991, AALAS.

Harkness J, Wagner J: *The biology and medicine of rabbits and rodents*, ed 3, Philadelphia, 1989, Lea & Febiger.

Questions

1. The genus and species names of the rabbit are
   a. *Oryctolagus cuniculus*
   b. *Mesocrietus auratus*
   c. *Meriones unguiculatus*
   d. *Cavia porcellus*

2. The genus and species names of the hamster are
   a. *Oryctolagus cuniculus*
   b. *Mesocrietus auratus*
   c. *Meriones unguiculatus*
   d. *Cavia porcellus*

3. The genus and species names of gerbils are
   a. *Oryctolagus cuniculus*
   b. *Mesocrietus auratus*
   c. *Meriones unguiculatus*
   d. *Cavia porcellus*

4. The genus and species names of guinea pigs are
   a. *Oryctolagus cuniculus*
   b. *Mesocrietus auratus*
   c. *Meriones unguiculatus*
   d. *Cavia porcellus*

5. The sex of juvenile guinea pigs is determined by
   a. Palpation of the pelvic region
   b. Behavioral traits
   c. Secondary sex characteristics
   d. Anogenital distance

6. The term for parturition in the guinea pig is
   a. Kindling
   b. Queening
   c. Farrowing
   d. Littering

Practice answer sheet is on page 327.

Correct answers are on pages 136–137.

7. The term for parturition in the rabbit is
   a. Kindling
   b. Queening
   c. Farrowing
   d. Littering

8. The laboratory animal species most likely to experience dystocia is a
   a. Rat
   b. Gerbil
   c. Hamster
   d. Guinea pig

9. The sex of juvenile mice is determined by
   a. Palpation of the pelvic region
   b. Behavior traits
   c. Secondary sex characteristics
   d. Anogenital distance

10. The cage type frequently used for housing nonhuman primates is
    a. Rack
    b. Squeeze
    c. Cabinet
    d. Metabolism

11. The scientific name of the mouse pinworm is
    a. *Eimeria*
    b. *Aspicularis*
    c. *Hymenolepis*
    d. *Oxyuris*

12. Which of the following is the most commonly used species in research?
    a. Rabbit
    b. Guinea pig
    c. Rat
    d. Mouse

13. The species with the shortest gestation period is the
    a. Hamster
    b. Gerbil
    c. Mouse
    d. Rabbit

14. What is the correct term for a female guinea pig?
    a. Doe
    b. Queen
    c. Bitch
    d. Sow

15. All of the following are rodents *except* the
    a. Guinea pig
    b. Rabbit
    c. Hamster
    d. Gerbil

16. A common problem resulting from incorrect restraint of a gerbil
    a. Prolapsed rectum
    b. Fractured back
    c. Proptosed eyes
    d. Tail slip

17. A common disease of juvenile hamsters is
    a. Wet tail
    b. Seizures
    c. Snuffles
    d. Leukemia

18. Seizures are a common problem in the
    a. Rabbit
    b. Hamster
    c. Mouse
    d. Gerbil

19. A male rabbit is called a
    a. Boar
    b. Bull
    c. Buck
    d. Barrow

20. The Animal Welfare Act is administered and enforced by the
    a. United States Department of Agriculture
    b. American Humane Society
    c. National Institutes of Health
    d. American Association for Laboratory Animal Science

21. The NIH *Guide for Care and Use of Laboratory Animals* recommends a ventilation rate of how many changes of 100% fresh air per hour?
    a. 5 to 10
    b. 10 to 15
    c. 15 to 20
    d. 20 to 25

22. The disease of rats and mice caused by low humidity is
    a. Sore hocks
    b. Wet tail
    c. Sore nose
    d. Ring tail

23. Ferrets are very susceptible to
    a. Canine distemper
    b. Feline panleukopenia
    c. Canine hepatitis
    d. Feline rhinotracheitis

24. A type of inbred albino mouse is
    a. DBA
    b. Swiss
    c. C57/BL
    d. BALB/C

25. Sacculus rotundus, appendix, and cecum are parts of which laboratory animal's gastrointestinal tract?
    a. Mouse
    b. Rabbit
    c. Hamster
    d. Guinea pig

26. Which type of guinea pig has long silky hair?
    a. Abyssinian
    b. English
    c. Peruvian
    d. Duncan-Hartley

27. Which laboratory animal species has a gestation period similar to that of cats?
    a. Gerbil
    b. Mouse
    c. Rabbit
    d. Guinea pig

28. Normal body temperature is highest in the
    a. Pigeon
    b. Hamster
    c. Rat
    d. Rabbit

29. Dutch and New Zealand are types of
    a. Guinea pigs
    b. Rabbits
    c. Hamsters
    d. Rats

30. The major causative agent of chronic respiratory disease in rats is
    a. *Pseudomonas*
    b. *Mycobacterium*
    c. *Pasteurella*
    d. *Mycoplasma*

31. Caudal paralysis, as a consequence of injury to the spinal cord from a fractured back, occurs commonly in the
    a. Gerbil
    b. Rabbit
    c. Hamster
    d. Guinea pig

32. Which organization's major focus is voluntary accreditation of laboratory animal facilities?
    a. American Association for Accreditation of Laboratory Animal Care
    b. American Society of Laboratory Animal Practitioners
    c. American Association for Laboratory Animal Science
    d. American College of Laboratory Animal Medicine

33. Which bedding material should *not* be used in a research facility?
    a. Pine
    b. Aspen
    c. Cedar
    d. Paper

Correct answers are on pages 136–137.

34. Which laboratory animal species has cheek pouches and callous pads on its buttocks?
    a. Hamster
    b. Guinea pig
    c. Rabbit
    d. Rhesus monkey

35. A rabbit with a purulent nasal discharge and conjunctivitis would most likely be affected by
    a. Kennel cough
    b. Venereal disease
    c. Ringworm
    d. Snuffles

36. A diet rich in vitamin C must be provided to which species because they *cannot* synthesize their own?
    a. Guinea pigs and nonhuman primates
    b. Hamsters and rabbits
    c. Rabbits and guinea pigs
    d. Nonhuman primates and gerbils

37. Which species normally has two types of feces, day feces and night feces?
    a. Hamster
    b. Gerbil
    c. Guinea pig
    d. Rabbit

38. Which laboratory animal species has ventral sebaceous glands?
    a. Gerbil
    b. Mouse
    c. Hamster
    d. Rat

39. All of the following are old-world monkeys *except* the
    a. Rhesus
    b. Squirrel
    c. Cynomolgus
    d. Stump tail

40. Offspring of which laboratory animal species are born fully furred and with open eyes?
    a. Guinea pig
    b. Mice
    c. Hamster
    d. Rabbit

41. Which caging material with high-impact strength is transparent and can withstand high temperatures?
    a. Polystyrene
    b. Polypropylene
    c. Polydextran
    d. Polycarbonate

42. Which group reviews animal research protocols to be sure the methods of care and use are appropriate and in compliance with federal and institutional guidelines?
    a. American Association for Laboratory Animal Science
    b. International Animal Care and Use Committee
    c. American Humane Society
    d. American Veterinary Medical Association

43. For a strain to be considered inbred, a minimum of how many generations of brother to sister or parent to offspring must occur?
    a. 20
    b. 16
    c. 10
    d. 8

44. The laboratory animal species with hip glands is the
    a. Gerbil
    b. Rat
    c. Hamster
    d. Mouse

45. The temperature of the rinse water in a cage washer should minimally reach
    a. 37.2° C (99° F)
    b. 62° C (143.6° F)
    c. 82.2° C (180° F)
    d. 105° C (221° F)

46. A greasy haircoat of a gerbil indicates that the ambient
    a. Humidity is too high
    b. Temperature is too low
    c. Humidity is too low
    d. Temperature is too high

47. All of the following are outbred stocks of rats *except* the
    a. Long Evans
    b. Sprague-Dawley
    c. Lewis
    d. Wistar

48. Animals that are free of absolutely all microorganisms and parasites are called
    a. Specific pathogen free
    b. Conventional
    c. Microbially defined
    d. Axenic

49. To sanitize a large piece of equipment, such as a sheep transport cage, you would use a
    a. Cabinet cage washer
    b. Rack cage washer
    c. Bottle washer
    d. Tunnel cage washer

50. Which laboratory animal species is most sensitive to bright light?
    a. Syrian hamster
    b. Long-Evans rat
    c. BALB/C mouse
    d. Dutch rabbit

51. Which zoonotic viral disease of primates produces a mild disease with ulcers on the mucous membranes and tongue in its natural host, the Macaca?
    a. Rabies
    b. Tuberculosis
    c. Measles
    d. Herpes B

52. Which animal is covered by the Animal Welfare Act?
    a. Rat specifically bred for research
    b. Sheep used for wool-production experiments
    c. Wild mouse used in research
    d. Chicken used in egg-production experiments

53. The best type of caging system for a near-term pregnant rat is
    a. Shoebox
    b. Suspended
    c. Metabolism
    d. Squeeze

54. Four of five mice housed together have large areas of alopecia on their muzzle. The most likely problem is
    a. Barbering
    b. Lice infestation
    c. Mite infestation
    d. Fighting

55. A detailed description of the procedures to be used in a research project that is reviewed by an appointed committee is called a
    a. Prospectus
    b. Report
    c. Protocol
    d. Summary

56. Which laboratory animal species hibernates?
    a. Rabbit
    b. Hamster
    c. Gerbil
    d. Guinea pig

57. A zoonotic disease of sheep is
    a. Psittacosis
    b. Orf
    c. Shigellosis
    d. Yellow fever

58. The most accessible vein for blood collection in the rabbit is
    a. Jugular
    b. Femoral
    c. Ear
    d. Orbital

Correct answers are on pages 136–137.

59. The best method for euthanizing a
    large group of mice is
    a. Decapitation
    b. Carbon dioxide
    c. Cervical dislocation
    d. Lethal injection

60. Use of penicillin is contraindicated in
    the
    a. Rabbit
    b. Mouse
    c. Guinea pig
    d. Gerbil

Answers

1. a

2. b

3. c

4. d

5. a The penis may be manually
   prolapsed. The opening of the female
   is shaped like a 'Y', and the male like a
   colon(:).

6. c

7. a

8. d Dystocia is a problem in guinea
   pigs, particularly those bred for the
   first time after the age of 6 months.

9. d The anogenital distance in male
   mice is twice that of female mice.

10. b

11. b

12. d

13. a A hamster has a 16-day gestation.

14. d

15. b Rabbits are actually lagomorphs,
    not rodents.

16. d Grasping the end of the gerbil's tail
    during restraint may separate the skin
    from the distal portion of the tail.

17. a

18. d

19. c

20. a

21. b

22. d

23. a

24. d

25. b

26. c

27. d

28. a

29. b

30. d

31. b

32. a

33. c Cedar chips stimulate hepatic
    enzyme systems that shorten
    anesthetic sleep times.

34. d

35. d

36. a Nonhuman primates and guinea
    pigs require supplementation with
    vitamin C.

37. d Rabbits have moist night feces,
    which are reingested, and dry day
    feces.

38. a

39. b Squirrel monkeys are new-world,
    nonhuman primates.

40. a

41. d

42. b

59. A box of reagents for blood chemistry analysis labeled for storage at 8° C can be safely stored
    a. In the freezer
    b. At room temperature
    c. In the incubator
    d. In the refrigerator

60. Which statement concerning collection of a plasma sample for blood chemistry analysis is *least* accurate?
    a. If a needle and syringe are used, hemolysis can be minimized by removing the needle from the syringe before discharging the blood into a sample tube.
    b. Volume changes caused by evaporation can be minimized by keeping the cap on the blood collection tube as much as possible.
    c. To separate, allow the sample to clot for approximately 30 minutes, gently remove the clot from the sides of the tube, and centrifuge and remove the plasma.
    d. Avoid lipemia by fasting the animal before collecting the sample.

61. Which sample condition *cannot* be minimized by preparing the animal or proper sample collection and handling?
    a. Hemolysis
    b. Icterus
    c. Lipemia
    d. Evaporation

62. The technology of dry chemistry differs from that of wet chemistry in that the reagents in dry chemistry are supplied
    a. In lyophilized pellets
    b. In liquid solutions
    c. Impregnated on slides, cards, or strips
    d. In powdered capsules

63. In wet chemistry technology, the amount of chemical substance in the blood is determined by measuring the
    a. Light passing through or absorbed by the final sample
    b. Heat generated by the end product
    c. Light reflected from the slide or card
    d. Volume, temperature, and pH of the final sample

64. In dry chemistry technology, the amount of chemical substance in the blood is determined by measuring the
    a. Light passing through or absorbed by the final sample
    b. Heat generated by the end product
    c. Light reflected from the slide, card, or strip
    d. Volume, temperature, and pH of the final sample

65. To help ensure the accuracy of spectrophotometers and other blood chemistry instruments, manufacturers recommend use of
    a. Standard solutions
    b. Quality-control sera
    c. Pooled samples
    d. A reference manual

66. To verify the accuracy of blood chemistry results in the laboratory, the technician should
    a. Keep a daily log of test results
    b. Repeat each procedure several times
    c. Analyze quality-control sera
    d. Send each sample tested to a reference laboratory for analysis

67. The aim of blood chemistry quality-control programs is to ensure that the method used will yield results that are
    a. Accurate
    b. Cost effective
    c. Within the reference range
    d. Credible

Correct answers are on pages 178–192.

68. Quality-control sera used in most laboratories are supplied in what form?
    a. Liquid
    b. Lyophilized
    c. Pellets
    d. Capsules

69. In blood chemistry assays, a reconstituted vial of control serum can be used most economically by
    a. Using the control serum only once a month
    b. Using the control serum only when the patient values are abnormal
    c. Separating the control serum into several aliquots, freezing and thawing one aliquot at a time
    d. Immediately refrigerating the vial after using it, to prevent deterioration

70. In regard to quality control in blood chemistry, which is *not* a source of a detectable error?
    a. Inconsistent or poor technique
    b. Equipment malfunction
    c. Reagent contamination or degeneration
    d. Random sampling errors

71. Quality-control sera used in blood chemistry testing can help ensure the accuracy of the method by evaluating all of the following *except* the
    a. Quality of reagents used
    b. Accuracy of equipment used
    c. Technique of the person performing the test
    d. Quality of the patient's sample

72. The calibrated glass tube used in spectrophotometry that contains the colored solution to be measured is called a
    a. Pipette
    b. Dilution vial
    c. Test tube
    d. Cuvette

73. The calibrated device used to deliver a specified volume of patient sample when performing blood chemistry analyses is called a
    a. Cuvette
    b. Dilut-o-mat
    c. Pipette
    d. Graduated cylinder

74. The group of values for a particular blood constituent, derived when a laboratory has repeatedly assayed samples from a significant number of clinically normal animals of a given species, is called the
    a. Reference range
    b. Biochemical profile
    c. Standard curve
    d. Quality control

75. In blood chemistry testing, the substance on which an enzyme acts is called a
    a. Substrate
    b. Sediment
    c. Proenzyme
    d. Product

76. The rate of an enzymatic reaction is measured while it is in progress in
    a. Endpoint reactions
    b. Kinetic reactions
    c. Thermocouple reactions
    d. Progressive reactions

77. Enzymes with similar catalytic activities but different physical and chemical properties, as well as different tissues of origin, are referred to as
    a. Isoenzymes
    b. Coenzymes
    c. Cofactors
    d. Activators

78. For clinical purposes, the isoenzymes separated and recognized most commonly include all of the following *except*
    a. Lactate dehydrogenase (LDH)
    b. Alkaline phosphatase (AP)
    c. Creatine kinase (CK)
    d. Aspartate aminotransferase (AST)

79. The blood chemistry units of measurement, including Bodansky units, Reitman-Frankel units, and Wroblewsky units, are all used in reporting the results of
    a. Electrolyte concentrations
    b. Enzyme concentrations
    c. Kidney assays
    d. Pancreas assays

80. The blood chemistry unit of measurement for the electrolytes sodium, potassium, and chloride is
    a. mg/dl
    b. g/dl
    c. IU/L
    d. mEq/L

81. Enzymes are proteins; most are found in highest concentration
    a. Inside cells
    b. Outside cells
    c. In the blood
    d. In the urine

82. Accuracy in blood chemistry kinetic enzymatic assays depends on all of the following *except*
    a. Temperature of reaction
    b. Time of reaction
    c. Sample volume
    d. Final color change of the reagents

83. Because anticoagulants can adversely affect results, serum is the preferred sample for assay of
    a. Lipids
    b. Enzymes
    c. Proteins
    d. Electrolytes

84. Radioimmunoassay (RIA) is used in measuring blood levels of
    a. Hormones
    b. Enzymes
    c. Electrolytes
    d. Gases

85. Flame photometry is used to measure blood levels of
    a. Electrolytes
    b. Hormones
    c. Enzymes
    d. Gases

86. The Azostix strip is a rapid quantitative test for blood levels of
    a. Aspartate aminotransferase
    b. Alanine transaminase
    c. Glucose
    d. Urea nitrogen

87. Dextrostix and Visidex strips are rapid quantitative tests for blood levels of
    a. Aspartate aminotransferase
    b. Alanine transaminase
    c. Glucose
    d. Urea nitrogen

88. Available technology for determination of blood electrolyte levels includes
    a. Electromagnetic fluctuation
    b. Scanning electronmicroscopy
    c. Ion selective electrode
    d. Immunoelectrophoresis

89. In dogs and cats the blood chemistry tests most commonly used to evaluate liver function are
    a. Alanine transaminase, and aspartate aminotransferase
    b. Electrolytes and blood urea nitrogen
    c. Gammaglutamyl transferase and sorbitol dehydrogenase
    d. Amylase and lipase

Correct answers are on pages 178–192.

90. In horses the blood chemistry tests most commonly used to evaluate liver function are
    a. Alanine transaminase and aspartate aminotransferase
    b. Electrolytes and blood urea nitrogen
    c. Gammaglutamyl transferase and sorbitol dehydrogenase
    d. Amylase and lipase

91. Blood chemistry assays, including dye excretion, ammonia tolerance, and bile acid concentrations, are used to evaluate function of the
    a. Pancreas
    b. Kidneys
    c. Heart
    d. Liver

92. Blood levels of cholesterol, triglycerides, and total protein are all used to evaluate function of the
    a. Kidneys
    b. Liver
    c. Pancreas
    d. Adrenal glands

93. Blood levels of total bilirubin generally are elevated in all of the following conditions *except*
    a. Hepatocellular damage
    b. Bile duct injury or obstruction
    c. Hemolytic disorders
    d. Acute pancreatitis

94. Blood levels of total bilirubin are used primarily to evaluate function of the
    a. Kidneys
    b. Liver
    c. Pancreas
    d. Adrenal glands

95. Serum chemistry tests for acute pancreatitis include
    a. Amylase and lipase
    b. Lipase and trypsin
    c. Amylase and trypsin
    d. Amylase, lipase, and trypsin

96. A common laboratory test for chronic pancreatitis is a fecal test for
    a. Amylase
    b. Lipase
    c. Trypsin
    d. Amylase, lipase, and trypsin

97. The principal *extracellular* cation that is commonly measured in a blood chemistry profile is
    a. Sodium
    b. Potassium
    c. Chloride
    d. Bicarbonate

98. The principal *intracellular* cation that is commonly measured in a blood chemistry profile is
    a. Sodium
    b. Potassium
    c. Chloride
    d. Bicarbonate

99. Arterial blood is the preferred sample for measurement of blood levels of
    a. Bicarbonate
    b. Chloride
    c. Sodium
    d. Magnesium

100. The term *A:G ratio* refers to the blood ratio of
    a. Alpha globulins to gamma globulins
    b. Albumin to globulin
    c. Ammonia to glucose
    d. Aspartate aminotransferase to gammaglutamyl transferase

101. A byproduct of muscle metabolism that is commonly used to evaluate glomerular filtration in a blood chemistry profile is
    a. Urea nitrogen
    b. Creatinine
    c. Alanine transaminase
    d. Aspartate aminotransferase

102. Serum electrolyte levels should be determined when evaluating function of the
    a. Liver
    b. Pancreas
    c. Kidneys
    d. Heart

103. Kidney disease leads to accumulation of metabolic waste in the blood, a condition known as
    a. Hematuria
    b. Hypernatremia
    c. Azotemia
    d. Hyperkalemia

104. In a diabetic animal, blood chemistry analysis is commonly performed to monitor insulin therapy by measuring blood levels of
    a. Sodium
    b. Potassium
    c. Glucose
    d. Insulin

105. In an animal with a history of bone resorption or convulsions, blood chemistry analysis is commonly performed to measure blood levels of
    a. Calcium and phosphorus
    b. Urea nitrogen and creatinine
    c. Aspartate aminotransferase and alanine transaminase
    d. Sodium and potassium

106. Which gland is the most active producer of corticosteroids measured in blood chemistry assays?
    a. Thyroid gland
    b. Pancreas
    c. Pituitary gland
    d. Adrenal glands

107. The gland that is evaluated by measurement of blood cortisol levels before and after administration of adrenocorticotropic hormone (ACTH) is the
    a. Thyroid gland
    b. Pancreas
    c. Liver
    d. Adrenal glands

108. The gland that is evaluated by measurement of blood levels of T_3 and T_4 is the
    a. Thyroid gland
    b. Pancreas
    c. Pituitary gland
    d. Adrenal glands

109. Measurement of blood levels of thyroid-stimulating hormone (TSH) and ACTH is used to evaluate function of the
    a. Thyroid gland
    b. Pancreas
    c. Pituitary gland
    d. Adrenal glands

110. In an animal showing lethargy, obesity, mild anemia, infertility, and alopecia, blood chemistry analysis commonly is performed to evaluate function of the
    a. Thyroid gland
    b. Pancreas
    c. Pituitary gland
    d. Adrenal glands

111. Chemistry evaluation of the kidney includes measurement of metabolic wastes in the blood in the form of
    a. Aspartate aminotransferase and alanine transaminase
    b. Urea nitrogen and creatinine
    c. Ammonia and pyruvic acid
    d. Bilirubin and urobilinogen

112. Ammonia is metabolized by the liver and eliminated by the kidneys. Levels of which metabolic byproduct are measured to assess kidney function?
    a. Phosphorus
    b. Creatinine
    c. Aspartate aminotransferase
    d. Urea nitrogen

113. Measurement of blood levels of amylase and lipase is used to evaluate function of the
    a. Kidneys
    b. Liver
    c. Pancreas
    d. Adrenal glands

Correct answers are on pages 178–192.

114. Measurement of blood levels of urea nitrogen (BUN) is used to evaluate function of the
    a. Kidneys
    b. Liver
    c. Pancreas
    d. Adrenal glands

115. Measurement of blood levels of creatinine is used to evaluate function of the
    a. Adrenal glands
    b. Liver
    c. Pancreas
    d. Kidneys

116. Assessment of liver function includes measurement of the two most abundant plasma proteins called
    a. Aspartate aminotransferase and alanine transaminase
    b. Fibrinogen and prothrombin
    c. Gammaglutamyl transferase and sorbitol dehydrogenase
    d. Albumin and globulin

117. An imbalance in blood calcium and phosphorus levels, measured in blood chemistry testing, would be expected in disorders of the
    a. Thyroid gland
    b. Parathyroid glands
    c. Liver
    d. Adrenal glands

118. A diagnosis of adrenal disease is determined by measurement of all of the following *except*
    a. Resting serum cortisol levels
    b. Serum cortisol levels following ACTH challenge
    c. Serum cortisol levels following dexamethasone suppression
    d. Resting serum ACTH levels

CYTOLOGY

119. *Exfoliative cytology* refers to the study of
    a. Cells shed from muscle tissue
    b. Cells shed from body surfaces
    c. Neoplastic cells exclusively
    d. Blood cells exclusively

120. *Pyknosis* is a term used to describe a
    a. Small, condensed, dark, fragmented nucleus
    b. Swollen, lacy nucleus
    c. Cell without a nucleus
    d. Nucleus without a cell

121. Which of the following is *not* a classification used to describe neoplastic cells?
    a. Bizarre and numerous nucleoli
    b. Increased mitotic index
    c. Uniform population of cells
    d. Basophilic cytoplasm with increased vacuolation

122. *Metaplasia* refers to
    a. An increase in cell numbers and mitotic activity in response to a stimulus
    b. An increase in cell size and/or functional activity in response to a stimulus
    c. An increase in cell growth and multiplication that is not dependent on a stimulus
    d. A reversible process in which one mature cell type is replaced by another

123. The sequence of microscopic evaluation of a cytologic specimen should proceed in which order after the smear has been properly stained and dried?
    a. Start with the oil-immersion lens because this allows better visualization of inclusions in the cells
    b. Scan the smear with 40X objective
    c. Scan with 4X to 10X objective for general impression and staining quality, then proceed to 40X and finally 100X for cellular morphology and inclusions
    d. The sequence has no significance

124. Tissue samples for histopathologic examination should be handled in all of the following ways *except*
    a. Placed in 10% formalin
    b. Cut into sections no more than 1 cm wide
    c. Placed in fluid-tight jars containing 10% formalin in a proportion 10 times the specimen's volume
    d. Preserved in formaldehyde

125. Which statement concerning cerebrospinal fluid is *least* accurate?
    a. Analysis is useful in diagnosis of some neurologic disorders.
    b. CSF is normally colorless and transparent.
    c. CSF normally has a very low protein concentration.
    d. CSF normally contains large numbers of blood cells.

126. Peritoneal fluid of horses
    a. Is frequently examined in cases of colic and weight loss
    b. Is normally malodorous
    c. Is normally very thick and viscid
    d. Normally contains bacteria

127. Chylothorax is
    a. An accumulation of yellow fluid in the abdomen
    b. A very "milky" fluid found in the abdomen
    c. An accumulation of "milky" fluid found in the pericardium
    d. A very "milky" fluid found in the pleural cavity

128. The viscosity of synovial fluid viscosity is attributable to
    a. Protein
    b. Hyaluronic acid
    c. Bacterial inflammation
    d. Hyaluronidase

129. Synovial fluid mucin forms a clot when added to
    a. Sodium bicarbonate
    b. Hyaluronic acid
    c. 3% potassium hydroxide
    d. Acetic acid

130. A transtracheal wash is performed by passage of a catheter through
    a. The mouth into an endotracheal tube
    b. The nasal passages
    c. The skin and trachea
    d. Any of the above

131. A 10-year-old male Laborador Retriever has a soft swelling approximately 10 cm in diameter on its rear leg. You obtain a fine-needle aspirate, make a smear, stain it with new methylene blue, and observe it microscopically. There are cells with numerous dark basophilic granules in the cytoplasm and a smudged appearance. Your cytology report should indicate the presence of what type of cells?
    a. Macrophages
    b. Mast cells
    c. Lymphocytes
    d. Basophils

Correct answers are on pages 178–192.

132. Which stain is used to confirm the presence of fat?
    a. New methylene blue
    b. Sudan III or IV
    c. Diff-Quik
    d. Giemsa

133. Which stain is referred to as a *supravital* stain?
    a. New methylene blue
    b. Camco Quik
    c. Eosin
    d. Sudan III or IV

134. Mrs. T brings her dog to your clinic for routine vaccinations and tells you she thinks her dog has ear problems. A smear from the ear reveals a yeast. What is the genus of the most common cause of mycotic (fungal) otitis externa?
    a. *Mucor*
    b. *Malassezia*
    c. *Dermatophilus*
    d. *Phycomycetes*

135. What is considered the minimal percentage of motile sperm in a normal canine ejaculate?
    a. 50 %
    b. 25 %
    c. 80 %
    d. 95 %

136. Which statement concerning queens and their reproductive behavior is most accurate?
    a. The average interval between estrous periods is 45 days.
    b. Queens are seasonally polyestrous and coitus is necessary for ovulation.
    c. Vaginal smears do not accurately predict estrus in the queen.
    d. The gestation period of the queen is 45 days.

137. The correct classification of vaginal epithelial cells from the deepest layer near the basement membrane, progressing superfically to the layer near the vaginal lumen, is
    a. Parabasal, basal, intermediate, superficial
    b. Superficial, intermediate, parabasal, basal
    c. Basal, parabasal, intermediate, superficial
    d. Intermediate, superficial, parabasal, basal

138. The largest cell seen in vaginal smears is
    a. Intermediate
    b. Basal
    c. Parabasal
    d. Superficial

139. Which stage of estrus exhibits the following changes on the vaginal smear? Epithelial cell type changes quickly to the noncornified cell, red blood cells disappear completely, and white blood cells come back in great numbers.
    a. Proestrus
    b. Estrus
    c. Diestrus
    d. Anestrus

140. Which cells predominate during anestrus?
    a. Parabasal and intermediate
    b. Neutrophils and superficial
    c. Intermediate and superficial
    d. Neutrophils and intermediate

141. In conjunctival and corneal scrapings, which cell combination suggests an allergic reaction?
    a. Lymphocytes and monocytes
    b. Neutrophils and monocytes
    c. Plasma cells and neutrophils
    d. Eosinophils and mast cells

142. Which cells are predominant in conjunctival smears from animals with conjunctivitis?
    a. Monocytes
    b. Neutrophils
    c. Mast cells
    d. Lymphocytes

143. Which of the following does *not* accurately describe the characteristics of a normal cell population?
    a. Equal distribution of cells
    b. Clearly differentiated cells
    c. Absence of foamy cytoplasm and nucleoli
    d. Pyknotic nuclei

144. Which statement concerning vaginal cytology is *least* accurate?
    a. Cytologic preparations made during the transition period from late estrus to early diestrus without benefit of prior preparations can appear very similiar to smears made in early or midproestrus.
    b. During proestrus, red blood cells may be abundant or absent, and bacteria are often present in large numbers.
    c. Parabasal cells are larger than anuclear cells.
    d. Vaginal smears from animals with pyometra or metritis usually contain large numbers of degenerated neutrophils.

145. Which stain should you use on a conjunctival scraping if you are interested in classifying bacteria?
    a. Diff-Quik
    b. New methylene blue
    c. Gram
    d. Eosin

146. Bone marrow cytologic evaluation *cannot* be used for
    a. Evaluation of the marrow's involvement in neoplastic conditions
    b. Identification of infectious agents, such as *Histoplasma capsulatum, Leishmania donovani,* and *Toxoplasma gondii*
    c. Evaluation of a patient with hyperproteinemia
    d. Differentiation of solid sarcomas from solid carcinomas

147. Which statement concerning the M:E ratio is *least* accurate?
    a. It is the ratio of nucleated erythroid cells to myeloid cells.
    b. Quantitative M:E ratios are determined by appropriately classifying 500 nucleated cells as myeloid or erythroid.
    c. Subjective evaluation of the M:E ratio is sufficient for diagnostic purposes.
    d. It is the ratio of myeloid cells to nucleated erythroid cells.

148. High-quality cytologic samples can be collected by any of the following methods *except*
    a. Swabbing
    b. Scraping
    c. Aspirating
    d. Debriding

149. Before making an impression smear from a specimen collected during surgery or necropsy,
    a. Blood and tissue fluids should be removed by blotting with clean absorbent material
    b. 70% alcohol should be used to blot the specimen
    c. The specimen should be soaked in formalin
    d. The specimen should be seared with a hot spatula

Correct answers are on pages 178–192.

150. Fine-needle aspirates should be collected using a preferred needle gauge of
    a. 14
    b. 16
    c. 21 or less
    d. 18

HEMATOLOGY

151. Eosinophilia is commonly seen with
    a. Bacterial infection
    b. Parasitic infection
    c. Viral infection
    d. Hormonal disorder

152. Which is the underlying cause of icterus?
    a. Anemia
    b. Hyperbilirubinemia
    c. Ketonemia
    d. Hemoglobinuria

153. Basophilic stippling is often associated with
    a. Lead poisoning
    b. Autoimmune disease
    c. Anemia
    d. Neoplasia

154. A common finding on a blood smear from an animal with autoimmune hemolytic anemia is
    a. Lymphocytosis
    b. Basophilic stippling
    c. Spherocytosis
    d. Leukemia

155. Denatured hemoglobin found in erythrocytes is known as
    a. A Heinz body
    b. A Howell-Jolly body
    c. An *Anaplasma* body
    d. A spherocyte

156. Yellow plasma is normal in
    a. Cattle
    b. Dogs
    c. Lipemia
    d. Hyperglycemia

157. Which cell produces antibodies?
    a. Hepatocyte
    b. Lymphocyte
    c. Eosinophil
    d. Spherocyte

158. Which of the following appears as a blue spheric nuclear remnant seen in some Wright-stained erythrocytes?
    a. Reticulocyte
    b. Howell-Jolly body
    c. Heinz body
    d. Leptocyte

159. An elevated hematocrit is most often associated with
    a. Hyperglycemia
    b. Anemia
    c. Dehydration
    d. Leukocytosis

160. Which of the following stimulates antibody production?
    a. Immunoglobulin
    b. Antigen
    c. T cell
    d. Plasma cell

161. Physiologic leukocytosis can be caused by
    a. Bacterial infection
    b. Parasite infection
    c. Toxemia
    d. Excitement

162. A normal leukocyte count with an increase in immature cells, which outnumber mature cells, is called
    a. Reticulocytosis
    b. Leukopenia
    c. A regenerative left shift
    d. A degenerative left shift

163. A leukocyte count can be falsely elevated by which of the following in the peripheral blood?
    a. Spherocytes
    b. Reticulocytes
    c. Metarubricytes
    d. Bands

164. What is the half life of neutrophils in the peripheral blood of dogs?
   a. 6 hours
   b. 1 day
   c. 7 days
   d. 110 days

165. Where is the storage pool of granulocytes found?
   a. Spleen
   b. Bone marrow
   c. Liver
   d. Capillaries

166. A variation in erythrocyte size is known as
   a. Polychromasia
   b. Anisocytosis
   c. Poikilocytosis
   d. Erythrocytosis

167. Which of the following is a nonnucleated, immature erythrocyte found in small numbers in the peripheral blood of dogs?
   a. Reticulocyte
   b. Metarubricyte
   c. Basophil
   d. Rubricyte

168. Which sample is recommended for hemoglobin testing?
   a. Serum
   b. Plasma
   c. Whole blood
   d. Blood smear

169. Which part of the complete blood count (CBC) is the most accurate procedure?
   a. Erythrocyte count
   b. Hemoglobin
   c. Leukocyte count
   d. Hematocrit

170. Which part of the manually performed CBC is the *least* accurate procedure?
   a. Erythrocyte count
   b. Leukocyte count
   c. Packed cell volume
   d. Hemoglobin

171. A neutrophil in which the cytoplasm is more basophilic than normal and contains vacuoles is also known as a
   a. Band cell
   b. Toxic neutrophil
   c. Metamyelocyte
   d. Hypersegmented neutrophil

172. Which of the following is *not* part of a stress leukogram?
   a. Leukocytosis
   b. Neutrophilia
   c. Monocytosis
   d. Eosinophilia

173. What is the normal packed cell volume of dogs?
   a. 35% to 55%
   b. 15% to 25%
   c. 45% to 65%
   d. 40% to 45%

174. Which of the following is *not* associated with responsive anemia?
   a. Poikilocytosis
   b. Reticulocytosis
   c. Anisocytosis
   d. Polychromasia

175. Which term describes a canine erythrocyte with a central rounded area of hemoglobin surrounded by a clear zone, with a dense ring of hemoglobin around the periphery?
   a. Plasma cell
   b. Spherocyte
   c. Reticulocyte
   d. Target cell

176. Which of the following is the *least* common granulocyte?
   a. Monocyte
   b. Basophil
   c. Eosinophil
   d. Metarubricyte

177. Which primary square(s) of the Neubauer hemocytometer is (are) used to count erythrocytes?
   a. All 9
   b. All 25
   c. Central primary square
   d. Four corner primary squares

Correct answers are on pages 178–192.

178. For what purpose are Unopettes used in hematology?

    a. Blood cell counting
    b. Hematocrit determination
    c. Hemoglobin determination
    d. Total protein determination

179. What term describes a subnormal neutrophil count?

    a. Leukocytosis
    b. Neutropenia
    c. Anemia
    d. Regenerative left shift

180. Which statement concerning quantitative buffy coat (QBC) analysis is *least* accurate?

    a. It determines the hematocrit.
    b. It determines the thrombocyte count.
    c. It can be used on the blood of any species.
    d. It determines the leukocyte count.

181. What causes plasma to appear red?

    a. Lipemia
    b. Lymphosarcoma
    c. Icterus
    d. Hemolysis

182. Approximately how much whole blood is needed to yield 1 milliliter of serum?

    a. 2 ml
    b. 3 ml
    c. 10 ml
    d. 20 ml

183. Reticulocytes are *never* found in the peripheral blood of

    a. Horses
    b. Cattle
    c. Dogs
    d. Cats

184. Which cell becomes a macrophage once it enters the tissues?

    a. Plasma cell
    b. Lymphocyte
    c. Neutrophil
    d. Monocyte

185. Which leukocyte count is in the range for a dog, cat, cow, or horse?

    a. 35,000/dl
    b. 5,750,000/dl
    c. 7,500/dl
    d. 275,000/dl

186. Which cell is produced by megakaryocytes?

    a. Erythrocyte
    b. Lymphocyte
    c. Neutrophil
    d. Thrombocyte

187. For which determination is a refractometer used?

    a. Leukocyte count
    b. Total protein level
    c. Hemoglobin level
    d. Erythrocyte indices

188. Bone marrow is *not* a major site of production for

    a. Erythrocytes
    b. Neutrophils
    c. Lymphocytes
    d. Monocytes

189. Leukemia is indicated by finding which cells in a peripheral blood smear?

    a. Bands
    b. Lymphoblasts
    c. Reticulocytes
    d. Plasma cells

190. Which species normally has the smallest erythrocytes?

    a. Horses
    b. Dogs
    c. Cattle
    d. Goats

191. Which of the following is an intracellular parasite of erythrocytes?

    a. *Babesia*
    b. *Ehrlichia*
    c. *Trypanosoma*
    d. *Toxoplasma*

192. Where is the buffy coat found in the spun microhematocrit tube?
    a. Beneath the packed red cells
    b. Above the packed red cells
    c. Above the plasma
    d. Buffy coats are not seen in microhematocrit tubes

193. What is the major difference between serum and plasma?
    a. Plasma has higher protein levels
    b. Serum is darker in color
    c. Plasma has a higher leukocyte count
    d. Serum has a higher yield for the same volume of blood

194. What is the term used to describe plasma that appears white or milky?
    a. Leukemia
    b. Lipemia
    c. Leukocytosis
    d. Icterus

195. What is the term used to describe the situation in which the many of the erythrocytes stain varying shades of blue?
    a. Anemia
    b. Anisocytosis
    c. Polychromasia
    d. Poikilocytosis

196. Which stain is used to visualize reticulocytes?
    a. Wright's
    b. Giemsa
    c. Gram's
    d. New methylene blue

197. Which of the following is a breakdown product of hemoglobin?
    a. Bilirubin
    b. Erythropoietin
    c. Urea
    d. Carotene

198. Which of the following is associated with clotting problems?
    a. Anemia
    b. Leukopenia
    c. Thrombocytopenia
    d. Reticulocytosis

199. How long must the typical microhematocrit tube be centrifuged for packed cell volume determination?
    a. 1 minute
    b. 5 minutes
    c. 10 minutes
    d. 15 minutes

200. Which measure determines the average size of an erythrocyte?
    a. Mean corpuscular volume
    b. Packed cell volume
    c. Mean corpuscular hemoglobin concentration
    d. Mean corpuscular hemoglobin

201. What is normally the most numerous leukocyte seen in bovine blood?
    a. Monocyte
    b. Neutrophil
    c. Lymphocyte
    d. Eosinophil

202. What is normally the most numerous leukocyte seen in canine blood?
    a. Monocyte
    b. Neutrophil
    c. Lymphocyte
    d. Eosinophil

203. Which blood cell resembles the mast cell found in tissues?
    a. Eosinophil
    b. Reticulocyte
    c. Neutrophil
    d. Basophil

204. Howell-Jolly bodies resemble which erythrocyte parasite?
    a. *Babesia*
    b. *Hemobartonella*
    c. *Trypanosoma*
    d. *Ehrlichia*

205. What is the name of the specialized slide on which diluted blood is placed for cell counting?
    a. Refractometer
    b. QBC-V
    c. Hemocytometer
    d. Leukometer

Correct answers are on pages 178–192.

206. Which term indicates an abnormally high lymphocyte count
    a. Lymphocytosis
    b. Leukosis
    c. Lymphocytopenia
    d. Lymphosarcoma

207. Which type of anemia is associated with icterus?
    a. Responsive
    b. Nonresponsive
    c. Hemolytic
    d. Megaloblastic

208. Which is the most immature erythrocyte that can be identified in bone marrow?
    a. Prorubricyte
    b. Rubriblast
    c. Erythrocytoblast
    d. Megakaryoblast

209. The abbreviation *seg* refers to which blood cell?
    a. Lymphocyte
    b. Monocyte
    c. Band
    d. Neutrophil

210. Which blood cell normally has vacuoles in its cytoplasm?
    a. Monocyte
    b. Lymphocyte
    c. Neutrophil
    d. Thrombocyte

211. The dark-staining material in the nuclei of lymphocytes and neutrophils is called
    a. Leukopoietin
    b. Chromatin
    c. Reticulum
    d. Vacuole

212. Which equine leukocyte normally has large, red-staining cytoplasmic granules?
    a. Basophil
    b. Monocyte
    c. Eosinophil
    d. Neutrophil

213. At what stage in granulopoiesis do the specific or definitive granules first appear?
    a. Metamyelocyte
    b. Progranulocyte
    c. Myeloblast
    d. Myelocyte

214. How does a band cell differ in appearance from a mature neutrophil?
    a. The mature neutrophil is larger
    b. The band nucleus has smooth, parallel sides
    c. The band cytoplasm does not contain granules
    d. The mature neutrophil has bluer cytoplasm

215. A canine erythrocyte that is smaller than normal, with no pale area in the center, is called a
    a. Rubricyte
    b. Metarubricyte
    c. Spherocyte
    d. Thrombocyte

216. Rouleaux formation is most commonly seen on blood smears from
    a. Horses
    b. Goats
    c. Dogs
    d. Cats

217. Which cells on a blood smear are frequently associated with disseminated intravascular coagulation (DIC)?
    a. Spherocytes
    b. Acanthocytes
    c. Basophils
    d. Schistocytes

218. If you count 40 reticulocytes per 1,000 erythrocytes, what is the observed reticulocyte count?
    a. 2%
    b. 4%
    c. 20%
    d. 40%

219. Which bovine erythrocyte parasite resembles *Hemobartonella felis* in cats?
    a. *Anaplasma*
    b. *Babesia*
    c. *Dirofilaria*
    d. *Ehrlichia*

220. What is indicated by a neutrophil with a nucleus with six lobes?
    a. Toxemia
    b. Female animal
    c. Old cell
    d. Leukemia

221. Which species normally has oval erythrocytes?
    a. Normal horses
    b. Normal llamas
    c. Anemic cats
    d. Toxemic dogs

222. What causes dark granules called Döhle bodies in the cytoplasm of canine neutrophils?
    a. Leukemia
    b. Parasitic infection
    c. Responsive anemia
    d. Toxemia

223. What is normally the largest blood cell in domestic species?
    a. Monocyte
    b. Neutrophil
    c. Eosinophil
    d. Lymphocyte

224. Mature erythrocytes are normally nucleated in
    a. Miniature horses
    b. Ferrets
    c. Camels
    d. Birds

225. Which leukocyte can normally have a bean-shaped nucleus?
    a. Lymphocyte
    b. Plasma cell
    c. Monocyte
    d. Band neutrophil

226. Which site is most commonly used for bone marrow collection in dogs?
    a. Proximal tibia
    b. Iliac crest
    c. Sternum
    d. Proximal humerus

227. Which neoplasm of plasma cells results in large numbers of immature or abnormal plasma cells in the bone marrow?
    a. Lymphosarcoma
    b. Lymphocytic leukemia
    c. Mast-cell tumor
    d. Multiple myeloma

228. Most cats in the United States have which blood type?
    a. A
    b. B
    c. C
    d. AB

229. What is tested in a major crossmatch?
    a. T-cell production
    b. Recipient serum against donor erythrocytes
    c. Recipient erythrocytes against donor serum
    d. Recipient urine against donor erythrocytes

230. Which anticoagulant is used most commonly in animal blood collection?
    a. Sodium heparin
    b. Potassium oxalate
    c. Potassium ethylenediaminetetraacetic acid (EDTA)
    d. Sodium citrate

231. Which anticoagulant is used to determine activated partial thromboplastin time and one-stage prothrombin time?
    a. Heparin
    b. Citrate
    c. Fluoride
    d. EDTA

Correct answers are on pages 178–192.

232. Which structure is normally found in the nuclei of immature blood cells?
    a. Nucleolus
    b. Golgi apparatus
    c. Heinz body
    d. Döhle body

233. A cat has a total leukocyte count of 15,000/dl. On the differential count, 65% of the cells are neutrophils. What is the absolute neutrophil count?
    a. 975/dl
    b. 975,000/dl
    c. 9,750/dl
    d. 5,250/dl

234. Certain oxidant drugs cause production of round structures in erythrocytes called
    a. Howell-Jolly bodies
    b. Russell's bodies
    c. Döhle bodies
    d. Heinz bodies

235. What causes hypochromia in erythrocytes?
    a. Hypertonic drugs
    b. Decreased hemoglobin
    c. Iron toxicity
    d. Increased erythrocyte production

236. What is the primary function of fibrinogen?
    a. Antibody production
    b. Phagocytosis
    c. Hemostasis
    d. Heinz body production

237. Which nucleated erythrocyte is seen most frequently on blood smears?
    a. Reticulocyte
    b. Metarubricyte
    c. Rubricyte
    d. Prorubricyte

238. *Hemobartonella felis* is seen most commonly in the erythrocytes of
    a. Cats
    b. Cattle
    c. Dogs
    d. Horses

239. An increased number of bands in the peripheral blood indicates
    a. Leukemia
    b. Autoimmune hemolytic anemia
    c. A left shift
    d. Neutropenia

240. When using the 100X oil immersion lens with the standard 10X ocular, what is the magnification of cells observed through the microscope?
    a. 90X
    b. 100X
    c. 110X
    d. 1000X

IMMUNOLOGY

241. Immunology is a branch of science dealing with all of the following *except*
    a. Resistance to infectious diseases
    b. Removal of wornout cells
    c. Recognition of abnormal cell mutants in the body
    d. Bacterial resistance to antibacterial drugs

242. Which white blood cells migrate through tissue and function to remove and destroy bacteria, damaged cells, and neoplastic cells?
    a. Lymphocytes
    b. Basophils
    c. Monocytes
    d. Eosinophils

243. Which immunoglobulin is the largest, having a molecular weight of approximately 900,000 daltons?
    a. IgG
    b. IgA
    c. IgM
    d. IgD

244. Which immunoglobulin is most abundant in the serum and plays the major role in humoral immunity?
    a. IgG
    b. IgM
    c. IgA
    d. IgD

245. Immunity that is generated by an animal's immune system following exposure to a foreign antigen is referred to as
    a. Passive immunity
    b. Active immunity
    c. Responsive immunity
    d. Celostral immunity

246. Mature macrophages found in connective tissue are known as
    a. Histiocytes
    b. Reticuloendothelial cells
    c. Monocytes
    d. Mast cells

247. Which of the following is *not* a major function of macrophages or a result of macrophage activity?
    a. Phagocytosis
    b. Fever
    c. Inflammation
    d. Production of peroxidase

248. Which of the following correctly lists the progressive stages of phagocytosis?
    a. Adherence, chemotaxis, ingestion, digestion
    b. Ingestion, adherence, chemotaxis, digestion
    c. Chemotaxis, adherence, ingestion, digestion
    d. Ingestion, digestion, chemotaxis, adherence

249. An attenuated vaccine is one in which
    a. Microorganisms have been killed
    b. Microorganisms are weakened but still alive
    c. Microorganisms are alive
    d. No microorganisms are found

250. Which statement concerning passive immunity is *least* accurate?
    a. It involves antibodies that have been produced in a donor animal.
    b. It provides immediate but short-lived immunity.
    c. It may be natural or artificial.
    d. It develops after exposure to a pathogen.

251. Cytokines are
    a. Chemicals that elicit a hormonal response
    b. Chemicals that attract white blood cells to an area and activate macrophages
    c. Chemicals secreted by monocytes
    d. Inclusions found in neutrophils

252. Anaphylactic shock is
    a. A mild reaction causing destruction of erythrocytes
    b. A moderate reaction causing hives
    c. A severe life-threatening reaction occurring seconds after an antigen enters the circulation
    d. A severe reaction caused by rapid loss of large volumes of blood or other body fluid

253. Which breed of horse is predisposed to combined immunodeficiency?
    a. Thoroughbred
    b. Appaloosa
    c. Quarter horse
    d. Arabian

254. Which of the following is *not* a malfunction of the immune system?
    a. Allergy
    b. Immunodeficiency
    c. Autoimmune disease
    d. Immunity conferred by vaccination

255. Which cells are chiefly concerned with production and secretion of antibodies?
    a. B-lymphocytes
    b. T-lymphocytes
    c. Neutrophils
    d. Monocytes

256. Which cells respond faster to a second exposure to an antigen than to the initial exposure?
    a. T-lymphocytes
    b. Monocytes
    c. Memory B-cells
    d. Memory T-cells

Correct answers are on pages 178–192.

257. Serology is the branch of science involved with detection of
    a. Bacteria
    b. Viruses
    c. Antibodies or antigens
    d. Parasites

258. ELISA is an acronym for
    a. Electro-linked immunosorbent assay
    b. Enzyme-linked immunosorbent assay
    c. Enzyme-linked immunoassay
    d. Electrolytic isoantibody assay

259. Which statement concerning ELISA testing is *least* accurate?
    a. The specificity is very high.
    b. Washing is a noncritical step in the methodology.
    c. It may be used to detect antibodies or antigen in the serum.
    d. It is now available in kit form.

260. Which serologic test is used for diagnosis of autoimmune hemolytic anemia?
    a. Coombs' test
    b. Zinc sulfate turbidity
    c. Intradermal testing
    d. Latex agglutination

261. Which statement concerning the tuberculin test is *least* accurate?
    a. Animals with tuberculosis show a delayed hypersensitivity reaction.
    b. Tuberculin is commonly injected into the caudal tail fold of cattle.
    c. Accidental self-injection is unlikely to cause tuberculosis.
    d. The response should be checked 1 hour after tuberculin injection.

262. Intradermal tests
    a. Detect allergies mediated by IgE antibody molecules
    b. Are not used in veterinary medicine
    c. Are interpreted in 5 minutes
    d. Detect allergies mediated by IgG antibody molecules

263. Vaccines may be given by any of the following routes *except*
    a. Subcutaneously
    b. Intramuscularly
    c. Intranasally
    d. Intraperitoneally

264. Which statement concerning antigen-antibody complexes is *least* accurate?
    a. They rapidly result in death.
    b. They resemble a lock and key in principle.
    c. They can be detected with serologic tests.
    d. They form only when a specific antigen meets its corresponding antibody.

265. Which of the following is *least* likely to cause vaccine failure?
    a. Improper storage
    b. Administration during anesthesia
    c. Interference by maternal antibodies
    d. Improper route of administration

266. A type of protein whose blood level may be elevated in some immunoproliferative diseases is
    a. Tamn-Horsfall
    b. Bence Jones
    c. Roberts
    d. Coombs

267. Damage produced by deposition of immune complexes in a local region is referred to as
    a. An Arthus reaction
    b. A Regis reaction
    c. Antibody deposition
    d. Complex precipitation

268. Pemphigus is
    a. Contagious
    b. A group of autoimmune disorders that affect the skin and oral mucosa
    c. Diagnosed exclusively by Coombs' test
    d. Seen only in Dalmatian dogs

269. Signs of immune-mediated thrombocytopenia include all of the following *except*
    a. Petechiae
    b. Ecchymoses
    c. Thrombocytosis
    d. Anemia

270. Which condition is associated with abnormal skin pigmentation, eye lesions, and cyclic neutropenia?
    a. Chédiak-Higashi syndrome
    b. Gray Collie syndrome
    c. Canine granulocytopathy syndrome
    d. Lupus erythematosus

271. Lymphocyte production occurs mainly in the
    a. Thymus and bone marrow
    b. Lymph nodes
    c. Spleen
    d. Liver

272. Which statement concerning monoclonal antibodies is *least* accurate?
    a. They are identical immunoglobulin molecules.
    b. They are formed by a single clone of plasma cells.
    c. They are most common in Abyssinian cats.
    d. They are commercially produced for use in immunoassays.

273. Cell-mediated hypersensitivity results from a reaction between an
    a. Antigen and a sensitized T-lymphocyte
    b. Antibody and a sensitized B-lymphocyte
    c. Antigen and antibody
    d. Antibody and a sensitized neutrophil

274. Acute anaphylaxis
    a. Is a generalized unusual or exaggerated systemic allergic reaction
    b. Is a localized reaction
    c. Typically does not cause shock
    d. Is treated with antibiotics

275. Most clostridial diseases are controlled by injection of
    a. Antitoxins
    b. Toxoids
    c. Live vaccines
    d. Immunostimulants

276. Which statement concerning feline immunodeficiency virus is most accurate?
    a. It is classified as a herpesvirus.
    b. It attacks only red blood cells.
    c. It causes pathologic changes similar to those caused by the human immunodeficiency virus.
    d. It can cause acquired immunodeficiency syndrome (AIDS) if a person becomes infected.

277. Hemagglutination is
    a. Clumping of erythrocytes
    b. Lysing of erythrocytes
    c. Crenation of erythrocytes
    d. Swelling of erythrocytes

278. Which test is routinely used to diagnose equine infectious anemia?
    a. Indirect fluorescent antibody test
    b. Coggins test
    c. Ford test
    d. Electrophoresis

279. Which statement concerning complement is *least* accurate?
    a. It is composed of a series of proteins that are activated to combine with antigen-antibody complexes, producing lysis when the antigen is an intact cell.
    b. Its activation is closely linked to inflammation and the clotting process.
    c. It is responsible for production of chemotactic substances that attract leukocytes to the site of inflammation.
    d. Complement activation signifies imminent death.

Correct answers are on pages 178–192.

280. Serum immunoglobulin levels are measured by
    a. The Coggins test
    b. Radioimmunodiffusion
    c. Enzyme-linked immunosorbent assay
    d. Clot retraction

281. Which factor is *least* likely to cause an immune disorder or dysfunction?
    a. Effects of aging
    b. Long-term use of corticosteroids
    c. Spaying and declawing during the same surgery
    d. Irradiation

282. Which factor is *least* likely to affect the performance of enzyme immunoassays?
    a. Time
    b. Temperature
    c. Hemolysis or lipemia
    d. Species

283. Seroconversion is
    a. A change in the color of serum
    b. A fourfold increase in the antibody titer
    c. A fourfold decrease in the antibody titer
    d. Indicative of no change in the antibody titer

284. After infection is eliminated, the immune response is reduced by
    a. B-lymphocytes
    b. B-memory lymphocytes
    c. Monocytes
    d. T-suppressor cells

285. What do sensitized cells produce in abnormal quantities when an allergen reappears after an initial exposure?
    a. Antihistamines
    b. Histamine
    c. Toxins
    d. Lysins

286. Which antibodies attract phagocytes and allow them to adhere to antigenic cells?
    a. Opsonins
    b. Precipitins
    c. Antitoxins
    d. Lysins

287. Nonspecific immunity is an important part of the body's defense mechanism in all of the following *except*
    a. Nasal passages
    b. Stomach acid
    c. Skin
    d. T-cells

288. Which cells are sensitized by IgE?
    a. Mast cells and basophils
    b. Eosinophils and basophils
    c. Monocytes and lymphocytes
    d. Neutrophils and eosinophils

289. T-killer cells function to
    a. Release histamine
    b. Recognize cancer cells as abnormal cells and eliminate them
    c. Coat cancer cells with antibody
    d. Release endorphin

290. Spherocytes are
    a. Macrocytic erythrocytes
    b. Neutrophils coated with complement
    c. Red blood cells destined for destruction by the immune system
    d. Degenerate lymphocytes

291. Cats exposed to feline leukemia virus typically respond in any of the following ways *except*
    a. Not becoming infected at all
    b. Becoming temporarily infected, developing immunity, and overcoming the infection
    c. Becoming infected and continuing to shed the virus indefinitely without becoming ill
    d. Becoming infected, becoming ill within 3 days, and dying within a week.

292. Which of the following is *not* a type of antibody?
    a. Lysin
    b. Precipitin
    c. Toxin
    d. Agglutinin

293. What is the predominant method of transmission of feline immunodeficiency virus in cats?
    a. Grooming
    b. Bite wounds
    c. Urine
    d. Feces

294. In assessing titers, how long after the first serum sample is collected should the second sample be collected?
    a. 7 days
    b. 3 days
    c. 2 to 6 weeks
    d. 14 weeks

295. Which statement concerning feline infectious peritonitis is *least* accurate?
    a. It is caused by a small RNA virus.
    b. It is widespread in nature.
    c. It is diagnosed by the coronaviral antibody test, IFA, and ELISA.
    d. It is fatal only in young kittens and very old cats.

Microbiology

296. Which microorganisms are the smallest and *not* free living?
    a. Algae
    b. Fungi
    c. Bacteria
    d. Viruses

297. What is the correct way to write the genus and species of bacteria?
    a. Streptococcus pyogenes
    b. Streptococcus *pyogenes*
    c. *Streptococcus* pyogenes
    d. *Streptococcus pyogenes*

298. The acid-fast stain is used to identify
    a. *Streptococcus*
    b. *Enterobacterium*
    c. *Microsporum*
    d. *Mycobacterium*

299. The main purpose of a simple stain is to
    a. Outline the shape of bacteria
    b. Differentiate between Gram-positive and Gram-negative organisms
    c. Identify organisms that grow individually
    d. Allow for a simplified way to recognize acid-fast organisms

300. *Escherichia coli* 0157 infections are obtained *most* likely from eating infected
    a. Steak
    b. Hamburger
    c. Frozen chicken
    d. Cold cuts

301. Gram-positive organisms appear as what color when stained with Gram's stain?
    a. Blue
    b. Red
    c. Green
    d. Clear

302. A well-organized glycocalyx is called a
    a. Slime layer
    b. Spore
    c. Fungus
    d. Capsule

303. Which of the following *best* describes what happens when a bacterial cell is placed in a solution containing 5% NaCl?
    a. No change is evident; the solution is isotonic
    b. The cell undergoes osmotic lysis
    c. Water moves out of the cell
    d. Water moves into the cell

304. Which of the following does *not* kill endospores?
    a. Autoclaving
    b. Incineration
    c. Hot-air sterilization
    d. Standard technique of pasteurization

Correct answers are on pages 178–192.

305. Which method is best to sterilize heat-sensitive medical equipment?

    a. Dry heat
    b. Autoclaving
    c. Gas sterilization
    d. Pasteurization

306. Viruses are *best* described as

    a. Free-living organisms
    b. Obligatory interstitial parasites
    c. Obligatory intracellular parasites
    d. Eukaryotic cells

307. Noncytopathic viruses release viral particles through

    a. Osmosis
    b. Diffusion
    c. Budding
    d. Lysis

308. A papilloma is a good example of

    a. A cytopathic virus
    b. A noncytopathic virus
    c. An oncogenic virus
    d. A noninfectious agent

309. A virus that maintains a state of equilibrium with a host that initially does *not* show any clinical signs of the infection is called a

    a. Slow virus
    b. Virion
    c. Prion
    d. Latent virus

310. A nosocomial infection is

    a. Always present but not apparent at the time of hospitalization
    b. Always acquired during the course of hospitalization
    c. Always caused by medical personnel
    d. Only the result of surgery

311. Proliferation of an organism such as *Bacillus anthracis* in the blood of cattle would be classified as a

    a. Blood dyscrasia
    b. Focal infection
    c. Local infection
    d. Septicemia

312. When normal flora prevent overgrowth of pathogens, it is called

    a. Commensalism
    b. Symbiosis
    c. Microbial antagonism
    d. Parasitism

313. The protein coating immediately surrounding the nuclear material in a virus is known as the

    a. Envelope
    b. Capsid
    c. Capsule
    d. Cell wall

314. A collection of viral particles in a cell is known as

    a. A viral accumulation
    b. Inclusion bodies
    c. A precipitate
    d. Granules

315. A low–molecular-weight protein that is produced by host cells in response to infection by a virus is known as

    a. Viral protein
    b. An inclusion body
    c. Interferon
    d. An antibiotic

316. Generally, endotoxins are products of

    a. Viruses
    b. Gram-negative bacteria
    c. Gram-positive bacteria
    d. Fungi

317. The microscopic morphology of *Staphylococcus* is described as a

    a. Coccus in chains
    b. Coccus in grape-like clusters
    c. Bacillus in chains
    d. Bacillus in no particular arrangement

318. Which organism is most likely grow on mannitol salt agar?

    a. *Streptococcus pyogenes*
    b. *Bacillus subtilis*
    c. *Clostridium perfringens*
    d. *Staphylococcus aureus*

414. Larvae enter the nasal cavity of sheep.

415. Which parasite spends its entire life cycle on or in its host?
   a. *Ctenocephalides*
   b. *Otodectes*
   c. *Hypoderma*
   d. *Dermacentor*

416. Which species is known as "walking dandruff?"
   a. *Trombicula*
   b. *Sarcoptes*
   c. *Demodex*
   d. *Cheyletiella*

417. Scabies is caused by
   a. *Trombicula*
   b. *Otodectes*
   c. *Melophagus*
   d. *Sarcoptes*

Questions 418 through 421

   a. *Bunostomum*
   b. *Ostertagia*
   c. *Trichostrongylus*
   d. *Hemonchus*

418. Hookworm.

419. Abomasal worm.

420. Brown stomach worm.

421. Barberpole worm.

422. Choose the correct size sequence, from largest adult form to smallest adult form.
   a. *Trichostrongylus, Nematodirus, Strongyloides, Eimeria*
   b. *Nematodirus, Trichostrongylus, Strongyloides, Eimeria*
   c. *Nematodirus, Trichostrongylus, Eimeria, Strongyloides*
   d. *Nematodirus, Strongyloides, Trichostrongylus, Eimeria*

Questions 423 through 426

   a. *Oesophagostomum*
   b. *Ostertagia*
   c. *Hemonchus*
   d. *Dictyocaulus*

423. Parasitizes the abomasal gastric glands.

424. Sucks blood in the abomasum.

425. Matures in the lungs.

426. Forms nodules in the intestinal mucosa.

427. The most common parasite found in pigs is
   a. *Ascaris*
   b. *Metastrongylus*
   c. *Oesophagostomum*
   d. *Trichuris*

428. The normal mode of infection by *Ancylostoma* is
   a. Ingestion of eggs
   b. Transmammary infection
   c. Transplacental infection
   d. Skin penetration

429. As a student extern at a humane society clinic, you observe many large worms in the feces lying on the bottom of a dog's pen. What is the most logical explanation?
   a. The dog has probably been treated for roundworms recently
   b. The dog has large numbers of roundworms, which are passed in the feces
   c. It is a period in the life cycle of roundworms that results in the passage of large numbers of worms
   d. The roundworms pass out in large numbers when the dog has diarrhea

430. Coughing and increased numbers of eosinophils in peripheral blood suggest
   a. *Trichuris* infection
   b. *Toxocara* infection
   c. *Dipylidium* infection
   d. *Giardia* infection

Correct answers are on pages 178–192.

431. Choose the correct size sequence, from smallest adult form to largest adult form.
  a. *Isospora, Uncinaria, Ancylostoma, Toxocara*
  b. *Isospora, Ancylostoma, Toxocara, Uncinaria*
  c. *Isospora, Ancylostoma, Uncinaria, Toxocara*
  d. *Ancylostoma, Isospora, Uncinaria, Toxocara*

432. Anemia is most likely associated with infection by
  a. *Isospora*
  b. *Paragonimus*
  c. *Strongyloides*
  d. *Ancylostoma*

433. A common sign of giardiasis is
  a. Chronic diarrhea
  b. Anemia
  c. Coughing
  d. Vomiting

Questions 434 through 437

  a. *Dioctophyma*
  b. *Fasciola*
  c. *Paragonimum*
  d. *Capillaria*

434. Liver fluke.

435. Lung fluke.

436. Kidney worm.

437. Lungworm.

438. *Trichuris* ova most resemble the ova of
  a. *Isospora*
  b. *Taenia*
  c. *Ancylostoma*
  d. *Capillaria*

Questions 439 through 442

  a. *Trichodectes*
  b. *Hematopinus*
  c. *Felicola*
  d. *Damalinia*

439. Chewing louse of dogs.

440. Chewing louse of cats.

441. Sucking louse of cattle.

442. Chewing louse of cattle.

443. The genus name for the spinose ear tick is
  a. *Otodectes*
  b. *Otobius*
  c. *Oestrus*
  d. *Oxyuris*

444. Which species is *not* parasitized by pinworms?
  a. Horses
  b. Dogs
  c. Rodents
  d. People

Questions 445 through 448

  a. *Alaria*
  b. *Fascioloides*
  c. *Stephanurus*
  d. *Metastrongylus*

445. Intestinal fluke.

446. Lungworm.

447. Kidney worm.

448. Large American liver fluke.

449. Which statement concerning *Ctenocephalides* is *least* accurate?
  a. "Flea dirt" is partially digested blood droppings (feces).
  b. Fleas are not host specific.
  c. Adults can survive months without feeding.
  d. Its eggs are sticky and can be seen adhering to the host's fur.

Questions 450 through 453

  a. *Ancylostoma*
  b. *Melophagus*
  c. *Notoedres*
  d. *Echinococcus*

450. Causes generalized pruritus.

451. Causes creeping eruption.

452. Causes hydatidosis.

453. Causes feline scabies.

Questions 454 through 457

    a. *Psoroptes*
    b. *Mallophaga*
    c. *Cryptosporidium*
    d. *Anoplura*

454. Protozoan.

455. Biting or chewing louse.

456. Sucking louse.

457. Mite.

URINALYSIS

458. The urine of an animal with hematuria is most likely to be
    a. Cloudy and red
    b. Clear and brown
    c. Red and clear
    d. Brown and cloudy

459. The specific gravity of a patient's urine is so high you cannot measure it. You dilute the sample 1:2 with distilled water. Now the specific gravity is 1.032. What is the sample's true specific gravity?
    a. 2.032
    b. 1.016
    c. 2.064
    d. 1.064

460. Specific gravity is
    a. The weight of urine compared with the weight of water
    b. Measured with a dipstick
    c. Another name for total protein
    d. The negative log of the pH

461. Calcium carbonate crystals are often seen in
    a. Dogs
    b. Horses
    c. Cats
    d. Cattle

462. In a urine sample, a red blood cell may be easily confused with
    a. A fat droplet
    b. A degenerate white blood cell
    c. A renal epithelial cell
    d. An amorphous crystal

463. All of the following are assessed in a routine urinalysis *except*
    a. pH
    b. Occult blood
    c. Urobilinogen
    d. Blood urea nitrogen

464. The *Ico* test of urine is used to detect
    a. Blood
    b. Fat
    c. Urobilinogen
    d. Bilirubin

465. What can you do if the specific gravity of a urine sample is greater than 1.065?
    a. Multiply the results by 2
    b. Dilute it 1:3 with distilled water
    c. Dilute it 1:2 with distilled water
    d. Read it using the total protein scale

466. When using dipsticks for urine chemical analysis, you should do all of the following *except*
    a. Check the expiration date
    b. Store them in the refrigerator
    c. Store them with desiccant
    d. Keep the bottle capped

467. A control should be run on the urine dipstick in all of the following instances *except*
    a. When the dipstick appears to be discolored
    b. When a new bottle is opened
    c. If one has been run previously during the same shift
    d. If there is a shift change in personnel

468. Which crystal is commonly described as having a *coffin lid* appearance?
    a. Bilirubin crystal
    b. Calcium oxalate crystal
    c. Cystine crystal
    d. Triple phosphate crystal

469. An ammonium biurate crystal is sometimes described as
    a. Shaped like an envelope
    b. Shaped like a pyramid
    c. Having a *thorny apple* appearance
    d. Looking like a bicycle wheel

Correct answers are on pages 178–192.

470. The best time to collect a sample for urinalysis is
    a. Late evening
    b. Afternoon
    c. Midmorning
    d. Morning

471. Urine samples collected in the morning tend to be
    a. Unacceptable for sediment analysis
    b. More concentrated, thus increasing the chances of observing abnormalities
    c. Bright orange
    d. The least concentrated sample

472. What are the two preferred methods of collecting a urine sample?
    a. Catheterization and voiding
    b. Expressing the bladder and cytocentesis
    c. Cytocentesis and catheterization
    d. Cytocentesis and voiding

473. Polyuria is
    a. Lack of urine production
    b. Production of excessive amounts of urine
    c. Excessive intake of water
    d. Excessive protein in the urine

474. Oliguria is
    a. Excessive eating
    b. Green urine
    c. Excessive bilirubin in the urine
    d. Decreased urine output

475. Anuria is
    a. Decreased urine output
    b. Excessive urination
    c. Complete lack of urine production
    d. Excessive drinking

476. Isosthenuria is urine with a specific gravity
    a. Of 1.010
    b. Below 1.010
    c. Of 1.000
    d. Above 1.065

477. How does the specific gravity of dilute, colorless urine compare with that of dark, yellow urine?
    a. Slightly higher
    b. Moderately higher
    c. Much Higher
    d. Lower

478. A urine pH above 7.0 is
    a. Characteristic of acidic urine
    b. Characteristic of alkaline urine
    c. Always abnormal
    d. Characteristic of a high-protein diet

479. Which statement concerning urine pH is *least* accurate?
    a. It is measured with a refractometer.
    b. It is a measure of hydrogen ion concentration.
    c. It depends on the animal's diet.
    d. It is a measure of acidity or alkalinity.

480. A urine specimen collected at 8 am and left at room temperature until the afternoon could be expected to have
    a. Decreased numbers of bacteria
    b. Increased numbers of bacteria
    c. Increased numbers of cells
    d. Decreased turbidity

Questions 481 through 483

    a. Dysuria
    b. Hematuria
    c. Pyuria
    d. Proteinuria

481. Blood in the urine.

482. Pus in the urine.

483. Painful urination.

484. Protein in the urine.

485. Specific gravity is a measure of
    a. Molecular weight
    b. Density
    c. Molarity
    d. Number of atoms present

486. Large quantities of calcium oxalate monohydrate crystals may indicate
    a. Renal disease
    b. Liver disease
    c. Dietary deficiencies
    d. Ethylene glycol toxicity

487. Dark yellow urine generally has a
    a. pH of 5.0 or below
    b. Low specific gravity
    c. High specific gravity
    d. pH of 8.0 or above

488. Which crystals are usually found in alkaline urine?
    a. Amorphous urates
    b. Bilirubin
    c. Cholesterol
    d. Calcium carbonate

489. All of the following crystals are generally found in acidic urine *except*
    a. Uric acid
    b. Calcium carbonate
    c. Calcium oxalate
    d. Bilirubin

490. Ammonium urate crystals are most commonly seen in
    a. Labrador Retrievers
    b. Persians
    c. Dalmatians
    d. Siamese

491. A urine with 3+ occult blood and that is red and clear is most likely to contain any of the following *except*
    a. Myoglobin
    b. Red blood cells
    c. Hemoglobin
    d. Almost no protein

492. When microscopically examining urine sediment, you should be sure to do all of the following *except*
    a. Report all elements per high-power field
    b. Resuspend the sediment in approximately 0.5 ml of urine
    c. Examine the urine sediment under both high and low powers
    d. Centrifuge the urine sample for 5 minutes

493. It is easier to observe the elements in urine sediment by
    a. Lowering the condenser to increase the light
    b. Raising the condenser to increase the light
    c. Lowering the condenser to reduce the light
    d. Raising the condenser to lower the light

494. Carnivores generally have
    a. Very high protein levels in urine
    b. Acidic urine
    c. Alkaline urine
    d. High glucose levels in urine

495. Vegetable diets generally yield
    a. Acidic urine
    b. High levels of ketones in urine
    c. Low levels of ketones in urine
    d. Alkaline urine

496. The sulfosalicylic acid test of urine is used to detect
    a. Bilirubin
    b. Protein
    c. Glucose
    d. Hemoglobin

497. Urine samples should be centrifuged at a
    a. Low speed (1,000 to 3,000 rpm) for 20 minutes
    b. High speed (6,000 to 10,000 rpm) for 20 minutes
    c. Low speed (1,000 to 3,000 rpm) for 5 minutes
    d. High speed (6,000 to 10,000 rpm) for 5 minutes

Correct answers are on pages 178–192.

Answers

Quality Control

1. **d**

2. **a**

3. **b**

4. **c**

5. **c** Controls are run for quality-control purposes only. They are not used to calibrate instruments.

6. **a**

7. **b**

8. **a**

9. **d**

10. **c**

11. **c**

12. **b**

13. **d** Shifts and trends indicate you have a problem and that you need to troubleshoot to determine the cause of the variability in the control results.

14. **c** Sampling errors are those that occur in obtaining and handling a specimen.

15. **d** Errors can occur with use of reagents and glassware.

16. **b** Equipment malfunctions are errors that can occur with instrumentation.

17. **a** Errors can be caused by the personnel conducting the test.

18. **d** Quality-control data should not change when the people conducting the tests are well trained and conscientious.

19. **b** It is not possible to tell through the use of quality-control measures whether the samples are of acceptable quality.

20. **b** Refractometers should be checked daily with distilled water to ensure that they zero to a specific gravity of 1.000. If the refractometer does not zero, it should be adjusted according to the manufacturer's instructions.

Sample Handling, Collection, and Storage

21. **d** Centrifuging a sample at too high a speed or for an extended period may cause hemolysis.

22. **b** The lid should be kept closed when the centrifuge is in use to prevent broken tubes from spinning out and samples from aerosolizing and evaporating.

23. **c** Transcription errors are clerical errors and do not require extra use of sample.

24. **a**

25. **c**

26. **a**

27. **b**

28. **d**

29. **c** Samples should not be mailed over the weekend because of the delayed delivery and because laboratory personnel are typically not present to process samples.

30. **b** Slides should not be sent in the same package as formalin samples because the fumes can affect the slides.

31. **b** Blood flow rate and withdrawal pressure can be controlled with a syringe but not with a vacuum tube system.

32. **a** Most anticoagulants work by forming insoluble complexes with calcium.

33. c

34. **d** Sodium citrate, because the anticoagulation is easily reversed by addition of ionized calcium.

35. **b**

36. **d**

37. **a**

38. **c**

39. **b**

40. **a**

Blood Chemistry

41. **d**

42. **a**

43. **b** Heparin interferes the least with chemical assays.

44. **d**

45. **b** Serum is usually preferred over plasma because some anticoagulants interfere with tests results. Fibrin clots in some plasma samples may also interfere but can be removed by further centrifugation. Whole blood is usually unacceptable because of the presence of blood cells and the potential for hemolysis.

46. **c** Technician, reagent, or equipment error may result in the need to repeat a test. Some results may require dilution of the sample and retesting. It is good practice to initially collect enough blood should repeat testing be necessary.

47. **a**

48. **b** Refrigeration is an acceptable means of preserving chemical constituents; the period or preservation varies for each constituent. Freezing prolongs the preservation of chemicals but may affect some test results. Samples stored at room temperature are not as stable; however, refrigerated or frozen samples should be allowed to warm to room temperature before analysis.

49. **a** General recommendation; chemicals in serum or plasma are least stable at room temperature.

50. **b** General recommendation; chemicals in serum or plasma are more stable when refrigerated than at room temperature.

51. **d** General recommendation; chemicals in serum or plasma are stable the longest when frozen, although freezing may affect some tests.

52. **c** Blood collected in this manner (without an anticoagulant), centrifuged, and separated after clotting will yield serum. Plasma is obtained when blood is collected in a tube containing anticoagulant, centrifuged, and separated.

53. **b** Hemolysis (rupture of erythrocytes) releases intracellular components into the surrounding fluid (serum or plasma). Among these intracellular components, potassium is the principal cation; levels of potassium in the serum or plasma therefore increase in hemolysis. Most of the phosphorus found in whole blood is organic phosphorus inside erythrocytes; inorganic phosphorus is found in the serum or plasma. Organic phosphorus released in hemolysis may interfere with the phosphorus assay performed on serum or plasma.

54. **a** Erythrocytes use glucose for energy; serum and plasma must be separated from cells as soon as possible after blood collection.

55. **b** Postprandial lipemia is common in a nonfasted animal.

56. **c**

57. **c**

58. **b** Icterus is caused by an increase in the total bilirubin in the blood; total bilirubin is a combination of conjugated and unconjugated bilirubin. Icteric (or yellow) serum or plasma is frequently seen in animals with liver disease or hemolytic anemia.

59. **d** 8° C is approximately 46° F, which is refrigerator temperature (F = 9/5 C + 32).

60. **c** A blood sample drawn for obtaining plasma should be collected using an anticoagulant; it should not clot.

61. **b** Icterus is a condition that cannot be corrected or prevented by proper sample collection or handling. It is frequently seen in animals with liver disease or hemolytic anemia. Hemolysis is most commonly attributed to technician error, although hemolysis may occur in some anemias. Lipemia can usually be prevented or minimized by fasting the animal before collection.

62. **c**

63. **a** Light passing through the sample is measured as the percent of transmittance (T), and light not passing through is measured as absorbance.

64. **c** Technology of reflective photometric principles are used in dry chemistry analyzers.

65. **b** Quality-control serum is freeze dried (lyophilized) and must be rehydrated before use. It contains specific quantities of chemical constituents; the range of acceptable values for each chemical constituent is provided by the manufacturer. It is analyzed as if it were patient serum, and the results are compared with the known values provided. Control serum is used for technician, reagent, and instrument assessment. Results within the acceptable ranges provided by the manufacturer help ensure the accuracy of test results.

66. **c** See answer 65. A daily log of test results should be kept by the technician, but this has nothing to do with the accuracy of the results. The results could still be wrong! Repeating each procedure several times does not demonstrate accuracy, only repeatable results. These results could also be wrong if the same technician errors are made, if the reagents are expired or improperly stored, or if the instrument is not functioning correctly.

67. **a** See answer 65. Accurate results are not always within the reference (normal) range for a species, nor are they always credible (believable). An extremely high or low result could very well be incredible.

68. **b** Quality-control sera are generally lyophilized (freeze dried) and must be reconstituted before use.

69. **c** Control sera should be used as recommended by the manufacturer, often each time a patient sample is analyzed. Reconstituted control serum is not stable for more than a few days when refrigerated, and an entire bottle is rarely used before it expires. After reconstituting one bottle, several aliquots are placed in small tubes and frozen. These aliquots can be thawed one at a time, thereby extending the use of the serum and cutting supply costs.

70. **d** Choices *a, b,* and *c* are each detectable through use of quality-control sera; random sampling errors are not.

71. **d** Quality-control sera are used to assess the reagents, equipment, and technician; it has nothing to do with the quality of the patient's sample.

72. **d** A cuvette is a precision optical instrument and requires special handling to achieve accurate results; test tubes are not an acceptable substitute.

73. **c** A pipette is usually automatic and delivers microliter volumes of patient sample.

74. **a**

75. **a** Each enzyme has a specific substrate; enzymes are often named for the substrate on which they act.

76. **b** Kinetic methods measure the rate of an enzymatic reaction while it is in progress and usually involve serial measurements of the product per unit of time. In endpoint reactions the product formed from enzyme activity is measured after the reaction has stopped.

77. **a** Some enzymes found in different tissues occur as isoenzymes. The serum concentration of an enzyme that occurs as isoenzymes is the total of the concentrations of all the isoenzymes present. The source of a particular isoenzyme can be identified by determining which isoenzyme is present in a patient's sample.

78. **d**

79. **b** These units of measurement derived their names from each investigator who developed a method of enzyme analysis.

80. **d**

81. **a**

82. **d** Kinetic reactions are measured while the reaction is in progress, not at the end. Temperature, time, and sample volume are all factors in a kinetic enzymatic assay.

83. **b**

84. **a** Radioimmunoassay (RIA) is one of the most sensitive tests available, making assay of minute quantities of hormones possible. Although highly sensitive, it is not suitable for routine diagnostic testing because of the short shelf life of the radioisotopes used, the expense and sophistication of the equipment, and the stringent safety and hazardous waste disposal considerations.

85. **a** The electrolytes sodium and potassium are commonly measured using flame photometry.

86. **d** These test strips estimate the amount of BUN.

87. **c** These test strips estimate the amount of blood glucose.

88. **c** Ion selective electrode and flame photometry are two methods of measuring electrolytes. Some electrolytes can also be measured using photometric or dry chemistry methods.

89. **a** These enzymes are found in hepatocytes and are used in small animals to evaluate liver function; GGT and SDH are primarily measured to evaluate liver function in horses.

90. **c** See answer 89.

91. **d**

92. **b**

93. **d**

94. **b** The liver conjugates bilirubin; it is a test of liver function.

95. **a** Although amylase, lipase, and trypsin are produced and secreted by the pancreas, only amylase and lipase are measured in the serum. Trypsin can be qualitatively measured in the feces as an assessment of chronic pancreatitis.

96. **c** See answer 95.

97. **a**

98. **b**

99. **a** Bicarbonate levels are often assayed in blood gas analysis to detect alterations in acid-base balance. The preferred sample is heparinized arterial whole blood.

100. **b** The A:G ratio is commonly determined as part of a liver profile.

101. **b**

102. **c** The kidneys play a role in electrolyte regulation.

103. **c** Elevated levels of nitrogenous waste products, especially urea nitrogen in the blood. Hypernatremia is an increase in sodium levels in the blood; hyperkalemia is an increase in potassium levels in the blood.

104. **c** Insulin's effect on blood glucose levels is monitored in a diabetic animal.

105. **a** Calcium plays a role in bone development, transmission of nerve impulses, and muscle contraction. Calcium concentrations are usually inversely related to phosphorus concentrations.

106. **d** The adrenal cortex produces numerous steroids; cortisol is the major steroidal hormone released in domestic animals.

107. **d** ACTH stimulates the adrenal cortex to secrete cortisol. In the ACTH response test, cortisol levels are measured before and after administration of ACTH.

108. **a** The thyroid gland secretes thyroid hormone (thyroxine), which is a combination of T_3 and T_4. T_4 is also converted to T_3 in the tissues.

109. **c** TSH and ACTH are both secreted by the anterior pituitary (adenohypophysis) gland, which is under the control of the hypothalamus. Blood levels of these hormones may be used to evaluate pituitary gland function.

110. **a** These are all signs of hypothyroidism.

111. **b** Urea nitrogen and creatinine are metabolic wastes measured to evaluate renal function.

112. **d** Ammonia is converted to urea by the liver; BUN is often decreased in hepatic disease and elevated in renal disease.

113. **c** The pancreas secretes these digestive enzymes; levels are elevated in acute pancreatitis.

114. **a** Urea nitrogen is the principal end product of protein catabolism. BUN levels are measured to evaluate the ability of the kidneys to excrete this waste.

115. **d** Creatinine is formed during normal muscle metabolism. Creatinine levels in the blood are used to evaluate the ability of the kidneys to excrete this waste.

116. **d** Albumin and globulin are the two most abundant plasma proteins. Fibrinogen and prothrombin are found in very small amounts in the blood.

117. **b** Parathyroid gland hormone (PTH) regulates blood levels of calcium and, indirectly, phosphorus.

118. **d** The adrenal gland secretes cortisol following stimulation by ACTH, released from the anterior pituitary (adenohypophysis). Resting cortisol levels and levels following ACTH stimulation and dexamethasone suppression are all used to evaluate adrenal function. Resting ACTH levels indicate secretion from the pituitary, which is under the control of the hypothalamus. Resting levels of ACTH do not usually evaluate adrenal function.

CYTOLOGY

119. **b**

120. **a** *Pyknosis* is a thickening and degeneration of a cell in which the nucleus shrinks and the chromatin condenses into a solid structureless mass.

121. **d** The common characteristics of malignant neoplastic cells include the following:

A. Cells are pleomorphic; they vary in size and shape.

B. Cells tend to be large.

C. Large nuclei vary in size and shape, with a high nucleus:cytoplasm ratio.

D. Nucleoi are often large, bizzare, and numerous.

E. Cytoplasm is basophilic, with vacuoles.

122. **c** *Metaplasia* is the change of a mature cell into a form that is abnormal for that tissue.

123. **c**

124. **d** Formaldehyde is a gaseous compound and is not used to preserve tissue samples for histopathologic examination.

125. **d**

126. **a**

127. **d**

128. **b** Hyaluronic acid is a mucopolysaccharide and is known as the cement substance of tissues; it forms a gel in intercellular spaces.

129. **d**

130. **d**

131. **b** Mast cells are sometimes referred to as *dirty* cells because of the dark basophilic granules found in their cytoplasm.

132. **a**

133. **a** New methylene blue is a supravital dye that precipitates basophilic material (RNA) and stains it blue.

134. **b**

135. **c**

136. **b**

137. **c**

138. **d**

139. **c**

140. **a**

141. **d**

142. **b** Neutrophils are essential for phagocytosis and proteolysis of bacteria, cellular debris, and solid particles, all of which may be present in association with conjunctivitis.

143. **d**

144. **c**

145. **c** The Gram stain is the classsic bacteriologic stain used to separate bacteria according to their Gram reaction, classified as Gram positive (blue) or Gram negative (red).

146. **d**

147. **a**

148. **d**

149. **a** Specimens that are to be used to make impression smears should be blotted with clean absorbent material to remove fresh blood, thus giving a more representative view of the cells making up the lesion.

150. **c**

HEMATOLOGY

151. **b**

152. **b**

153. **a**

154. **c**

155. **a**

156. **a** Cattle normally have yellow plasma caused by carotenoids in their diet.

157. **b** Lymphocytes transform to plasma cells, which produce antibodies.

158. **b**

159. **c**

160. **b**

161. **d**

162. **d** A degenerative left shift is seen when the leukocyte count is normal or low and when bands outnumber mature neutrophils.

163. **c** Metarubricytes (nucleated erythrocytes) in the peripheral blood falsely elevate the leukocyte count.

164. **a**

165. **b**

166. **b**

167. **a**

168. **c**

169. **d**

170. **a**

171. **b**

172. **d** Absolute eosinopenia is seen in a stress leukogram.

173. **a** Although it may vary slightly in some laboratories, the normal PCV for dogs is 35% to 55%.

174. **a**

175. **d**

176. **b**

177. **c** When using the Neubauer hemocytometer, erythrocytes are counted in five secondary squares within the central primary square.

178. **a**

179. **b**

180. **c** The quantitive buffy coat method is used only on the blood of dogs, cats, and horses.

181. **d**

182. **b**

183. **a** The horse does not release immature erythrocytes into the peripheral blood.

184. **d**

185. **c** Although the upper limit of normal leukocyte counts varies from species to species, 7500/dl is well within the normal range.

186. **d**

187. **b**

188. **c** Lymphoid tissue, not bone marrow, is the major site of lymphocyte production.

189. **b** Lymphoblasts may be seen in the peripheral blood in lymphocytic leukemia.

190. **d**

191. **a** *Babesia* is an intracellular parasite of erythrocytes in dogs, cattle, and horses.

192. **b** The buffy coat layer is found between the packed red cells and plasma.

193. **a**

194. **b**

195. **c** Polychromasia occurs when the erythrocytes vary in color from blue to red.

196. **d** The reticulum in reticulocytes stains blue with new methylene blue.

197. **a** Hemoglobin breaks down to bilirubin, iron, and globin.

198. **c**

199. **b** The standard microhematocrit centrifuge takes 5 minutes to run the PCV.

200. **a** Mean corpuscular volume is the average size of an erythrocyte.

201. **c**

202. **b**

203. **d** Basophils that contain blue granules resemble mast cells.

204. **b**

205. **c**

206. **a**

207. **c** Hemolytic anemia, especially if acute and massive, produces icterus.

208. **b**

209. **d** A *seg* is another name for the segmented neutrophil.

210. **a**

211. **b**

212. **c**

213. **d**

214. **b** The band nucleus has smooth, parallel sides compared with the irregular, twisted nucleus of the mature neutrophil.

215. **c** A spherocyte is a densely stained erythrocyte smaller than the others.

216. **a**

217. **d**

218. **b** Forty is 4% of 1,000.

219. **a**

220. **c** Hypersegmented neutrophils containing more than five nuclear lobes occur as the cells age.

221. **b** Members of the camel family, which include the llama, have oval erythrocytes.

222. **d**

223. **a**

224. **d** Birds, reptiles, and fish normally have mature nucleated erythrocytes.

225. **c** The classic monocyte has a bean-shaped nucleus.

226. **b** The iliac crest and the proximal femur are the most common sites used for bone marrow collection in dogs.

227. **d**

228. **a**

229. **b** In a major crossmatch, donor red cells are mixed with serum from the recipient.

230. **c** Potassium or sodium EDTA is the most common anticoagulant used in blood collection.

231. **b**

232. **a**

233. **c** 65% of 15,000 is 9,750.

234. **d**

235. **b**

236. **c** Fibrinogen functions in the last step in the hemostatic process.

237. **b** Metarubricytes are the most common immature erythrocytes seen in the peripheral blood of dogs and cats.

238. **a** *Hemobartonella felis* is a common feline blood parasite.

239. **c**

240. **d** Multiply the 10X by 100X to get 1000X magnification with the oil-immersion lens.

IMMUNOLOGY

241. **d**

242. **c** Monocytes are derived from promonocytes, which are bone marrow stem cells. Once monocytes enter the bloodstream, they remain there for only a few days before entering tissues and developing into macrophages.

243. **c** IgM is the first antibody produced in the primary immune response and represents about 20% of the serum antibodies.

244. **a** IgG is the most abundant of the five classes of immunoglobulins, representing about 80% of serum immunoglobulin protein. It is the only immunoglobulin that can cross the placenta and therefore is the major component of passive maternal antibody transfer.

245. **b**

246. **a**

247. **d** Peroxidase is an enzyme found in granulocytes, not in monocytes.

248. **c**

249. **b** Attenuation is a process that reduces the virulence of an organism until, although still alive, it is no longer capable of producing disease. Methods of attenuation include heating organisms to sublethal temperatures, exposing microorganisms to marginally sublethal concentrations of inactivating chemicals, and adapting organisms to unusual conditions so that they lose their adaptation to their usual host. Viruses may be attenuated by growing them in species that are not a natural host. Whatever method is used, the microorganism still retains its ability to produce an immune response.

250. **d**

251. **b** Cytokines are soluble biologic messenger proteins controlling macrophages and lymphocytes taking part in the cell-mediated immune reaction.

252. **c**

253. **d** Combined immunodeficiency occurs in approximately 2% to 3% of Arabian foals. The foals fail to produce functional T or B cells. They may receive maternal immunoglobulins as they suckle successfully, but when the maternal immunoglobulins have been used, the foal cannot produce its own antibodies. All foals stricken usually die within 4-6 months as a result of infection.

254. **d**

255. **a**

256. **c**

257. **c**

258. b

259. b Complete washing of test wells used in ELISA is the critical step to ensure accurate results. Follow the manufacturer's instructions explicitly regarding washing procedures.

260. a Coombs' tests are used to detect certain antigen-antibody reactions, one of which is used for diagnosis of autoimmune hemolytic anemia.

261. d Tuberculin is the name given to extracts of *Mycobacterium tuberculosis*, *Mycobacterium bovis*, or *Mycobacterium avium*. The extracts are used to identify animals with tuberculosis.

262. a IgE-mediated allergic reactions include urticaria, atopy and anaphylactic shock.

263. d

264. a

265. b

266. b Bence Jones proteins (monoclonal immunoglobulin) may precipitate when heated to 60° C but redissolve as the temperature is raised to 80° C. These proteins may be found in the urine and are suggestive of multiple myeloma, a malignant neoplasm of plasma cells.

267. a The Arthus reaction is a local antibody-mediated hypersensitivity reaction in which antibody-antigen complexes that fix complement are deposited in the walls of small vessels, causing acute inflammation.

268. b

269. c

270. b Grey collie syndrome is also known as canine cyclic hematopoiesis. This abnormality of hematopoietic stem cells results in detectable, cyclic fluctuations in numbers of neutrophils. Dogs affected are susceptible to infection.

271. a

272. c

273. a

274. a

275. b

276. c

277. a

278. b The Coggins test is an agar-gel, double diffusion, immunodiffusion test used to detect antibodies against equine infectious anemia.

279. d

280. b

281. c

282. d

283. b

284. d T-suppressor cells are a type of lymphocyte that suppresses B-lymphocyte activity.

285. b Histamine is released in allergic and inflammatory reactions and causes dilatation of capillaries, decreased blood pressure, increased release of gastric juices, and constriction of the smooth muscles of the bronchi and uterus.

286. a An opsonin is an antibody or complement split product that binds to particles and facilitates their phagocytosis.

287. d

288. a Mast cells and basophils normally produce a small quantity of histamine, but when they are sensitized by IgE, they react abnormally, producing large quantities of histamines and other chemicals. These chemicals cause allergic attacks (such as runny noses, and swollen tissues).

289. b

290. c

291. d

292. **c** Toxins are poisons produced from certain animals, plants, or pathogenic microorganisms.

293. **b** Because FIV is found in saliva, bite wounds serve as a means of transmission.

294. **c** Titer is a measure of antibody units per unit volume of serum. Titer testing is performed immediately after infection (acute phase) and 2 to 6 weeks after collection of the first serum sample (convalescent phase).

295. **d**

MICROBIOLOGY

296. **d** Viruses are not free living because they are obligatory intracellular parasites. They use host cell structures for reproduction.

297. **d** Genus and species names are both italicized (underlined when using a typewriter).

298. **d** *Mycobacterium* has a waxy component in its cell wall structure that allows this stain to identify it.

299. **a** Simple stains use only one color and, therefore, can be used only to identify microscopic morphology.

300. **b** *E coli* 0157 may contaminate meat during slaughter. Grinding the meat increases the chances of infection by introducing the organism into the center of the meat. Improper cooking does not destroy the organism.

301. **a**

302. **d**

303. **c** 0.9% NaCl is isotonic; 5% NaCl is hypertonic. Water moves toward the higher solute concentration, which in this case is outside the cell.

304. **d** The standard technique for pasteurization heats a liquid to 63° C for 30 minutes. To kill endospores, the temperature must reach 121° C and be maintained for 15 minutes.

305. **c** Ethylene oxide can be used.

306. **c**

307. **c**

308. **c** Papillomas are warts.

309. **d**

310. **b**

311. **d** Septicemia is the presence of pathogenic bacteria in the blood.

312. **c**

313. **b**

314. **b**

315. **c**

316. **b**

317. **b**

318. **d**

319. **c** *Staphylococcus aureus* ferments the mannitol, resulting in a color change of yellow in the medium. *Staphylococcus epidermidis* does not ferment mannitol, and hence causes no color change.

320. **a**

321. **c**

322. **c**

323. **a**

324. **b**

325. **c**

326. **b**

327. **d**

328. **a**

329. **d**

330. **d** *Clostridium botulinum* causes flaccid paralysis.

331. **b**

332. **c**

333. **d**

334. **d**

335. **d**

336. **d**

337. **c**

338. **b**

339. **d**

340. **d** Parvoviruses are resistant to most common disinfectants except sodium hypochlorite.

341. **b** Many cases of cystitis are caused by retrograde infections by Gram-negative enteric organisms.

342. **d**

343. **b**

344. **d**

345. **b**

346. **b**

347. **d** Gram stain is a differential stain.

348. **d**

349. **a** All the other answers are examples of acquired passive immunity.

350. **b**

351. **b** *E coli* is among the normal flora of the intestines.

352. **c**

353. **c**

354. **b** Alpha is incomplete hemolysis, beta is complete hemolysis, and gamma is no hemolysis.

355. **c** Catalase causes the release of O_2 from hydrogen peroxide (H_2O_2).

PARASITOLOGY

356. **a**

357. **d** Cestodes refer to the subclass Cestoda, the tapeworms.

358. **c** Trematodes refer to the class Trematoda, the flukes.

359. **a** *Dirofilaria immitis* is a nematode; the others are protozoans.

360. **d**

361. **b** Direct smears use only a small amount of feces. The other techniques increase the chances of seeing ova by concentrating the ova from a large amount of feces in a small sample, such as under the cover slip or in the top or bottom layer of flotation solution.

362. **a** Some fluke ova have a higher specific gravity than many other ova and therefore do not float in flotation solutions.

363. **d**

364. **b** Pinworm eggs are deposited on the skin around the anus and are not normally seen in the feces.

365. **a**

366. **d** Trophozoites may collapse in nonisotonic flotation solutions and may be difficult to recognize.

367. **d** Occult means hidden and refers to the absence of microfilariae in the other three situations.

368. **b**

369. **c**

370. **a**

371. **b** Microfilaremia in a 4-month-old puppy is a result of transplacental infection from an infected bitch. Four months is too brief a time for infective larvae to develop into adult worms and release microfilariae. Adult heartworms are killed with a different medication. The principal host of *Dirofilaria immitis* is the dog, but other, more rare, hosts are cats, horses, and people.

372. **d** The infective stage of *Dipylidium caninum* is found in the flea. Rabbits are hosts for *Taenia pisiformis*, another tapeworm of dogs and cats.

373. **b** A spurious infection is not a true parasite infection. The ova are present because the dog has ingested ruminant feces that contained *Moniezia*.

374. **b**

375. **d**

376. **b**

377. **a** *Taenia* and *Echinococcus* ova are so similar that definitive diagnosis can be made only by examination of the adult worms.

378. **c**

379. **d** Serologic tests detect antigens, whereas concentration tests detect microfilariae. Concentration tests, therefore, do not detect occult infections. There are other species of *Dirofilaria*, but they are thought to be innocuous (harmless), as is *Dipetalonema reconditum*.

380. **c** Trophozoites are more fragile than cysts and ova.

381. **d** These are all zoonotic diseases. Visceral larva migrans is caused by ingestion of *Toxocara*; creeping eruption is caused by skin penetration by *Ancylostoma*; hydatodosis is infection with the hydatid cyst of *Echinococcus*.

382. **a** All are protozoans. *Giardia* and *Trichomonas* are flagellates.

383. **a** Smegma is a secretion found within the prepuce, where the protozoan lives. *Thelazia* species are eyeworms whose larvae may be found in tears. Embryonated ova or hatched larvae from the lungworm *Dictyocaulus* may be found in feces. *Stephanurus* passes eggs that are found in urine.

384. **a** *Tritrichomonas foetus* is a protozoan parasite of cattle.

385. **b** *Dictyocaulus* species are lungworms found in the trachea and bronchi of cattle and sheep.

386. **c** *Dioctophyma renale* is the giant kidney worm of wild carnivores and other species. Its eggs are found in urine sediment.

387. **d** *Anaplasma* is an intracellular parasite of bovine red blood cells.

388. **a**

389. **d**

390. **c**

391. **b**

392. **d**

393. **c**

394. **a**

395. **b**

396. **b** There are 3 species of large strongyles and more than 40 species of small strongyles of horses.

397. **b** Tapeworm infections are usually not a widespread problem in horses. According to some references, treatment is seldom needed.

398. **c**

399. **b**

400. **a**

401. **d**

402. **a** *Echinococcus granulosus* produces larvae that form hydatid cysts in the intermediate hosts, such as people.

403. **c**

404. **d**

405. **a**

406. **b**

407. **a** The second intermediate host of *Diphyllobothrium latum* is the broad fish tapeworm.

408. **c** Ova of *Paragonimus kellicotti*, the lung fluke, are found in the sputum or feces of dogs and cats.

409. **b**

410. **d**

411. **d**

412. **a**

413. **b**

414. **c**

415. **b** Mites may live off their host for a short time, but they propagate only while on their host.

416. **d**

417. **d**

418. **a**

419. **c**

420. **b**

421. **d**

422. **b**

423. **b**

424. **c**

425. **d**

426. **a**

427. **a**

428. **d**

429. **a**

430. **b** Larvae migrate to the liver and then to the lungs.

431. **c**

432. **d** Hookworms feed on blood from the intestinal wall and can produce profound anemia.

433. **a** *Giardia* is a flagellate protozoan that invades the small intestine and causes chronic diarrhea.

434. **b**

435. **c**

436. **a**

437. **d**

438. **d** Both *Trichuris vulpis* and *Capillaria aerophila* ova have bipolar plugs, but the *Capillaria* ovum is smaller and tends to be more asymmetric than the *Trichuris* ovum.

439. **a**

440. **c**

441. **b**

442. **d**

443. **b**

444. **b**

445. **a**

446. **d**

447. **c**

448. **b**

449. **d** Flea eggs are not sticky and drop off into the environment.

450. **b** *Melophagus ovinus* bites cause pruritus over much of the sheep's body.

451. **a** *Ancylostoma* larvae penetrate the skin of people but can develop no further.

452. **d** *Echinococcus granulosus* larvae form a fluid-filled hydatid cyst in people. The fluid is toxic and may produce anaphylactic shock and death if spilled into body cavities.

453. **c** *Notoedres cati* is the cause of feline scabies, also known as notoedric mange.

454. **c** *Cryptosporidium* is a small protozoan that is associated with chronic diarrhea.

455. **b** Biting or chewing lice are members of the order Mallophaga.

456. **d** The order Anoplura includes sucking lice.

457. **a** *Psoroptes ovis* causes common mange in cattle and sheep.

URINALYSIS

458. **a** Because of the presence of red blood cells.

459. **d** Only multiply the last two digits of the specific gravity by the dilution factor. Specific gravity is always in the range of $1.0\times\times$.

460. **a**

461. **b**

462. **a** Red blood cells and fat droplets are often the same size. However, fat droplets come in various sizes.

463. **d** BUN is not part of a routine urinalysis.

464. **d**

465. **c** Dilute the urine 1:2 with distilled water and multiply the last two digits of the specific gravity by 2.

466. **b**

467. **c** Controls only need to be run once a shift unless a problem occurs.

468. **d**

469. **c**

470. **d** Morning urine is concentrated and allows for detection of substances that may not be present in a more dilute sample.

471. **b**

472. **c** Cystocentesis and catheterization both provide good samples for urinalysis that are free of contamination from the distal genital tract and external areas.

473. **b**

474. **d**

475. **c**

476. **a**

477. **d**

478. **b**

479. **a**

480. **b** Bacterial numbers continue to increase if the sample is left at room temperature.

481. **b**

482. **c**

483. **a**

484. **d**

485. **b**

486. **d**

487. **c** Dark yellow urine is generally more concentrated; therefore, the specific gravity is higher.

488. **d**

489. **b**

490. **c**

491. **d** Urine containing blood typically has a high protein content.

492. **a** Not all elements are reported per high-power field. Some casts and crystals, for example, are reported per low-power field.

493. **c** If the light is too bright, it is hard to see some of the elements in the urine.

494. **b**

495. **d** Vegetable diets may cause the urine to be alkaline.

496. **b** Sulfosalicylic acid is used to detect protein in the urine.

497. **c** Urine samples should be centrifuged at low speed for 5 minutes.

Medical Calculations

Douglas E. N. Bach, DVM   *Karl M. Peter, DVM*
Richard N. Thwaits, DVM, PhD

Recommended Reading

Bayley AJ: *Compendium of veterinary products*, Port Huron Mich, 1991, North American Compendiums.
Bill RP: *Pharmacology for veterinary technicians*, St Louis, 1993, Mosby.
Boyer MJ: *Math for nurses*, ed 2, Philadelphia, 1991, JB Lippincott.
Curren A, Munday L: *Math for meds*, ed 6, San Diego, 1990, Walcur.
Janney C, Timpke J: *Calculation of drug dosages*, ed 3, Long Beach Calif, 1991, TJ Designs.

Questions

1. A 25% solution of sulfamethazine contains how many milligrams of sulfamethazine per milliliter?
   a. 2500 mg/ml
   b. 250 mg/ml
   c. 25 mg/ml
   d. 2.5 mg/ml

2. How much sodium chloride is required to produce 5 L of 0.85% saline solution?
   a. 42.5 mg
   b. 4.25 kg
   c. 425 mg
   d. 42.5 g

3. What volume of a 1.2% sodium hydroxide (NaOH) solution can be made from 600 mg of NaOH?
   a. 50 ml
   b. 5 ml
   c. 250 ml
   d. 500 ml

4. What volume of distilled water must be added must a 5-g vial of thiopental sodium to create a 2.5% solution?
   a. 40 ml
   b. 200 ml
   c. 250 ml
   d. 500 ml

Practice answer sheet is on page 333.

Correct answers are on pages 202–204.

5. A stock solution was diluted 1:5, then 1:3, then 1:2, and finally 1:6 to produce a final concentration of 0.4 mg/ml. The original concentration of the stock solution was
   a. 0.025%
   b. 6.4 mg/ml
   c. 7.2%
   d. 7.2 mg/ml

6. What volume of water must be added to 12.5 ml of a 6% stock solution to produce a 0.5% solution?
   a. 150 ml
   b. 137.5 ml
   c. 37.5 ml
   d. 6.25 ml

7. A 30% stock solution of potassium permanganate ($KMnO_4$) was diluted 4 times as follows: 0.1 ml of stock was added to 0.4 ml of distilled water; 4.5 ml of distilled water was added; the resulting solution was diluted 1:3; the resulting solution was again diluted, to 0.06 L. The final concentration of the solution was
   a. 1.36%
   b. 50 mg/ml
   c. 5 mg/ml
   d. 0.05%

8. What volume of 4.5% potassium chloride (KCl) solution is needed to prepare 0.75 L of a 9-mg/ml KCl solution?
   a. 15 ml
   b. 375 ml
   c. 1.5 ml
   d. 150 ml

9. The concentration of a culture medium produced by dissolving 2.5 g in 0.4 L of distilled water is
   a. 0.15%
   b. 0.625%
   c. 0.16%
   d. 6.25%

10. The amount of glucose to be weighed out to produce 500 ml of a 4.5% solution is
    a. 22.5 g
    b. 2.25 g
    c. 0.225 kg
    d. 22.5 mg

11. A stock solution was diluted 4 times as follows: 18 ml of distilled water was added to 2 ml of stock; the resulting solution was diluted 1:3; 240 ml of distilled water was added; the resulting solution was diluted to 0.9 L. If the final concentration of the diluted solution was determined to be 100 μg/ml, the original concentration of the stock solution was
    a. 4.5 mg/ml
    b. 4.5%
    c. 60 mg/ml
    d. 0.21%

12. What volume of sulfuric acid (H_2SO_4)is in 275 ml of a 12% v/v solution?
    a. 33 ml
    b. 22.9 ml
    c. 3.3 ml
    d. 4.36 ml

13. The concentration of a glucose solution produced when 4500 mg of glucose is dissolved in 3.6 L of water is
    a. 0.8%
    b. 0.008%
    c. 0.125%
    d. 1.25%

14. The basic unit of mass in the metric system is the
    a. Kilogram
    b. Gram
    c. Milligram
    d. Microgram

15. 50 g is equal to
    a. 0.005 kg
    b. 0.05 kg
    c. 500,000 mg
    d. 5,000,000 µg

16. The mean cellular hemoglobin (MCH) for a particular blood sample is calculated to be 24.3 pg. This is equal to
    a. 24,300 mg
    b. 2,430 µg
    c. 24.3×10^{12} g
    d. 24.3×10^{-12} g

17. The mean corpuscular volume (MCV) for a particular blood sample is calculated to be 66.5 fl. This is equal to
    a. 66.5×10^{-15} L
    b. 66.5×10^{15} ml
    c. 66.5×10^{-3} µl
    d. 66.5×10^{-9} L

18. The basic unit of length in the metric system is the
    a. Millimeter
    b. Centimeter
    c. Meter
    d. Kilometer

19. 485 km is equal to
    a. 4.85×10^3 m
    b. 485×10^4 mm
    c. 4.85×10^8 mm
    d. 48,500 cm

20. 250 cc is equal to
    a. 25 ml
    b. 0.25 L
    c. 25,000 µL
    d. 2.5 L

21. One ton of livestock feed is equal to
    a. 1,000 lb
    b. 10,000 g
    c. 2,204 lb
    d. 1,000,000 mg

22. One centimeter is
    a. Greater than 1 mm but shorter than 1µ (1 micron)
    b. Shorter than both 1m and 1mm
    c. Greater than both 1mm and 1µ
    d. Shorter than 1 km but greater than 1m

23. A dog weighs 55 lb. Its weight can also be stated as
    a. 121 kg
    b. 25 g
    c. 121 mg
    d. 25 kg

24. 8 oz is equal to approximately
    a. 227,200 mg
    b. 454 g
    c. 227 mg
    d. 2.27 kg

25. 10 inches is equal to approximately
    a. 25 mm
    b. 4 cm
    c. 25 cm
    d. 0.04 m

26. The volume of a stock solution required to prepare 3.5 L of a 1:40 dilution is
    a. 0.14 L
    b. 87.5 ml
    c. 630 ml
    d. 0.875 L

27. A stock solution of atropine sulfate has a concentration of 2.2 mg/ml. It may also be used clinically as a 0.05% solution. The volume of the more concentrated atropine solution required to prepare 40 ml of the dilute solution is
    a. 17.6 ml
    b. 9.1 ml
    c. 4.4 ml
    d. 0.91ml

Correct answers are on pages 202–204.

28. The volume of a 1:25 dilution that can be prepared from 150 ml of stock solution is
    a. 3,750 ml
    b. 6 L
    c. 6,000 ml
    d. 375 ml

29. If a 0.75% solution results from addition of 380 ml of water to 20 ml of stock solution, the concentration of the stock solution is
    a. 15%
    b. 0.375 mg/ml
    c. 14.25%
    d. 300 mg/ml

30. If you are asked to administer 0.1 mg of epinephrine to an animal with threatened cardiac collapse, how much of a 1:10,000 solution should you inject?
    a. 10 ml
    b. 0.01 ml
    c. 0.1 ml
    d. 1 ml

31. When the doctor orders an intravenous infusion, you need three pieces of information to calculate the flow rate in drops per minute. Which of the following is *not* relevant to this calculation?
    a. Total volume to be infused
    b. Type of fluid to be delivered
    c. Calibration of the administration set being used (in drops per milliliter)
    d. Duration of the infusion

32. The doctor orders an intravenous infusion to run at 20 ml/hr. Calculate the flow rate using an administration set that delivers 60 drops per milliliter.
    a. 30 drops/min
    b. 33 drops/min
    c. 20 drops/min
    d. More information is needed

33. Calculate the flow rate for an intravenous infusion of 1 L of fluid to run over 8 hours with a set calibrated at 20 drops per millileter.
    a. 20 drops/min
    b. 42 drops/min
    c. 50 drops/min
    d. 125 drops/min

34. Calculating drug dosages involves routine conversion between units of measure within the metric system. Which of the following conversions is *not* correct?
    a. 3 cc = 3 ml
    b. 1 μg = 1,000 mg
    c. 1 kg = 1,000 g
    d. 1 L = 1,000 ml

35. Which metric conversion is *not* correct?
    a. 3,500 ml = 3.5 L
    b. 520 mg = 0.52 g
    c. 950 µg = 9.5 mg
    d. 750 cc = 0.75 L

36. Which common equivalent is *not* correct?
    a. 1 T = 3 t = 15 ml
    b. 1 oz = 30 ml = 2 Tbl
    c. 1/2 gr = 64 mg
    d. 1 L of H_2O = 1,000 g of H_2O

37. Which equivalent is *not* correct?
    a. 1 T = 1 Tbl = "1 tablespoonful" = 15 ml
    b. 1 t = 1 tsp = "1 teaspoonful" = 5 ml
    c. 1 gt = 1 drop
    d. 1 gr = "1 gram" = 30 ml

38. A doctor's order calls for prednisone at a dosage of 2 mg/kg to be delivered orally to a 7.5-kg cat. How many 5-mg tablets of prednisone would you give the cat?
    a. 1/4
    b. 1
    c. 2
    d. 3

39. You are asked to give a patient phenobarbital PO at 2.2 mg/kg. The medication is available in $^1/_2$-gr tablets. How many tablets should you give a 35-lb dog?
    a. 1/4
    b. 1/2
    c. 1
    d. 2

40. A prescription reads *Amoxicillin, 750 mg, PO BID, X 10 days*. The drug is available in 500-mg tablets. How many tablets must you count out to fill this prescription?
    a. 30
    b. 60
    c. 90
    d. 120

41. 25 mg of diphenhydramine elixir *PO* is ordered for a $12^1/_2$-year-old, 12.5-kg Beagle. The solution contains 12.5 mg/5 ml. What volume should you give to this patient?
    a. 0.5 ml
    b. 2 ml
    c. 10 ml
    d. 20 ml

42. You are asked to give a head trauma patient 20% mannitol at 0.5 g/kg by slow intravenous injection. You check the record and see that the dog weighs 44 lb. What volume should you give?
    a. 10 ml
    b. 25 ml
    c. 50 ml
    d. 250 ml

43. How much drug does 100 ml of a 10% solution contain?
    a. 0.1 g
    b. 1 g
    c. 10 g
    d. More information is needed

44. You are asked to draw up 2 ml of 50% dextrose in water to give to a hypoglycemic kitten. What volume should you draw into the syringe?
    a. 1 ml
    b. 2 ml
    c. 10 ml
    d. More information is needed

45. To mix a 4% solution in a bottle that contains 5 g of drug powder, how much water should you add?
    a. 12.5 ml
    b. 50 ml
    c. 125 ml
    d. 500 ml

46. To prepare a dose of 0.2 mg of atropine using a solution containing 400 µg/ml, how much do you draw into the syringe?
    a. 0.05 ml
    b. 0.2 ml
    c. 0.5 ml
    d. 2 ml

47. You are asked to give 20 mg of furosemide intravenously. The solution contains 25 mg/ml. What volume should you draw into the syringe?
    a. 0.8 ml
    b. 1.25 ml
    c. 2.5 ml
    d. The weight of the patient must be known

48. You are asked to prepare 20 mEq of KCl for addition to a 1-L bag of lactated Ringer's solution. The solution contains 30 mEq/15 ml. How much should you draw into a syringe to add to the fluid bag?
    a. 10 ml
    b. 20 ml
    c. 30 ml
    d. 40 ml

Correct answers are on pages 202–204.

49. You are asked to infuse fluids intravenously at 50 ml/hr. The administration set is calibrated at 60 drops/ml. How fast should you set the drip rate?
    a. 1 drops/min
    b. 10 drops/min
    c. 50 drops/min
    d. 60 drops/min

50. You are asked to infuse 3 L of 0.9% saline intravenously during 24 hours. The administration set is calibrated at 15 drops/ml. How fast should you set the drip rate.
    a. 200 drops/min
    b. 125 drops/min
    c. 31 drops/min
    d. 15 drops/min

51. You are asked to infuse fluids intravenously at 60 drops/min. The drip rate is currently at 7 drops/15 sec. What adjustment in the drip rate is necessary
    a. No adjustment is necessary
    b. Double the flow rate
    c. Reduce the flow rate by 50%
    d. Increase the flow rate by 25%

52. You are asked to infuse 1 L of fluids intravenously at 25 drops/min during 10 hours. After 5 hours you observe that 650 ml has been given. What adjustment in the drip rate is necessary?
    a. No action is necessary; the IV infusion will be completed on schedule
    b. The rate must be slowed from 25 drops/min to 18 drops/min to complete the infusion as ordered
    c. The rate must be increased from 25 drops/min to 32 drops/min to complete the infusion as ordered
    d. Rate must be slowed from 100 ml/hr to 60 ml/hr to complete the infusion as ordered

53. You are asked to infuse 750 ml of fluids, intravenously during 6 hours. The administration set is calibrated at 20 drops/ml. After 2 hours you observe that 300 ml has been infused. What should the adjusted drip rate be?
    a. 8 drops/min
    b. 19 drops/min
    c. 27 drops/min
    d. 38 drops/min

54. You are asked to infuse 500 ml of fluids intravenously during 6 hours. The administration set is calibrated at 20 drops/ml. After 4 hours you observe that only 150 ml has been given. What should the adjusted drip rate be?
    a. 19 drops/min
    b. 25 drops/min
    c. 39 drops/min
    d. 58 drops/min

55. How much 50% dextrose must be added to 1 L of lactated Ringer's solution to make a solution containing 5% dextrose?
    a. 5 ml
    b. 50 ml
    c. 55 ml
    d. 110 ml

56. Diphenhydramine elixir is prescribed at 12.5 mg PO q8h. The drug is available in 30-ml bottles containing 25 mg/5 ml. How long will one bottle last?
    a. 2 days
    b. 4 days
    c. 6 days
    d. 1 week

57. You are asked to prepare a bottle of heparinized saline with a concentration of 4 IU heparin/ml to flush indwelling catheters. The stock sodium heparin solution contains 1,000 IU/ml. How much of heparin must be added to each 250-ml bottle of sterile physiologic saline (0.9% NaCl) to make the flushing solution?
   a. 1 ml
   b. 2 ml
   c. 3 ml
   d. 4 ml

58. You are asked to prepare a solution containing potassium chloride at 20 mEq/L. How much of a 2 mEq/ml solution of KCl should be added to a 500-ml bag of fluids to comply with this order?
   a. 5 ml
   b. 10 ml
   c. 20 ml
   d. 30 ml

59. What is the fluid deficit for a 50-lb dog estimated to be approximately 8% dehydrated?
   a. 500 ml
   b. 1 L
   c. 2 L
   d. 4 L

60. A 1-L sample contains
   a. 1 ml
   b. 10 ml
   c. 100 ml
   d. 1,000 ml

61. A 10-cc syringe can hold
   a. 1 ml
   b. 10 ml
   c. 100 ml
   d. 1,000 ml

62. A 5-kg dog weighs approximately
   a. 2.5 lb
   b. 5 lb
   c. 7.5 lb
   d. 11 lb

63. A 354-g rat weighs
   a. 0.0354 kg
   b. 0.354 kg
   c. 3.54 kg
   d. 35.4 kg

64. A 450-µg sample contains
   a. 4.5 g
   b. 0.45 g
   c. 0.045 g
   d. 0.00045 g

65. A 3,700-cc sample contains
   a. 370 ml
   b. 37 L
   c. 0.37 L
   d. 3.7 L

66. An 11-lb cat weighs approximately
   a. 22 kg
   b. 5 kg
   c. 500 g
   d. 5,000 g

67. A 6.2-g sample contains
   a. 3 kg
   b. 3,100 mg
   c. 6,200,000 µg
   d. 6,200 µg

68. A 0.5-g/cc sample contains
   a. 5 mg/cc
   b. 50 g/100 ml
   c. 5 g/100 ml
   d. 500 mg/100 ml

69. A 500-kg horse weighs approximately
   a. 250 lb
   b. 750 lb
   c. 1,100 lb
   d. 1,000 lb

70. A 20-dr vial of digitalis contains approximately
   a. 1.5 oz
   b. 2 oz
   c. 2.5 oz
   d. 4 oz

Correct answers are on pages 202–204.

71. A 120-gr aspirin contains approximately
    a. 7.8 mg
    b. 78 mg
    c. 780 mg
    d. 7,800 mg

72. A 45-gr/30 ml solution contains approximately
    a. 100 mg/ml
    b. 450 mg/ml
    c. 10 g/ml
    d. 1 g/100 ml

73. A 12-fl dr bottle contains approximately
    a. 36 ml
    b. 45 ml
    c. 68 ml
    d. 120 ml

74. A 1/120-gr tablet contains approximately
    a. 0.005 mg
    b. 0.05 mg
    c. 0.5 mg
    d. 5 mg

75. A 2-qt container holds
    a. 12 oz
    b. 18 oz
    c. 32 oz
    d. 64 oz

76. A 14-oz bottle contains approximately
    a. 420 ml
    b. 210 ml
    c. 105 ml
    d. 56 ml

77. A 6-T dose given BID requires
    a. 2 oz/day
    b. 240 ml/day
    c. 1.8 L for a 10-day supply
    d. 2.6 L for a 2-wk supply

78. A dosage of 1 T daily requires
    a. 2 oz for a 14-day supply
    b. 5 oz for a 14-day supply
    c. 7 oz for a 14-day supply
    d. 10 oz for a 14-day supply

79. A dosage of 2 tablespoons BID requires approximately
    a. 16 oz for a 16-day supply
    b. 1 qt for a 16-day supply
    c. 36 oz for a 16-day supply
    d. 2.5 pt for a 16-day supply

80. A dosage of 1.5 tsp BID requires
    a. 8 T for a 2-wk supply
    b. 1 oz for a 2-wk supply
    c. 10 T for a 2-wk supply
    d. 14 T for a 2-wk supply

81. A dosage of 5 ml TID equals approximately
    a. 1 tsp/day
    b. 2 tsp/day
    c. 3 tsp/day
    d. 5 tsp/day

82. A dosage of 1 T every other day requires approximately
    a. 45 ml for a 2-wk supply
    b. 90 ml for a 2-wk supply
    c. 105 ml for a 2-wk supply
    d. 210 ml for a 2-wk supply

83. A 554-kg mare needs sulfadimethoxine at 10 mg/lb daily. It is available as a 40% solution. How much sulfadimethoxine should be administered daily?
    a. 13.85 ml
    b. 138.5 ml
    c. 45.32 ml
    d. 30.5 ml

84. Fenbendazole liquid is available as a 22.2% concentration, and a 45-lb German Shorthaired Pointer needs 50 mg/lb. How many teaspoons does it require?
    a. 1 tsp
    b. 1.5 tsp
    c. 2 tsp
    d. 3 tsp

85. Procaine penicillin is available in a concentration of 300,000 IU/ml and is administered at 20,000 IU/kg. How much do you give a 900-lb Arabian gelding?
    a. 2.7 ml
    b. 27 ml
    c. 60 ml
    d. 132 ml

86. Altrenogest for horses is available as a 0.22% solution. The daily dosage is 0.044 mg/kg. If you treated a 990-lb Morgan mare for 15 days, how much would you dispense for the owner?
    a. 9 ml
    b. 135 ml
    c. 165 ml
    d. 254 ml

Questions 87 through 89

A 9-month-old female Great Dane is admitted for a routine ovariohysterectomy. The animal weighs 65 lb and the veterinarian wants to use the following preanesthetic regimen: butorphanol (10 mg/ml) IM at 0.2 mg/kg; acepromazine (10 mg/ml) IM at 0.05 mg/kg; and atropine (0.02% solution) SC at 0.02 mg/kg.

87. How much butorphanol should be administered?
    a. 0.6 ml
    b. 1.3 ml
    c. 2.9 ml
    d. 6 ml

88. How much acepromazine should be administered?
    a. 0.15 ml
    b. 0.3 ml
    c. 0.7 ml
    d. 1.5 ml

89. How much atropine should be administered?
    a. 1.43 ml
    b. 3.0 ml
    c. 6.5 ml
    d. 14.3 ml

Questions 90 through 92

A yearling paint gelding is admitted for castration. The animal weighs 700 lb and the veterinarian wants to use the following regimen: butorphanol (10 mg/ml) IV at 0.02 mg/kg; xylazine (10 mg/ml) IV at 0.2 mg/kg; and ketamine (100 mg/ml) IV at 2.2 mg/kg.

90. How much butorphanol should be administered?
    a. 0.6 ml
    b. 1.4 ml
    c. 3.1 ml
    d. 6 ml

91. How much xylazine should be administered?
    a. 3.2 ml
    b. 6.4 ml
    c. 14 ml
    d. 31 ml

92. How much ketamine should be administered?
    a. 2.8 ml
    b. 7.0 ml
    c. 15.4 ml
    d. 34 ml

Correct answers are on pages 202–204.

Answers

1. **b**   25% solution = 25 g/100 ml = 250 mg/ml.

2. **d**   0.85% solution = 0.85 g/100 ml × 5,000 ml = 42.5 g.

3. **a**   1.2% solution = 1.2 g/100 ml = 1,200 mg/100 ml = 600 mg/50 ml.

4. **b**   2.5% solution = 2.5 g/100 ml = 5 g/200 ml.

5. **c**   Total dilution = (1:5) × (1:3) × (1:2) × (1:6) = 1:180.

   Total dilution factor (DF) = 180.

   [O] = [F] × DF = 0.4 mg/ml × 180 = 72 mg/ml = 7.2%.

6. **b** $C_1V_1 = C_2V_2$; 6% × 12.5 ml = 0.5% × V_2.

   V_2 (final volume) = 150 ml.

   150 ml − 12.5 ml stock = 137.5 ml water.

7. **d**   Total dilution = (1:5) × (1:10) × (1:3) × (1:4) = 1:600.

   [F] = [O] × 1/D = 30% × 1/600 = 0.05%.

8. **d** $C_1V_1 = C_2V_2$; 45 mg/ml × V_1 = 9 mg/ml × 750 ml.

   V_1 (volume of stock) = 150 ml.

9. **b**   2.50 g/400 ml = 0.625 g/100 ml = 0.625%.

10. **a**   4.5% solution = 4.5 g/100 ml × 500 ml = 22.5 g.

11. **b**   Total dilution = (1:10) × (1:3) × (1:5) × (1:3) = 1:450.

    Total dilution factor = 450.

    [O] = [F] × DF = 100 μg/ml × 450 = 45,000 μg/ml = 45 mg/ml = 4.5%.

12. **a**   12% V/V solution = 12 ml/100 ml × 275 ml = 33 ml.

13. **c**   4,500 mg/3.6 L = 4.5 g/3,600 ml = 0.125 g/100 ml = 0.125%.

14. **b**   Gram is the basic unit of mass; 1 kg = 10^3 g; 1 mg = 10^{-3} g; 1 mg = 10^{-6} g.

15. **b**   1 kg = 1,000 g.

16. **d**   1 pg = 10^{-12} g (pico = 10^{-12}).

17. **a**   1 fl = 10^{-15} L (femto = 10^{-15}).

18. **c**   Meter is the basic unit of length; 1 mm = 10^{-3} m; 1 cm = 10^{-2} m; 1 km = 10^3 m.

19. **c**   1 km = 10^3 m = 10^6 mm; 485 km = 485 × 10^6 mm = 4.85 × 10^8 mm.

20. **b**   250 cc = 250 ml = 0.25 L.

21. **c**   1 ton = 1,000 kg; 1 kg = 2.204 lb.

22. **c**   1 cm = 10 mm = 10,000 μ(microns).

23. **d**   2.204 lb = 1 kg.

24. **a**   1 oz = 28.4 g; 1 g = 1,000 mg.

25. **c**   1 in = 2.5 cm.

26. **b**   1/40:87.5 ml/3,500 ml.

27. **b** $C_1V_1 = C_2V_2$; 2.2 mg/ml × V_1 = 0.5 mg/ml × 40 ml; V_1 = 9.1 ml.

28. **a**   1/25:150 ml/3,750 ml.

29. **a**   20 ml + 380 ml = 400 ml; dilution = 20:400 = 1:20.

    [O] = [F] × DF = 0.75% × 20 = 15%.

30. **d**   1:10,000 = 0.01% = 0.1 mg/ml; volume = 1.0 ml.

31. **b**   The calculation is performed similarly regardless of the type of fluid.

32. **c**   20 ml/hr × 1 hr/60 min × 60 drops/ml.

33. **b**   125 ml/hr × 1 hr/60 min × 20 drops/ml.

34. **b**   Know your metric conversions and watch your decimal places! 1 mg = 1,000 μg.

35. **c** 1 mg = 10^3 µg.

36. **c** Study apothocary and household measurements, as well as the metric system.

37. **d** Do not confuse abbreviations: g = gram; gr = grain.

38. **d** 7.5 kg × 2 mg/kg × 1 tablet/5 mg.

39. **c** 35 lb × 1 kg/2.2 lb × 2.2 mg/kg; 1/2-gr tab = 32 mg.

40. **a** 750 mg × 1 tab/500 mg; 1-1/2 tab twice daily = 3 tabs/day × 10 days = 30 tabs.

41. **c** 25 mg × 5 ml/12.5 mg.

42. **c** 44 lb × 1 kg/2.2 lb × 0.5 g/kg/200 mg/ml (20% = 200 mg/ml).

43. **c** "%" means "grams per hundred milliliters."

44. **b** Just do it!

45. **c** 4% = 4 g/100 ml = 5 g/X = 125 ml.

46. **c** 0.2 mg × 1,000 µg/ml × 1 ml/400 µg.

47. **a** 20 mg × 1 ml/25 mg.

48. **a** 20 mEq/L × 15 ml/30 mEq.

49. **c** 50 ml/hr × 1 hr/60 min × 60 drops/ml.

50. **c** 3,000 ml/24 hr × 1 hr/60 min × 15 drops/ml.

51. **b** 17 drops/15 sec = X/60 sec.

52. **b** 1,000 – 650 = 350 ml remain; 10 – 5 = 5 hr remain; 350 ml/5 hr × 1 hr/60 min × 15 drops/ml.

53. **d** 112.5 ml/hr × 1 hr/60 min × 20 drops/ml.

54. **d** 350 ml remain to be delivered in 2 hr; 175 ml/hr × 1 hr/60 min × 20 drops/ml.

55. **d** 5 (X + 1,000) = 50X; solve for X.

56. **b** 12.5 mg × 5 ml/25 mg = 2.5 ml per dose = 7.5 ml per day; 30 ml/7.5.

57. **a** 4 IU/ml × 250 ml × 1 ml/1,000 IU = ml heparin per 250-ml bottle.

58. **a** 20 mEq/L × 1 ml/2 mEq = 10 mEq/L; thus, add 5 ml/500-ml bag.

59. **c** 55 lb × 1 kg/2.2 lb × 1 L/1 kg × 0.08 (1 kg = 1 L; 8% = 0.08).

60. **d** 1 L = 1,000 ml.

61. **b** Cubic centimeters and milliliters are equivalent.

62. **d** 1 kg = 2.2 lb.

63. **b** 1 kg = 1,000 g.

64. **d** 1,000,000 mg = 1 g.

65. **d** 1 L = 1,000 ml = 1,000 cc.

66. **b** 1 kg = 2.2 lb.

67. **c**

68. **b**

69. **c**

70. **c** 1 dr = 1/8 oz.

71. **d** 1 gr = 65 mg.

72. **a** 1 gr = 65 mg.

73. **b** 1 fl dr = 3.7 ml.

74. **c** 1 gr = 65 mg.

75. **c** 1 qt = 32 oz.

76. **a** 1 oz = 30 ml.

77. **c** 1 T = $^1/_2$ oz = 15 ml.

78. **c** 1 T = $^1/_2$ oz.

79. **b** 1 T = $^1/_2$ oz; 16 oz = 1 pt; 32 oz = 1 qt.

80. **d** 3 tsp = 1 T = $^1/_2$ oz.

81. **c** 1 tsp = 5 ml.

82. **c** 1 T = 15 ml.

83. **d** Example of percent calculations:

In performing percent calculations, the important aspect to remember is that % is equal to grams per 100 ml. Therefore, in this case, sulfadimethoxine is 40% or 40 mg/100 ml, or 400 mg/ml. The mare weighs 554 kg, which is equal to 1218.8 lb (554 kg × 2.2 lb/kg), and the dosage is 10 mg/lb. Thus, the mare requires 12,188 mg of sulfadimethoxine/day (1218.8 lb/mare × 10 mg/lb). We know that 40% sulfadimethoxine is equal to 400 mg/ml, so the mare needs a daily dose of 30.5 ml (12,188 mg ÷ 400 mg/ml).

84. c

85. b

86. b

87. a Sample calculation:

The problem should be divided into 3 parts.

1. Calculate the correct weight. The dog weighs 65 lb or 29.5 kg (2.2 lb/kg).

2. Calculate the total amount of medication needed. The dosage for butorphanol is 0.2 mg/kg. Thus, a 29.5-kg animal needs 5.9 mg of butorphanol (29.5 kg × 0.2 mg/kg) for the total dose.

3. Calculate the actual dose to be administered, which requires knowing the concentration of the medication. In this case, butorphanol is available in a concentration of 10 mg/ml. Thus, the animal needs approximately 0.6 ml (5.9 mg ÷ 10 mg/ml).

88. a

89. b

90. a

91. b

92. b

Notes

Medical Nursing

Kerry L. Coombs, DVM
Ed Gordon, DVM
Jean Holzen, CVT

Lori Renda-Francis, LVT
Mary Lou Shea, CAHT
S. Randall Vanderhurst, DVM

Recommended Reading

Arighe M: Drains, dressings, and external coaptation devices. In Auer JA, editor: *Equine surgery*, Philadelphia, 1992, WB Saunders.

Blood DC, Studdert VP: *Ballière's comprehensive veterinary dictionary*, London, 1988, Ballière Tindall.

Colville J: *Diagnostic parasitology for veterinary technicians*, St. Louis, 1991, Mosby.

McCurnin DM: *Clinical textbook for veterinary technicians*, ed 3, Philadelphia, 1994, WB Saunders.

The Merck veterinary manual, ed 7, Rahway NJ, 1989, Merck & Co.

Pasquini C, Spurgeon T: *Anatomy of domestic animals*, Pilot Point Tex, 1989, Sudz Publishing.

Reece WO: *Physiology of domestic animals*, Philadelphia, 1991, Lea & Febiger.

Stashak TS, editor: *Equine wound management*, Philadelphia, 1991, Lea & Febiger.

Stashak TS, editor: *Adams' lameness in horses*, Philadelphia, 1987, Lea & Febiger.

Practice answer sheet is on page 335.

Questions

PHYSICAL EXAMINATION

1. Long-handle neck tongs can be used to grasp a pig to apply a
   a. Harness
   b. Snout rope
   c. Dental speculum
   d. Halter

2. A struggling sheep rapidly becomes hyperthermic in hot weather because its normal body temperature is
   a. 98° F (36.6° C)
   b. 101° F (38.3° C)
   c. 103° F (39.4° C)
   d. 105° F (40.5° C)

3. The easiest large domestic animal to handle is the
   a. Sheep
   b. Goat
   c. Cow
   d. Pig

4. What is the most important skill that a restrainer can develop?
   a. Hypnosis
   b. Firm voice
   c. Slow movements
   d. Self-confidence

5. Clinical signs of *hyperthermia* include
   a. Decreased heart rate
   b. Increased respiratory rate
   c. Decreased temperature
   d. Increased urine output

6. Clinical signs of *hypothermia* include
   a. Increased body temperature
   b. Increased cardiac output
   c. Decreased blood pressure
   d. Bright red mucous membrane

7. What is a clinical sign of shock?
   a. Increased blood pressure
   b. Pale mucous membranes
   c. Decreased heart rate
   d. Increased cardiac output

8. What is the best method of handling an extremely agitated cat?
   a. Apply firm restraint
   b. Use a cat bag
   c. Use a cat muzzle
   d. Back off and allow the cat to calm down

9. When restraining a domestic cat, the best rule to remember is
   a. Always wear gloves
   b. Use the least amount of restraint possible for the procedure
   c. Always grasp the cat with your fingers encircling its head
   d. Always use a cat bag or towel

10. When setting a sheep up on its haunches, you should *never*
    a. Lift the head over the neck
    b. Grasp the flank area
    c. Twist the sheep's head to the side
    d. Try to set the animal up if it weighs more than 200 lb

11. Pigs naturally pull back when pressure is applied around their
    a. Lower jaw (mandible)
    b. Tail
    c. Midsection
    d. Upper jaw (maxilla)

12. The first concern when dealing with any animal should be the
    a. Safety of the animal
    b. Safety of the handlers
    c. Protection of the equipment
    d. Time the procedure will take

13. The normal temperature, pulse rate, and respiration rate (TPR) of swine are
    a. 102° F to 103.6° F, 60 to 80/min, 8 to 18/min
    b. 99.5° F to 101.5° F, 28 to 45/min, 8 to 16/min
    c. 101.5° F, 110 to 140/min, 26/min
    d. 99.5° F, 66 to 114/min, 330 to 480/min

14. The normal cloacal temperature of a chicken is
    a. 98° F (36.6° C)
    b. 101° F (38.3° C)
    c. 103° F (39.4° C)
    d. 107° F (41.6° C)

15. What are the normal temperature, pulse rate and respiratory rate of a cow?
    a. 100° F, 30/min, 50/min
    b. 101.5° F, 60/min, 20/min
    c. 102.5° F, 30/min, 50/min
    d. 102.5° F, 60/min, 20/min

16. Causing an animal to lie on its side with pressure exerted on its muscles and nerves by a series of carefully placed and tightened ropes is called
    a. Casting
    b. Chuting
    c. Haltering
    d. Hog tieing

17. From what area is it best to approach a horse?
    a. The rear
    b. Directly in the front
    c. At a 45° angle from the left shoulder
    d. Any direction

18. What is the basic tool of restraint for the horse?
    a. Leg hobbles
    b. Nose twitch
    c. Casting
    d. Halter

19. What is the normal capillary refill time in a dog?
    a. 1 to 2 seconds
    b. 5 to 6 seconds
    c. 1 minute
    d. 10 minutes

20. Which is *not* a route of injection?
    a. Intravenous
    b. Anteroposterior
    c. Intramuscular
    d. Subcutaneous

21. Which needle has the largest interior diameter?
    a. 27 gauge
    b. 22 gauge
    c. 20 gauge
    d. 16 gauge

22. Which site is *not* usually used to collect blood in a dog?
    a. Saphenous
    b. Cephalic
    c. Tail
    d. Jugular

23. Which vein is found on the lateral aspect of the back leg?
    a. Saphenous
    b. Cephalic
    c. Femoral
    d. Jugular

24. Which vein is located on the cranial (dorsal) surface of the front leg?
    a. Saphenous
    b. Cephalic
    c. Femoral
    d. Jugular

25. Which agent should *not* be used to control blood flow from a nail that was cut too short?
    a. Styptic powder
    b. Alcohol
    c. Silver nitrate
    d. Cornstarch

26. What are the normal temperature, pulse rate and respiratory rate of a dog?
    a. 101.5° F, 90/min, 20/min
    b. 101.5° F, 180/min, 25/min
    c. 100° F, 90/min, 20/min
    d. 100° F, 180/min, 25/min

27. Which lymph node may be palpated caudal to the stifle?
    a. Axillary
    b. Inguinal
    c. Popliteal
    d. Mandibular

Correct answers are on pages 224–231.

28. Which instrument is used to examine the ear canal?
    a. Ophthalmoscope
    b. Fluoroscope
    c. Microscope
    d. Otoscope

29. An animal in sternal recumbency is
    a. On its side
    b. Sitting on its rump
    c. Positioned with its back on the table or floor
    d. Positioned with its abdomen on the table or floor

30. When collecting blood using a needle and syringe, how should the bevel of the needle be positioned?
    a. Up
    b. Down
    c. Pointing to the side
    d. It does not matter

31. When giving an intramuscular injection, it is good practice to withdraw on the syringe plunger after the needle is inserted to
    a. Draw air into the syringe
    b. See if the needle has been inserted into a blood vessel
    c. Make the plunger easier to depress
    d. Provide stability to the syringe

32. When using isopropyl alcohol as a disinfectant, what is the recommended concentration?
    a. 25%
    b. 50%
    c. 70%
    d. 99%

33. Which muscle located cranial to the femur can be used for intramuscular injections?
    a. Quadriceps
    b. Triceps brachii
    c. Semitendinosus
    d. Trapezius

34. Before medicating a patient, there are five "rights" (questions) you should ask yourself. Which of the following is *not* one of those questions?
    a. Right patient?
    b. Right medication?
    c. Right route?
    d. Right temperature?

35. What type of preparation is a biologic?
    a. Antibiotic
    b. Vaccine
    c. Anesthetic
    d. Fluid

36. What does a tonometer measure?
    a. Venous pressure
    b. Arterial pressure
    c. Intraocular pressure
    d. Speed of blood flow

37. Where are the anal sacs located?
    a. Ventral to the mandible
    b. Cranial to the scapula
    c. In the inguinal area
    d. On either side of the anus

38. When examining a patient, you count 7 pulses in 10 seconds. How should you record this animal's pulse rate?
    a. 7 beats/min
    b. 42 beats/min
    c. 28 beats/min
    d. 70 beats/min

39. When using a mercury thermometer to measure rectal temperature, what is the *minimum* time the thermometer should be left in the rectum?
    a. 10 seconds
    b. 60 seconds
    c. 2 minutes
    d. 5 minutes

NORMAL VALUES

40. The blood smear of a normal dog should have what percentage of eosinophils?
    a. 60% to 77%
    b. 35% to 75%
    c. 2% to 10%
    d. 12% to 30%

41. The blood smear of a normal dog should have what percentage of lymphocytes?
    a. 12% to 30%
    b. 60% to 70%
    c. 2% to 8%
    d. 25% to 60%

42. The packed cell volume of a normal dog is
    a. 10% to 21%
    b. 37% to 55%
    c. 10 to 21 g/dl
    d. 35 to 55 g/dl

43. The white blood cell count of a normal dog is
    a. 1,000 to 3,000/μl
    b. 30,000 to 50,000/μl
    c. 4,000 to 1,000/μl
    d. 6,000 to 17,000/μl

44. The hemoglobin level of a normal dog is
    a. 12% to 18%
    b. 12 to 18 g/dl
    c. 100 g/dl
    d. 20% to 80%

45. The red blood cell count of a normal dog is
    a. 5.5 to 8.5 × 10^6/μl
    b. 3,000 to 5,000/μl
    c. 1.1 to 6.4 × 10^6/μl
    d. 10,000 to 20,000/μl

46. The blood urea nitrogen of a normal dog is
    a. 10 to 28 mg/dl
    b. 1 to 2 mg/dl
    c. 10% to 28%
    d. 1% to 2%

47. The serum creatinine level of a normal dog is
    a. 55% to 93%
    b. 1 to 2 mg/dl
    c. 10 to 30 mg/dl
    d. 1% to 2%

48. The serum lipase level of a normal dog is
    a. 13 to 200 IU/L
    b. 1 to 2 g/dl
    c. 200 to 400 IU/L
    d. 1 to 2 IU/L

49. The blood glucose level of a normal dog is
    a. 45 to 70 mg/dl
    b. 1,000 to 2,000 mg/dl
    c. 70 to 100 mg/dl
    d. 10 to 30 g/dl

50. The total plasma protein level of a normal dog is
    a. 6 to 7 g/dl
    b. 10% to 40%
    c. 10 to 30 g/dl
    d. 1 to 2 g/dl

51. Which of the following would *not* be seen in a peripheral blood smear from a normal dog?
    a. Erythrocytes
    b. Platelets
    c. Leukocytes
    d. Megakaryoblast

52. The normal mean corpuscular volume of a dog is
    a. 300 to 345 fl
    b. 1 to 2 fl
    c. 60 to 77 fl
    d. 103 to 400 fl

53. The normal mean corpuscular hemoglobin concentation of a dog is
    a. 32 to 36 g/dl
    b. 1 to 2 g/dl
    c. 135 to 234 g/dl
    d. 60 to 98 g/dl

Correct answers are on pages 224–231.

54. The normal packed cell volume of a horse is
    a. 20% to 39%
    b. 48% to 58%
    c. 12% to 30%
    d. 32% to 52%

55. The normal white blood cell count of a horse is
    a. 5,000 to 12,500/μl
    b. 10,000 to 20,000/μl
    c. 4,000 to 5,000/μl
    d. 10,500 to 30,000/μl

56. How much urine does a dog normally produce in 24 hours?
    a. 5 ml/kg
    b. 15 ml/kg
    c. 30 ml/kg
    d. 45 ml/kg

57. How much urine does a cat normally produce in 24 hours?
    a. 5 ml/kg
    b. 15 ml/kg
    c. 30 ml/kg
    d. 45 ml/kg

58. How many white blood cells may be found in normal canine urine?
    a. 0 to 3/hpf
    b. 2 to 8/hpf
    c. 10 to 14/hpf
    d. 1 to 8/hpf

59. The most common type of leukocyte found in the peripheral blood of dogs is the
    a. Monocyte
    b. Basophil
    c. Eosinophil
    d. Neutrophil

60. Which of the following are both agranulocytes?
    a. Monocytes and neutrophils
    b. Lymphocytes and monocytes
    c. Eosinophils and basophils
    d. Lymphocytes and eosinophils

Drug Administration

61. Which route of drug administration produces the *fastest* onset of action?
    a. Topical
    b. Oral
    c. Intramuscular
    d. Intravenous

62. Which of the following is *not* a parenteral route of drug administration?
    a. Subcutaneous
    b. Intramuscular
    c. Oral
    d. Intravenous

63. Agents used to induce vomiting are called
    a. Pyrethrins
    b. Emetics
    c. Sulfonamides
    d. Diuretics

64. Another term for a *laxative* is
    a. Relaxant
    b. Diuretic
    c. Adjuvant
    d. Cathartic

65. Which drug is used as an anthelmintic?
    a. Penicillin
    b. Piperazine
    c. Pyrethrin
    d. Streptomycin

66. Which drug is *not* an antibiotic?
    a. Chloramphenicol
    b. Amoxicillin
    c. Tetracycline
    d. Furosemide

67. Which type of drug is used to stimulate urine production?
    a. Depressant
    b. Relaxant
    c. Emetic
    d. Diuretic

68. How often should controlled substances be inventoried?
    a. Monthly
    b. Continously, with use
    c. Annually
    d. Every other month

69. An intraarticular injection is given into
    a. A blood vessel
    b. The eye
    c. The skin
    d. A joint

Questions 70 through 73

    a. PO
    b. IC
    c. IV
    d. IM

70. Intracardiac route.

71. Intramuscular route.

72. Intravenous route.

73. Oral route.

Questions 74 through 77

    a. q
    b. prn
    c. Rx
    d. dd

74. Abbreviation meaning *treatment*.

75. Abbreviation meaning *divided*.

76. Abbreviation meaning *every*.

77. Abbreviation meaning *as needed*.

FLUID THERAPY

78. The higher the hematocrit and total protein values, the greater the degree of
    a. Anemia
    b. Hypoglycemia
    c. Dehydration
    d. Hyperkalemia

79. What is the approximate degree of dehydration in a patient showing increased skin tugor, prolonged capillary refill time, dry mucous membranes, and eyes sunken into the orbits?
    a. 0.5%
    b. 10% to 12%
    c. 2% to 3%
    d. 5% to 6%

80. Which of the following is *not* a sign of fluid volume overload?
    a. Restlessness
    b. Hyperpnea
    c. Serous nasal discharge
    d. Dry mucous membranes

81. What is the best route of fluid administration for a slightly dehydrated patient that can drink water and is not vomiting?
    a. Oral
    b. Intravenous
    c. Intraosseus
    d. Intramuscular

82. Use of a cephalic catheter for intravenous fluid administration is usually limited to
    a. 2 to 4 hours
    b. 7 to 14 days
    c. 48 to 72 hours
    d. 30 days

83. Normal daily fluid maintenance requirements are approximately
    a. 10 to 15 mg/kg
    b. 40 to 60 mg/kg
    c. 100 to 300 mg/kg
    d. 1 to 2 mg/kg

Correct answers are on pages 224–231.

84. Which statement concerning subcutaneous administration of fluids is *least* accurate?
    a. Fluids should be infused with a large-bore needle.
    b. Fluids should first be warmed to body temperature.
    c. Fluids should be physiologically isotonic.
    d. 50% dextrose can be safely infused subcutaneously.

85. Isotonic solutions
    a. Must be given only intravenously
    b. Must be given only subcutaneously
    c. Must be given only intraperitoneally
    d. May be given intravenously, subcutaneously, or intraperitoneally

86. Hypertonic solutions
    a. Must be given only intravenously
    b. Must be given only subcutaneously
    c. Must be given only intraperitoneally
    d. May be given intravenously, subcutaneously, or intraperitoneally

87. The principal cation in extracellular fluid is
    a. Na^+
    b. Mg^{++}
    c. K^+
    d. Fe^{++}

88. The principal anion in extracellular fluid is
    a. SO_4^{--}
    b. NO_3^-
    c. Cl^-
    d. HCO_3^-

89. Lactated Ringer's solution is
    a. Slightly hypertonic
    b. Very hypertonic
    c. Hypotonic
    d. Isotonic

90. Sterile water is
    a. Hypotonic
    b. Isotonic
    c. Slightly hypertonic
    d. Very hypertonic

BANDAGING AND SPLINTS

91. Bandaging provides all the following *except*
    a. Keeps the wound warm
    b. Promotes an alkaline environment
    c. Minimizes postoperative edema
    d. Absorbs wound exudate

92. Bandaging promotes wound healing by all the following *except*
    a. Protecting the wound from additional trauma and contamination
    b. Preventing desiccation
    c. Immobilizing the wound to prevent cellular disruption
    d. Decreasing oxygen availability

93. Fiberglass cast materials have all of the following advantages *except*
    a. Slow setting time
    b. Light weight
    c. Good ventilation
    d. Extreme rigidity

94. Which bandage is most commonly used for temporary immobilization of fractures distal to the elbow or stifle before surgery?
    a. Full-leg Stack
    b. Robert Jones
    c. Modified Robert Jones
    d. Military field

95. The most common splint material used in veterinary practice is
    a. Wooden slats
    b. Metal bars
    c. Plastic (PVC) pipe
    d. Low-temperature thermoplastics

96. How frequently should splints be adjusted on foals?
    a. Once a day
    b. Twice a day
    c. Every other day
    d. Three times a day

97. The major functions of a stent bandage include all the following *except*
    a. Used in regions that are difficult to cover
    b. Applies direct pressure and decreases motion
    c. Reduces the tension on the primary incision line
    d. Provides good absorption of exudate

98. The equine joint on which a cast is most effective for preventing flexion is the
    a. Carpus
    b. Hock
    c. Fetlock
    d. Stifle

99. Failure to use adequate padding in bandages on limbs can produce any of the following *except*
    a. Tendonitis
    b. Pressure sores
    c. Severe edema
    d. Instability

100. The ties of the many-tailed spider bandage are positioned on which aspect of the affected limb?
    a. Dorsal
    b. Palmar/plantar
    c. Medial
    d. Lateral

101. Which splint is used on simple closed fractures of the radius and ulna or tibia and fibula in young dogs and occasionally used on large animals (mostly the rear limbs of cattle)?
    a. Kimzey
    b. Schroeder-Thomas
    c. Board
    d. Plastic (PVC)

102. The Robert Jones bandage is *not* appropriate for stabilizing fractures of the
    a. Femur or humerus
    b. Radius or carpus
    c. Tibia or third metacarpal bone
    d. Third metacarpal bone

103. The toes of a bandaged limb should be monitored daily for all of the following *except*
    a. Warmth
    b. Sensitivity
    c. Color
    d. Swelling

104. A compression bandage used to immobilize a structure aids in all the following *except*
    a. Controlling swelling
    b. Reducing movement
    c. Supporting damaged structures
    d. Containing an infectious inflammatory condition

105. A chest or abdominal bandage, when applied firmly for compression, should *not* remain in place on a small animal for longer than
    a. 4 hours
    b. 1 hour
    c. 6 hours
    d. 8 hours

WOUND HEALING

106. Select the correct order for the processes of wound healing.
    a. Inflammation, debridement, repair, maturation
    b. Maturation, debridement, repair, inflammation
    c. Debridement, inflammation, maturation, repair
    d. Repair, inflammation, maturation, debridement

107. Which phase of healing begins immediately after tissue injury?
    a. Debridement
    b. Repair
    c. Inflammation
    d. Maturation

Correct answers are on pages 224–231.

108. Which phase of healing begins approximately 6 hours after tissue injury?
    a. Debridement
    b. Repair
    c. Inflammation
    d. Maturation

109. Which phase of healing begins 3 to 5 days after tissue injury?
    a. Debridement
    b. Repair
    c. Inflammation
    d. Maturation

BREED IDENTIFICATION

110. The breed of dog that is considered "barkless" is the
    a. Pug
    b. Basenji
    c. Pomeranian
    d. Lhasa apso

111. The breed of cat known for its stubby tail is the
    a. Persian
    b. Maine coon cat
    c. Siamese
    d. Manx

112. The breed of dog that frequently has urate crystals in its urine is the
    a. Dalmatian
    b. German shepherd
    c. Chihuahua
    d. Cocker spaniel

113. The breed of dog most likely to be affected by hip dysplasia is the
    a. Wirehaired fox terrier
    b. Brittany spaniel
    c. Whippet
    d. Labrador retriever

114. The breed of goat with long, wide, pendulous ears and a Roman nose is the
    a. Toggenburg
    b. Nubian
    c. Saanen
    d. French alpine

115. The breed of goat with almost no external ears is the
    a. Oberhasli
    b. French alpine
    c. La Mancha
    d. Saanen

116. The all-white breed of goat is the
    a. Saanen
    b. French alpine
    c. La Mancha
    d. Toggenburg

117. The breed of pig that is red is the
    a. Berkshire
    b. Duroc
    c. Yorkshire
    d. Landrace

118. The breed requiring a *smaller* dose of thiobarbiturate anesthetic per pound than that calculated by its weight is the
    a. Whippet
    b. Labrador retriever
    c. Collie
    d. Newfoundland

119. The breed of pig that is white and has erect ears is the
    a. Landrace
    b. Hampshire
    c. Yorkshire
    d. Berkshire

120. The breed of dairy cow whose milk contains the highest percentage of butterfat is the
    a. Holstein
    b. Ayrshire
    c. Guernsey
    d. Jersey

121. The breed of dairy cow that is usually black and white is the
    a. Holstein
    b. Guernsey
    c. Ayrshire
    d. Jersey

122. The breed of dog commonly affected with intervertebral disc disease is the
    a. Dalmatian
    b. Dachshund
    c. Great Dane
    d. Irish setter

123. The breed of dog in which gastric dilatation–volvulus (bloat) is frequently seen is the
    a. Pug
    b. Saint Bernard
    c. Lhasa apso
    d. Shar pei

124. The breed of dog frequently exhibiting inherited idiopathic epilepsy is the
    a. Great Dane
    b. Miniature schnauzer
    c. Miniature poodle
    d. Siberian husky

125. The breed of chicken known for its white eggs is the
    a. Rhode Island red
    b. Leghorn
    c. White Plymouth rock
    d. New Hampshire

126. The breed of dog frequently affected by entropion is the
    a. Basset hound
    b. Samoyed
    c. Shar pei
    d. Saint Bernard

127. The breed of dog that is brachycephalic is the
    a. Pekingese
    b. Collie
    c. Greyhound
    d. Malamute

128. The breed of dog that commonly has its tail docked is the
    a. Dachshund
    b. Siberian husky
    c. Newfoundland
    d. Old English sheep dog

129. The breed of dog that commonly has its ears cropped is the
    a. Borzoi
    b. Keeshond
    c. Doberman pinscher
    d. Cocker spaniel

130. Which breed of cattle is a beef breed?
    a. Guernsey
    b. Holstein
    c. Jersey
    d. Angus

131. A long-coated guinea pig is the
    a. Peruvian
    b. Abyssinian
    c. American
    d. Crested

132. Which breed of guinea pig has a rough haircoat?
    a. Crested
    b. American
    c. Peruvian
    d. Abyssinian

133. Which breed of rabbit is commonly used in research?
    a. Angora
    b. Minilop
    c. Netherland dwarf
    d. New Zealand white

134. The long-haired breed of cat that resembles the Siamese in color is the
    a. Manx
    b. Burmese
    c. Himalayan
    d. Persian

Correct answers are on pages 224–231.

135. The breed of beef cattle that is black and polled is the
    a. Limousin
    b. Angus
    c. Charolais
    d. Hereford

136. The breed of cat that frequently has crossed eyes and a kinked tail is the
    a. Siamese
    b. Himalayan
    c. Persian
    d. Maine coon cat

137. The breed of dog known for its ability to track scents is the
    a. Boston terrier
    b. Welsh corgi
    c. Bedlington terrier
    d. Bloodhound

138. An ideal breed of dog to be kept as a blood donor is the
    a. Greyhound
    b. Basset hound
    c. Dachshund
    d. Chihuahua

139. The breed of cat with uniquely folded ears is the
    a. Persian
    b. Burmese
    c. English flop
    d. Scottish fold

140. Which breed of sheep is used predominantly for meat?
    a. Merino
    b. Romney marsh
    c. Suffolk
    d. Karakul

141. Which type of cat is most likely to be deaf?
    a. Calico
    b. Orange tiger
    c. Tortoiseshell
    d. White

142. The breed of dog particularly prone to parvoviral infection after 4 months of age is the
    a. German shorthaired pointer
    b. Rottweiler
    c. Yorkshire terrier
    d. Afghan hound

143. The breed of dog known for its predisposition to retinal problems is the
    a. Pekingese
    b. Dalmatian
    c. Doberman pinscher
    d. Collie

144. The dairy breed with the highest average milk yield is the
    a. Holstein
    b. Guerney
    c. Jersey
    d. Ayrshire

145. The breed of dog prized for its lack of shedding is the
    a. Collie
    b. Labrador retriever
    c. Poodle
    d. Pug

146. Which breed of cat is most likely to develop hairballs?
    a. Domestic shorthair
    b. Burmese
    c. Persian
    d. Siamese

147. Of the following horse breeds, which is in the pony class?
    a. Arabian
    b. Welsh
    c. Morgan
    d. Suffolk

148. Which horse breed is considered a draft horse?
    a. Clydesdale
    b. Standardbred
    c. Thoroughbred
    d. American saddlehorse

149. Which horse breed is used for harness racing?
    a. Standardbred
    b. Thoroughbred
    c. Percheron
    d. Palomino

150. Which dog breed would probably require the *smallest* amount of thiobarbiturate anesthetic per pound of body weight?
    a. Jack Russell terrier
    b. Lhasa apso
    c. Great Pyrenees
    d. Keeshond

151. The breed of dog particularly susceptible to heat stroke is the
    a. Beagle
    b. English bulldog
    c. Italian greyhound
    d. Schipperke

152. Which breed of dog is most commonly born by cesarean section?
    a. Collie
    b. Beagle
    c. Pomeranian
    d. Boston terrier

153. The breed of beef cattle noted for its heat tolerance is the
    a. Angus
    b. Longhorn
    c. Hereford
    d. Brahman

154. The breed of dog born with no tail is the
    a. Old English sheepdog
    b. Schipperke
    c. Miniature poodle
    d. Miniature schnauzer

155. The breed of cat most likely to be a wool sucker is the
    a. Siamese
    b. Manx
    c. Persian
    d. Domestic longhair

156. Which dog breed is most likely to exhibit destructive behavior?
    a. Chihuahua
    b. Pomeranian
    c. Malamute
    d. Shih tzu

157. Which breed of dog is most likely to exhibit aggressive behavior?
    a. Irish setter
    b. Labrador retriever
    c. Golden retriever
    d. Chow chow

158. The breed of chicken bred for meat is the
    a. Cornish
    b. Leghorn
    c. Rhode Island red
    d. Wyandotte

159. Which dog breed is most likely to have zinc-responsive dermatosis?
    a. Bichon frise
    b. Australian shepherd
    c. Alaskan malamute
    d. Akita

DISEASE CONTROL

160. High mountain or brisket disease of cattle is caused by
    a. Parasitic infection of the lung
    b. *Pasteurella* infection
    c. Hypoxia from low oxygen pressure
    d. Cardiotoxic plants

Correct answers are on pages 224–231.

161. A previously nonvaccinated mature horse that receives a traumatic wound that becomes contaminated should be given
    a. Tetanus antitoxin only
    b. Tetanus toxoid only
    c. Both tetanus antitoxin and tetanus toxoid
    d. Neither tetanus toxoid nor tetanus antitoxin; only local wound therapy is required

162. Colostrum is important for the newborn because it provides
    a. Passive immunity from the dam
    b. Protection against internal parasites
    c. Protection against hypothermia
    d. Active immunity from the sire

163. Which statement concerning newborn foals is *least* accurate?
    a. Equine encephalitis vaccine should be given soon after birth.
    b. An injection of tetanus antitoxin is recommended soon after birth.
    c. Tetanus toxoid should be given soon after birth.
    d. As soon as the foal is delivered, the umbilical cord should be severed and the foal helped to stand.

164. The scientific name for *heaves* in horses is
    a. Chronic obstructive pulmonary disease
    b. Acute bronchopneumonia
    c. Tracheobronchitis
    d. Pulmonary embolism

165. Equine infectious anemia is diagnosed by
    a. Fecal examination
    b. Coggins test
    c. Bacterial culture of blood
    d. Nasal swab analysis

166. The term *sleeping sickness* in horses refers to
    a. Strangles
    b. Distemper
    c. Encephalitis
    d. Tetanus

167. Which statement concerning scours in calves is most accurate?
    a. Scours are caused only by *E coli.*
    b. An important part of treatment for scours is to replenish electrolytes.
    c. Scours usually occur at about 3 months of age.
    d. Scours is seldom fatal.

168. What area of the bovine body does *hardware disease* affect?
    a. Foot
    b. Abomasum
    c. Reticulum
    d. Intestine

169. Signs of *snuffles* in rabbits include
    a. Vomiting
    b. Diarrhea
    c. Splayed legs
    d. Chronic rhinitis

170. Contagious ecthyma (orf) is an infectious viral dermatitis of
    a. Swine
    b. Horses
    c. Cattle
    d. Sheep

171. *Blue eye,* or corneal edema, can occur with which canine disease or after vaccination against that disease?
    a. Toxocariasis
    b. Canine adenovirus infection
    c. Kennel cough
    d. Rabies

172. The most common viral infections of dogs include
    a. Rickets and scurvy
    b. Pasteurellosis and staphylococcosis
    c. Canine distemper and canine hepatitis
    d. Toxoplasmosis and coccidioidomycosis

173. Feline infectious peritonitis is caused by a
    a. Bacterium
    b. Rickettsia
    c. Fungus
    d. Virus

174. Which of the following is *not* an infectious disease of small animals?
    a. Distemper
    b. Leptospirosis
    c. Patent ductus arteriosus
    d. Pneumonitis

175. What canine bacterial disease can be transmitted through the air by aerosolization of urine?
    a. Infectious hepatitis
    b. Leptospirosis
    c. Parvovirus infection
    d. Salmonellosis

176. Which disease of monkeys causes small sores around the mouth and can be fatal to people?
    a. Tuberculosis
    b. B-virus encephalitis
    c. Salmonellosis
    d. Coccidiosis

177. Which animal is most likely to transmit rabies virus to people?
    a. Marmot
    b. Fox
    c. Mule deer
    d. Bear

178. At what age should a dog or cat first be vaccinated against rabies?
    a. 8 weeks
    b. 10 weeks
    c. 12 weeks
    d. 16 weeks

179. Against which disease should ferrets be vaccinated?
    a. Feline panleukopenia
    b. Feline rhinotracheitis
    c. Canine distemper
    d. Canine parvovirus infection

180. Which organism causes *diamond skin disease* in pigs?
    a. Transmissible gastroenteritis virus
    b. *Erysipelothrix rhusiopathiae*
    c. *Haemophilus suis*
    d. *Bordetella bronchiseptica*

181. Which disease is most dangerous in a herd of breeding horses?
    a. Influenza
    b. Strangles
    c. Rhinopneumonitis
    d. Chronic obstructive pulmonary disease

182. Which canine disease responds to antibiotic therapy?
    a. Canine distemper
    b. Parvovirus infection
    c. Canine adenovirus infection
    d. *Bordetella bronchiseptica* infection

183. Which respiratory disease of cats causes ulcerative stomatitis?
    a. Rhinotracheitis
    b. Calicivirus infection
    c. Pneumonitis
    d. Distemper

184. Purpura hemorrhagica is a complication of which disease in horses?
    a. Rhinopneumonitis
    b. Infectious anemia
    c. Influenza
    d. Strangles

185. Which disinfectant is most effective against parvovirus?
    a. Chlorhexidine
    b. Povidone iodine
    c. Alcohol
    d. Sodium hypochlorite

186. Why are intranasal vaccines so effective against respiratory diseases?
    a. They kill all viruses as they are inhaled
    b. Immunoglobulin A is produced at the site of virus entry
    c. Given intranasally, they work with nasal mucus to increase protection
    d. It is much easier to give them intranasally than subcutaneously or intramuscularly

Correct answers are on pages 224–231.

187. Which disease of cats interferes with production of immunoglobulins during vaccination?
    a. *Toxascaris leonina* infection
    b. Cheyletiellosis
    c. Feline leukemia virus infection
    d. Coccidiosis

188. Bacterins are commonly used to vaccinate animals against all of the following *except*
    a. Blackleg
    b. Feline distemper
    c. Leptospirosis
    d. Borreliosis

189. What tissue should be submitted for rabies diagnosis?
    a. Heart
    b. Lung
    c. Brain
    d. Lymph node

190. Which disease of cattle *cannot* be prevented by vaccination?
    a. Blackleg
    b. Botulism
    c. Malignant edema
    d. Brucellosis

191. *Campylobacter fetus,* which can cause abortion in cattle, is transmitted by
    a. Oral ingestion
    b. Inhalation
    c. Venereal contact
    d. Penetrating wounds

192. For what disease is the Coggins test used in diagnosis?
    a. Brucellosis
    b. Equine infectious anemia
    c. Tuberculosis
    d. Bovine leukemia

193. Glanders (farcy) is a bacterial disease of horses that causes nodules in the lungs and skin. It is caused by
    a. Arteriovirus
    b. *Pseudomonas mallei*
    c. *Escherichia coli*
    d. *Actinobacillus*

194. Rabies virus introduced by a bite from an infected animal travels from the bite area to the brain via
    a. Venous blood
    b. Lymph vessels
    c. Tissue diffusion
    d. Peripheral nerves

195. Of those listed, probably the most prevalent serious virus infection of cats is
    a. Feline panleukopenia
    b. Leptospirosis
    c. Toxoplasmosis
    d. Cat-scratch fever

196. The two most common agents involved in feline respiratory disease complex for which vaccines exist are
    a. Papovavirus and reovirus
    b. Herpesvirus and calicivirus
    c. Calicivirus and myxovirus
    d. Herpesvirus and myxovirus

197. Infertility and abortion in cattle can be caused by
    a. *Staphylococcus aureus*
    b. Foot and mouth disease
    c. *Campylobacter fetus*
    d. Coronavirus diarrhea of calves

198. What are the signs of ear mite infestation in cats?
    a. Pruritus ani
    b. Serosanguineous discharge from the ear
    c. Ear hematomas from head shaking
    d. Persistent cough

PUBLIC HEALTH AND ZOONOSES

199. What is an effect of toxoplasmosis in people?
    a. Cutaneous tracts develop
    b. Furunculosis
    c. Abortion during first trimester
    d. Chronic diarrhea

200. *Yersinia pestis* is most pathogenic to
   a. Dogs
   b. Cattle
   c. Horses
   d. People

201. Which vaccine is used to vaccinate people against rabies?
   a. Modified-live canine virus
   b. Bacterin from monkeys
   c. Human diploid cell vaccine
   d. Killed chimpanzee virus

202. Rabbits can transmit which disease to people?
   a. Syphilis
   b. Herpesvirus infection
   c. Leukemia
   d. Tularemia

203. Which statement concerning zoonotic diseases is most accurate?
   a. Cat-scratch fever produces high temperatures in affected cats.
   b. Common ringworm is not transmitted from cats to people.
   c. Human pinworms are not found in dogs or cats.
   d. Rabies does not affect skunks.

204. Which statement concerning zoonotic diseases is most accurate?
   a. Tuberculosis is never transmitted from dogs to people.
   b. Histoplasmosis is seldom transmitted from dogs to people.
   c. Animals with toxoplasmosis are always visibly ill.
   d. Blastomycosis occurs only in reptiles and amphibians.

205. The incidence of trichinosis *(Trichina)*, which can infect people, is *decreased* by
   a. Feeding cooked garbage to hogs
   b. Applying hydrated lime to the premises
   c. Autoclaving at 250 psi
   d. Eliminating rabbits from the farm

206. Which of the following is considered a potential vector for Lyme disease (borreliosis), which can cause severe human illness?
   a. Flea
   b. Mite
   c. Tick
   d. Louse

207. Which is an example of a disease transmitted by an arthropod vector?
   a. Lice infestation transmitted by community use of a saddle blanket
   b. Toxoplasmosis transmitted by contact with infective cat feces
   c. Malaria transmitted from one person to another by a mosquito
   d. Ascariasis transmitted by eating contaminated dirt

208. Which species is the rodent flea that can transmit plague to people through its bite?
   a. *Xenopsylla*
   b. *Pulex*
   c. *Ctenocephalides felis*
   d. *Ctenocephalides canis*

209. What condition is produced by a migrating *Toxocara canis* larva if it moves into a human brain?
   a. Encephalitis
   b. Elephantiasis
   c. Strabismus
   d. Brain tumor

210. A person ingesting *Toxocara canis* ova is most likely to develop
   a. Visceral larva migrans
   b. Cutaneous larva migrans
   c. Creeping eruption
   d. Anal pruritus

211. What area of the human body does creeping eruption affect?
   a. Skin
   b. Eye
   c. Liver
   d. Lung

Correct answers are on pages 224–231.

212. Which tapeworm has people as its definitive host?
     a. *Dipylidium caninum*
     b. *Echinococcus granulosus*
     c. *Taenia pisiformis*
     d. *Taenia solium*

213. Which tapeworm uses people as an intermediate host and causes the disease known as *hydatid disease*?
     a. *Taenia pisiformis*
     b. *Echinococcus granulosus*
     c. *Dipylidium caninum*
     d. *Taenia solium*

214. What defect can be produced in the fetus of a pregnant woman exposed to *Toxoplasma*?
     a. Hydrocephalus
     b. Down's syndrome
     c. Spina bifida
     d. Dwarfism

215. If you are advising a pregnant woman to avoid *Toxoplasma*, which of the following would you tell her?
     a. Store cat feces in an open container
     b. Wear gloves while gardening to avoid contact with cat feces
     c. Wash your hands after handling your dog
     d. Avoid procedures involving horses

216. How are people commonly exposed to *Giardia* from wild or domestic animals?
     a. Undercooked beef
     b. *Giardia*-infected urine
     c. Water supplies
     d. Infected animal blood

217. Which condition must be reported to the Department of Health?
     a. Toxocariasis
     b. Ancylostomiasis
     c. Strongylosis
     d. Echinococcosis

218. People infected with *Dirofilaria immitis* via a mosquito would most likely have lesions of the
     a. Myocardium
     b. Glomeruli
     c. Alveoli of the lungs
     d. Cerebral cortex

219. Which statement concerning parasitism is most accurate?
     a. *Demodex* is the tapeworm of people.
     b. Equine pinworms have major significance in people.
     c. *Toxocara canis* larvae can imbibe blood from the human intestine.
     d. *Echinococcus multilocularis* can use people as an intermediate host.

220. Which canine parasite can cause the disease called visceral larva migrans in children?
     a. *Toxocara canis*
     b. *Isospora*
     c. *Toxascaris leonina*
     d. *Trichuris vulpis*

221. People who own cats can be exposed to *Toxoplasma* oocysts from cat feces in a litterbox. After being passed in the feces, the oocyst is
     a. Infectious immediately
     b. Infectious after 2 to 4 days
     c. Infectious after 24 hours
     d. Changed to a zygote

222. Which disease can cause cyclic fever in people and can be contracted from cattle?
     a. Borreliosis
     b. Brucellosis
     c. Tetanus
     d. Malignant edema

223. Bubonic or pneumonic plague *(Yersinia pestis)* can be transmitted to people by the bite of
     a. Mosquitoes
     b. Rodent fleas
     c. Biting flies
     d. Ticks

224. Erysipeloid of people, caused by *Erysipelothrix rhusiopathiae,* is the result of wound infection with contaminated material. Which farm animal is most likely to carry this organism?
   a. Horses
   b. Cattle
   c. Sheep
   d. Pigs

225. Psittacosis (ornithosis) is a chlamydial disease that people can develop from contact with infected animals. Which species is most likely to transmit psittacosis to people?
   a. Ferret
   b. Cockatiel
   c. Llama
   d. Horse

226. People can contract tetanus, caused by *Clostridium tetani,* by
   a. Contact with sheep
   b. Wound infection from fecal contaminated soil
   c. Performing a necropsy on a hawk
   d. Performing a fecal examination on a dog

227. Which fungus can cause ringworm in people?
   a. *Malassezia*
   b. *Cryptococcus*
   c. *Microsporum*
   d. *Brucella*

228. Tularemia, caused by *Francisella tularensis,* could infect people performing which activity?
   a. Examining cat feces
   b. Vaccinating cattle
   c. Deworming horses
   d. Skinning rabbits

229. How can a person develop sarcocystosis?
   a. Eating contaminated beef
   b. Contact with avian blood samples
   c. Contact with llama saliva
   d. Bite by an infected mosquito

230. Which species is the most likely source of tuberculosis *(Mycobacterium tuberculosis)* for people?
   a. Sheep
   b. Parrots
   c. Nonhuman primates
   d. Dogs

231. African sleeping sickness (trypanosomiasis) can be transmitted to people by which vector?
   a. Mosquito
   b. Tsetse fly
   c. Flea
   d. Tick

232. Eating raw or partially cooked salmon can infect people with which tapeworm?
   a. *Taenia*
   b. *Echinococcus*
   c. *Dipylidium*
   d. *Diphyllobothrium*

233. Eating raw or rare meat from which wild animal can cause trichinosis in people?
   a. Deer
   b. Bear
   c. Squirrel
   d. Antelope

234. Equine encephalomyelitis (EEE, WEE, VEE) is a viral disease that can be transmitted to people by the bite of an infected
   a. Tick
   b. Mite
   c. Louse
   d. Mosquito

235. Which animal is the most likely reservoir for infectious hepatitis (A-virus) for people contacting the animal's feces?
   a. Dog
   b. Horse
   c. Monkey
   d. Snake

Correct answers are on pages 224–231.

236. Rabies is a fatal viral disease that is most likely to be transmitted to people by the bite of a
    a. Guinea pig
    b. Macaw
    c. Rhesus monkey
    d. Bat

237. Which disease causes abortions in cattle, fistulous withers in horses, and undulant fever in people?
    a. Campylobacteriosis
    b. Leptospirosis
    c. Erysipelas
    d. Brucellosis

238. Which coccidian is most likely to infect people drinking contaminated water?
    a. *Sarcocystis*
    b. *Eimeria*
    c. *Cryptosporidium*
    d. *Isospora*

Answers

PHYSICAL EXAMINATION

1. **b** Long-handle neck tongs can be used to help apply a snout rope, which is a better means of restraint.

2. **c** The normal body temperature of a sheep is about 103° F, with a range of 102 to 104° F.

3. **a** The sheep is usually the easiest to handle because it is less aggressive than the others listed.

4. **d** Although all are good skills, self-confidence is the most important.

5. **b** The other signs indicate hypothermia.

6. **c** The other signs indicate hyperthermia.

7. **b**

8. **d** Attempts to control an extremely agitated cat often end with injury to the cat through use of excessive force.

9. **b** Cats respond best when the least amount of restraint is applied to the extent necessary for the procedure being performed.

10. **a** Lifting the head over the neck may cause injury, whereas turning the head to the side helps set the animal on its haunches.

11. **d** When pressure is applied to the upper jaw, a pig will pull back, which can be used to guide the animal.

12. **b** Safety of the people working on the animal should always be the primary concern, although the safety of the animal must also be taken into consideration.

13. **a** (b—horse, c—cat, d—rat).

14. **d** The average temperature of a chicken is about 107° F.

15. **b**

16. **a** Casting is a means of restraint by applying ropes to pull the animal down on its side and is used mainly when a chute is not available.

17. **c** It is best to approach the horse at a 45-degree angle from the left shoulder, because this is what most horses are accustomed to.

18. **d** A halter is the most common horse restraint and the first tool usually used; the others may be used if more restraint is needed to perform a procedure.

19. **a** Normal capillary refill time is 1 to 3 seconds for a dog.

20. **b**

21. **d** Needle circumference *decreases* as the gauge number increases.

22. **c** The tail vein is rarely used to draw blood from a dog.

23. **a** The saphenous vein is found lateral to the hock.

24. **b** The cephalic is found on the front leg.

25. **b** Alcohol prolongs bleeding time.

26. **a**

27. **c** The popliteal lymph node is located behind the stifle.

28. **d** An otoscope is used to examine ears.

29. **d** In sternal recumbency, the animal's chest and abdomen are adjacent to the table.

30. **a** The bevel of the needle should be pointed upward.

31. **b** Before administering any injection, you should aspirate to check for blood.

32. **c**

33. **a** The quadriceps muscle is a good choice for intramuscular injections.

34. **d** The right temperature is not one of the five questions, although the other answers are correct, in addition to the right dose and frequency.

35. **b**

36. **c**

37. **d**

38. **b**

39. **b** 60 seconds is the minimum, or until the mercury stops rising.

Normal Values

40. c
41. a
42. b
43. d
44. b
45. a
46. a
47. b
48. a
49. c
50. a
51. d
52. c
53. a
54. d
55. a
56. c
57. b
58. a
59. d
60. b

Drug Administration

61. d
62. c
63. b
64. d
65. b
66. d
67. d
68. b
69. d

70. **b**

71. **d**

72. **c**

73. **a**

74. **c**

75. **d**

76. **a**

77. **b**

FLUID THERAPY

78. **c**

79. **b**

80. **d** Dry mucous membranes are a sign of dehydration.

81. **a** Oral fluid administration is the preferred method because of reduced expense, ease of administration, and safety.

82 **c** Beyond 3 days, the patency of the catheter decreases and the risk of infection increases.

83. **b**

84. **d** A dextrose solution with a concentration greater than 2.5% given subcutaneously could cause sloughing of skin and abscess formation.

85. **d**

86. **a**

87. **a**

88. **c**

89. **d**

90. **a**

BANDAGING AND SPLINTS

91. **b** Bandaging promotes an acidic environment at the wound surface by preventing carbon dioxide loss and absorbing ammonia produced by bacteria.

92. **d** Covering a wound provides an acidic environment, which increases oxygen dissociation from hemoglobin and thus oxygen availability in the wound.

93. **a** Fiberglass is known for its rapid setting time.

94. **b** A Robert Jones bandage provides stability through compression of many cotton layers; a modified Robert Jones is less bulky and provides little or no splinting capabilities.

95. **c** It is used because of its light weight and strength.

96. **b**

97. **d**

98. **b** Because the hock is angled, PVC application is impractical, and the carpus and fetlock would be splinted by other less costly materials because they have no angulation. Stifles are never splinted.

99. **d**

100. **d**

101. **b**

102. **a**

103. **b**

104. **d** If the infection is not under control, a compression bandage may force bacteria and associated toxic products deeper into the tissues.

105. **a**

WOUND HEALING

106. **a**

107. **c**

108. **a**

109. **b**

BREED INDENTIFICATION

110. **b** A Basenji can make a sound, but that sound is not considered a bark.

111. **d** Manx; all the other breeds listed have a long tail.

112. **a** Urate crystals are seen more abundantly in the urine of Dalmatians than of other breeds.

113. **d** Hip dysplasia is most commonly seen in dogs whose mature weight is greater than 40 pounds.

114. **b** The Nubian has long, wide, pendulous ears and a Roman nose.

115. **c** The La Mancha has almost no external ears (*gopher* ears) or extremely short ears (*elf* ears).

116. **a** The Saanen is a large, all-white breed of goat.

117. **b**

118. **a** The whippet and other thin breeds of dog require much less thiobarbiturate because they lack body fat.

119. **c**

120. **d** The jersey produces milk with an average butterfat content of 4.73%.

121. **a**

122. **b** The dachshund, a chondroplastic breed, is commonly affected with intervertebral disc disease.

123. **b** The Saint Bernard, a large, deep-chested breed, is highly susceptible to gastric dilatation and torsion (bloat).

124. **c** The miniature poodle is frequently affected by inherited idiopathic epilepsy.

125. **b** The leghorn lays white eggs, whereas the other three breeds lay brown eggs.

126. **c** Entropion, or infolding of the eyelid, is frequently seen in the shar pei.

127. **a** The Pekingese is a brachycephalic or short-nose breed.

128. **d** Of the four breeds listed, only the old English sheep dog has its tail docked.

129. **c** Of the breeds listed, only the Doberman pinscher has its ears cropped.

130. **d** The Angus is a breed of beef cattle. All others are breeds of dairy cattle.

131. **a** The Peruvian guinea pig is long coated; all others are short coated.

132. **d** The Abyssinian is the only rough-coated breed of guinea pig.

133. **d**

134. **c** The Himalayan has the full coat of the Persian, with the pale coloring and darker parts of the Siamese.

135. **b** a—the limousin is gold; c—the Charolais is white; d—the Hereford is red with a white face.

136. **a** The Siamese frequently has genetically induced crossed eyes and a bend at the distal end of the tail.

137. **d** The bloodhound is frequently used in tracking.

138. **a** The greyhound makes an ideal blood donor because of its short hair and long straight veins and because most lack the A factor.

139. **d** The Scottish fold first appeared in Scotland as a result of a spontaneous mutation in the 1960s. It has folded ears, a short nose, and large round eyes.

140. **c** The Suffolk is a meat breed, whereas the others are used for their wool or pelt.

141. **d** The dominant gene for white coat also predisposes to deafness.

142. **b**

143. **d** The collie has a high incidence of an underdeveloped retina.

144. **a** The holstein has an average milk yield of over 20,000 lb per year.

145. **c** The poodle, while shedding, retains loose hair within its hair coat, which predisposes it to mat formation.

146. **c** The Persian cat, as a result of its long hair, is most likely to develop hairballs.

147. **b** The Welsh is a pony.

148. **a** The Clydesdale is a draft horse used for pulling.

149. **a**

150. **c** The larger the animal, the lower its basal metabolic rate and, consequently, the anesthetic agent is more slowly metabolized.

151. **b** The English bulldog, because of respiratory difficulty, is especially prone to heat stroke.

152. **d** The Boston terrier, because of its large head, is frequently born by cesarean section.

153. **d**

154. **b**

155. **a**

156. **c** The malamute and other northern breeds are considered to have the greatest tendency to exhibit destructive behavior.

157. **d**

158. **a** The Cornish is a meat breed, whereas the others are bred primarily for eggs.

159. **c** The Alaskan malamute has a decreased ability to absorb zinc from the intestinal tract.

Disease Control

160. **c** Hypoxia from low oxygen pressure is seen in cattle living at high altitudes.

161. **c** Tetanus antitoxin and tetanus toxoid are given together. The antitoxin supplies immunoglobulins against tetanus immediately; the toxoid causes the equine lymphocytes to produce immunoglobulin for long-term protection.

162. **a** Passive immunity from the dam protects the newborn against diseases to which the dam has developed immunity.

163. **b** Tetanus toxoid is given at 4 months. Encephalitis vaccine is given at 6 to 8 months. Never sever an umbilical cord, as it will keep hemorrhaging and could exsanguinate (bleed out) the foal.

164. **a**

165. **b**

166. **c** a—Bacterial respiratory infection; b—viral infection; d—causes rigidity and convulsions.

167. **b** Electrolytes are used to treat scours from almost any cause. Specific treatment for bacterial infection and supportive treatment for viral scours are also needed.

168. **c** Metal objects can lodge in the reticulum and penetrate to the liver and pericardium of ruminants, especially cattle.

169. **d** Snuffles is an acute, subacute, or chronic inflammation of the nasal passages of rabbits. It is caused by *Pasteurella*.

170. **d**

171. **b** Canine adenovirus infection (infectious canine hepatitis) or vaccination with a modified-live virus can result in corneal edema.

172. **c**

173. **d** Feline infectious peritonitis is caused by a virus but is also associated with immunodeficiencies caused by feline leukemia virus or feline immunodeficiency virus infection.

27. Which antibiotic is a bacteriostatic drug that readily penetrates the blood-brain barrier and achieves therapeutic concentrations of antibiotic in the central nervous system?
    a. Amoxicillin
    b. Enrofloxacin
    c. Oxytetracycline
    d. Chloramphenicol

28. Chloramphenicol is metabolized by specific enzymes in the liver. Consequently, it interferes with or influences how rapidly other drugs metabolized by the same liver enzymes are eliminated from the body. This is important to remember to prevent accidental overdose of a simultaneously administered drug. Metabolism of which drug is affected by simultaneous use of chloramphenicol?
    a. Phenobarbital
    b. Aspirin
    c. Sulfadimethoxine
    d. Enrofloxacin

29. Why is chloramphenicol used with extreme caution in cats and neonates?
    a. It can bind with dietary calcium (milk) and become deactivated
    b. The liver is unable to metabolize chloramphenicol effectively in these animals
    c. It can alter developing bone, enamel, and cartilage
    d. It may drastically alter gut bacterial flora, resulting in fatal diarrhea

30. What fatal reaction to chloramphenicol has been reported in cats and people?
    a. Kidney failure
    b. Aplastic anemia
    c. Pulmonary edema (fluid-filled lungs)
    d. Liver failure

31. Which antimicrobial is banned from use in any food animal because of the risk to human health?
    a. Oxytetracycline
    b. Dicloxacillin
    c. Chloramphenicol
    d. Sulfadimethoxine

32. When are drugs like sulfadimethoxine, sulfadiazine, and other sulfa drugs most likely to cause kidney problems?
    a. When an animal is receiving intravenous fluids and these are having a diuretic effect on the kidneys
    b. When an animal is dehydrated
    c. When an animal has only one functional kidney
    d. When an animal has a bladder infection

33. What are trimethoprim and ormetoprim?
    a. Insect growth regulators
    b. Agents that enhance bactericidal activity of sulfa drugs
    c. Agents that enhance the spectrum of activity of penicillins
    d. Agents that reduce the risk of liver damage from hepatotoxic drugs

34. Within the past few years there have been reports of dogs having an adverse reaction to sulfadiazine, a very commonly used sulfonamide. For which reaction should clients and the veterinary professional watch?
    a. Cardiac arrest
    b. Sudden liver failure
    c. Decreased tear production
    d. Increased urination

35. Which bactericidal antimicrobial is also effective against important protozoa (e.g., *Giardia*) and is considered the drug of choice in chronic diarrhea associated with giardiasis?
    a. Clindamycin
    b. Griseofulvin
    c. Metronidazole

Correct answers are on pages 254–262.

d. Sulfasalazine

36. Ketoconazole, miconazole, and griseofulvin are effective against
    a. Viruses
    b. Flukes
    c. Intestinal nematodes
    d. Fungi

37. What is the drug of choice for long-term maintenance of an epileptic dog in a seizure-free state?
    a. Primidone
    b. Phenytoin
    c. Diazepam
    d. Phenobarbital

38. Which anticonvulsant drug is converted by the liver primarily to phenobarbital, which accounts for most of its anticonvulsant activity?
    a. Diazepam
    b. Primidone
    c. Phenytoin
    d. Clonazepam

39. Which traditional anticonvulsant is now being used simultaneously with phenobarbital in dogs that are nonresponsive to phenobarbital alone?
    a. Diazepam
    b. Potassium bromide
    c. Phenytoin
    d. Strychnine

40. Which drug is a respiratory stimulant?
    a. Oxytocin
    b. Dobutamine
    c. Propranolol
    d. Doxapram

41. Drugs that effectively block the cough reflex are called
    a. Mucolytics
    b. Expectorants
    c. Antitussives
    d. Antihistamines

42. Drugs that reduce the viscosity and stickiness of secretions in the respiratory tree are called
    a. Mucolytics
    b. Expectorants
    c. Antitussives
    d. Antihistamines

43. Drugs that increase the volume of watery secretions within the respiratory tree as a means to make a dry cough productive are called
    a. Mucolytics
    b. Expectorants
    c. Antitussives
    d. Antihistamines

44. Butorphanol and hydrocodone are examples of
    a. Mucolytics
    b. Expectorants
    c. Antitussives
    d. Antihistamines

45. Drugs that are described as β_2-receptor stimulators have what effect on the respiratory tree?
    a. Increase the volume of watery secretions
    b. Increase the volume of sticky mucoid secretions
    c. Cause bronchoconstriction
    d. Cause bronchodilatation

46. Terbutaline, albuterol, and metaproterenol are described as selective β_2-agonists. They are used in veterinary medicine to
    a. Treat feline asthma or other bronchoconstrictive diseases
    b. Treat low blood pressure caused by shock
    c. Suppress a productive cough, such as in bronchopneumonia
    d. Stimulate secretions within the respiratory tree to aid the mucociliary apparatus

47. Methylxanthines are often used to improve breathing in cardiac patients and patients with respiratory disease. Which drugs are methylxanthines used for this purpose?
    a. Theophylline and aminophylline
    b. Codeine and dextromethorphan
    c. Hydrocodone and butorphanol
    d. Guaifenesin and propranolol

48. Most drugs that control arrhythmias of the heart are said to be *negative inotropes*. What does this mean?
    a. They increase the heart rate
    b. They decrease the heart rate
    c. They increase the force of contractions
    d. They decrease the force of contractions

49. What is the drug of choice for emergency intravenous administration to control ventricular arrhythmias that may be observed during anesthesia?
    a. Propranolol
    b. Lidocaine
    c. Procainamide
    d. Digoxin

50. Hyperthyroid cats have heart rates of over 200 beats per minute because of large numbers of β_1-sympathetic receptors in their heart (making the heart more sensitive to epinephrine and norepinephrine). This high heart rate is an anesthetic risk. What drug is used to slow the heart rate and decrease arrhythmias associated with β_1-receptor stimulation?
    a. Lidocaine
    b. Propranolol
    c. Quinidine
    d. Digoxin

51. Digoxin is said to have a *narrow therapeutic index*. What does this mean?
    a. Plasma drug concentrations that produce toxicity are very low
    b. Plasma drug concentrations required to achieve a beneficial effect are very high
    c. Plasma drug concentrations that produce toxicity are very close to the minimum concentration at which a beneficial effect occurs
    d. Plasma drug concentrations are extremely variable from animal to animal

52. Because digoxin has a narrow therapeutic index, veterinary technicians and owners of animals receiving digoxin must be able to detect early signs of digoxin toxicity, such as
    a. Increased urination and increased water consumption
    b. Increased coughing and difficulty breathing
    c. Decreased appetite, anorexia, diarrhea, and/or vomiting
    d. Wobbly gait, fainting (syncope), and disorientation

53. Some drugs commonly used to treat veterinary patients with cardiovascular disease alter the electrolyte levels (Na^+, K^+, Cl^-) within the body. Which electrolyte change greatly enhances the risk of digoxin toxicity?
    a. Increased sodium (hypernatremia)
    b. Increased potassium (hyperkalemia)
    c. Decreased chloride (hypochloremia)
    d. Decreased potassium (hypokalemia)

Correct answers are on pages 254–262.

54. Which alteration in body function requires changing the digoxin dose? How should the dose be changed?
    a. Decreased liver function; increase digoxin dose
    b. Decreased liver function; decrease digoxin dose
    c. Decreased kidney function; increase digoxin dose
    d. Decreased kidney function; decrease digoxin dose

55. Drugs classified as *ACE inhibitors* or α_1- *antagonists* have what effect on the body?
    a. Increase the strength of heart contractions
    b. Cause vasodilatation
    c. Cause bronchodilatation
    d. Increase the heart rate

56. Hydralazine, prazosin, and captopril are examples of
    a. Positive inotropes
    b. Antiarrhythmics
    c. Bronchodilators
    d. Vasodilators

57. Nitroglycerin is sometimes used as a paste applied to the pinna or to the abdominal skin in dogs with cardiovascular disease. Nitroglycerin has what beneficial effect?
    a. Increases strength of heart contractions
    b. Causes vasodilatation
    c. Causes bronchodilatation
    d. Decreases the heart rate

58. Spironolactone, chlorothiazide, and furosemide are classified as?
    a. Diuretics
    b. Positive inotropes
    c. Antiarrhythmics
    d. Vasodilators

59. What role does aspirin play in treating diseases like feline dilative cardiomyopathy or similar cardiovascular diseases?
    a. Increases the diuretic effect of drugs like furosemide
    b. Decreases the risk of abnormal platelet clumping and subsequent thrombus formation
    c. Increases the ability of vasodilators to keep the coronary arterioles fully dilated
    d. Decreases oxygen consumption by the weakened cardiac muscle

60. Which controlled substance rating indicates the drug with the greatest potential for abuse?
    a. C-III
    b. C-II
    c. C-V
    d. C-IV

61. For what reason is apomorphine used in canine patients in emergency veterinary medicine?
    a. To keep blood pressure elevated in animals in shock
    b. To alleviate pain
    c. To produce emesis after ingestion of a toxin
    d. To maintain kidney function during periods of reduced blood flow to the kidneys

62. Which drug is most likely to be prescribed to prevent *motion sickness*?
    a. Apomorphine
    b. Syrup of ipecac
    c. Atropine
    d. Dimenhydrinate

63. For what is syrup of ipecac used?
    a. To stimulate defecation to flush out poisons from the distal bowel
    b. To induce vomiting
    c. To stimulate duodenal movement to overcome constipation
    d. To increase blood supply to the gastrointestinal tract

64. Why should syrup of ipecac and activated charcoal (universal antidote) *not* be given simultaneously?
   a. The resultant vomiting is too severe and too prolonged
   b. They cancel out the beneficial effect of each other
   c. Neither is absorbed in sufficient quantity to be of any benefit
   d. Severe diarrhea and intestinal cramping result.

65. Anticholinergic drugs like atropine, aminopentamide (Centrine), or isopropamide (Darbazine) are expected to have what effect on the gastrointestinal tract?
   a. Increase secretions by the bowel
   b. Increase movement of feces through the bowel
   c. Decrease ability of compounds to irritate the bowel wall
   d. Decrease bowel motility

66. Narcotics like paregoric, diphenoxylate, and loperamide are used to treat gastrointestinal disease. What effect do they have on the gastrointestinal tract?
   a. Decrease diarrhea by decreasing peristaltic waves
   b. Decrease diarrhea by relaxing segmental mixing contractions
   c. Decrease diarrhea by increasing segmental mixing contractions
   d. Decrease constipation by increasing intestinal secretions

67. Bismuth subsalicylate is the active ingredient in a common over-the-counter (OTC) preparation used for some types of gastrointestinal disease. For what is it used?
   a. Mild laxative
   b. Antiemetic
   c. Antidiarrheic
   d. Emetic

68. Drugs like flunixin meglumine, ibuprofen, and other nonsteroidal antiinflammatory drugs (NSAIDs) often produce side effects in the gastrointestinal tract with long-term use or high-dosage use (especially in dogs). What are these side effects?
   a. Increased bowel motility, resulting in fluid diarrhea
   b. Decreased ability to digest fat, resulting in fatty stool (steatorrhea)
   c. Ulcers or gastritis from decreased mucus production
   d. Decreased bowel motility, resulting in constipation

69. Cimetidine and ranitidine are often called H_2 blockers, traditionally referred to as histamine receptors. For what are they used?
   a. Antidiarrheal
   b. Laxative
   c. Rumen stimulant
   d. Antiulcer

70. What type of medication is sucralfate (Carafate)?
   a. Antiulcer
   b. Antidiarrheal
   c. Antibloat
   d. Anticonstipation

71. The most appropriate drug to use in treating animals with hypothyroidism is
   a. Thyroid-stimulating hormone (TSH)
   b. Thyroid extract
   c. Synthetic levothyroxine (T_4)
   d. Synthetic liothyronine (T_3)

72. For what disease are methimazole and propylthiouracil used?
   a. Hypothyroidism in dogs
   b. Cushing's disease (hyperadrenocorticism) in dogs
   c. Hyperthyroidism in cats
   d. Addison's disease (hypoadrenocorticism) in dogs

Correct answers are on pages 254–262.

73. Which drug is used to return a mare to proestrus from diestrus through lysis of the corpus luteum?
    a. Progesterone
    b. Estrogen
    c. Prostaglandin
    d. Gonadotropin

74. Which hormone group is marketed as a way to bring transitional anestrous mares into proestrus to begin cycling? The hormone is given for several days to mimic diestrus and then withdrawn to mimic natural lysis of the corpus luteum and a return to proestrus.
    a. Estradiol cypionate (ECP)
    b. Prostaglandin-F_2-alpha (dinoprost tromethamine)
    c. Human chorionic gonadotropin (hCG)
    d. Progestin (altrenogest)

75. Which reproductive hormone can produce pyometra in dogs if used at high dosages for several days? It is also used in the pregnant mare in an attempt to keep it from prematurely aborting its fetus.
    a. Estrogen
    b. Progesterone
    c. Gonadotropin
    d. Prostaglandin

76. Which reproductive hormone can cause severe (and sometimes fatal) aplastic anemia or open-cervix pyometra several weeks after it has been given at supraphysiologic dosages (higher than normally found in the body)?
    a. Estradiol cypionate
    b. Prostaglandin-F_2-alpha (dinoprost tromethamine)
    c. Human chorionic gonadotropin
    d. Progestin (altrenogest)

77. Which drug is used as a contraceptive in dogs and sometimes for correction of behavioral problems in cats (e.g., inappropriate urination)?
    a. Altrenogest
    b. Megestrol acetate
    c. Estradiol cypionate
    d. Dinoprost tromethamine

78. Which drug is *not* a nonsteroidal antiinflammory drug (NSAID) and does *not* cause gastrointestinal upset as do most NSAIDs?
    a. Aspirin (salicylate)
    b. Flunixin meglumine
    c. Acetaminophen
    d. Phenylbutazone

79. Glucocorticoids have different durations of activity, a fact that plays an important role in their risk of side effects with long-term use. Which glucocorticoid has the longest duration of activity?
    a. Hydrocortisone
    b. Prednisolone
    c. Triamcinolone
    d. Dexamethasone

80. A very predictable short-term side effect of glucocorticoid therapy of which every client should be aware is
    a. Polyuria and polydipsia
    b. Cough and nasal discharge
    c. Anorexia and diarrhea
    d. Dry skin and skin irritations

81. Commonly used glucocorticoids affect the complete blood count (CBC). What are the effects of glucocorticoid use on the CBC?
    a. Neutrophils decreased, eosinophils increased, lymphocytes decreased
    b. Neutrophils increased, eosinophils increased, lymphocytes increased
    c. Neutrophils increased, eosinophils decreased, lymphocytes decreased
    d. Neutrophils decreased, eosinophils decreased, lymphocytes increased

82. Continuous administration of glucocorticoids can change
    a. Teratogenic renal failure
    b. Estregenic Addison's disease
    c. Iatrogenic Cushing's disease
    d. Telogenic Johne's disease

83. In what species might glucocorticoid administration lead to abortion during the last few weeks of gestation?
    a. Horses and cattle
    b. Pigs and dogs
    c. Dogs and cats
    d. Horses and cats

84. Nonsteroidal antiinflammatory drugs are most likely to cause side effects in what two organ systems?
    a. Renal and pulmonary
    b. Renal and gastrointestinal
    c. Pulmonary and cardiac
    d. Cardiac and hepatic

85. Which nonsteroidal antiinflammatory drug, when given perivascularly in horses, can cause skin necrosis and sloughing?
    a. Phenylbutazone
    b. Flunixin meglumine
    c. Ketoprofen
    d. Meclofenamic acid

86. One of the following antiinflammatory drugs is sometimes applied topically. Care must be taken to clean the area where it is applied; however, it readily penetrates the skin and can carry bacterial toxins or other chemicals with it into the body. Which drug is this?
    a. Dexamethasone
    b. Dimethyl sulfoxide
    c. Flunixin meglumine
    d. Hydrocortisone

87. Which common insecticide (flea products, dips) must be administered cautiously because it can produce toxicity when used with carbamate flea powders or oral flea tablets, such as cythioate (Proban)?
    a. Pyrethrin
    b. Chlorpyrifos
    c. Ivermectin
    d. Piperonyl butoxide

88. A drug package insert states that the drug is an anticestodal. Against what type of parasite will this drug be effective?
    a. Ascarids (*Toxocara, Toxascaris*)
    b. Tapeworms (*Taenia*)
    c. Protozoa (*Eimeria, Giardia*)
    d. Flukes (liver fluke, lung fluke)

89. Which breed of dog has a blood-brain barrier that allows ivermectin to reach toxic concentrations within the brain more readily than in other breeds?
    a. German shepherd
    b. Collie
    c. Schnauzer
    d. Cocker spaniel

90. Which drug is used most commonly as a *microfilaricide* in treatment of heartworm disease?
    a. Thiacetarsamide
    b. Diethylcarbamazine
    c. Ivermectin
    d. Piperazine

91. If an animal or person receives an overdose of organophosphate insecticide (from dips, powders, sprays), what is the treatment of choice?
    a. Diphenhydramine (Benadryl)
    b. Corticosteroids (glucocorticoids)
    c. Intravenous fluids to aid elimination of the compound through the urine
    d. Atropine

Correct answers are on pages 254–262.

92. Which insecticide is effective in treating demodectic mange?
    a. Fenoxycarb
    b. Amitraz
    c. Pyrethrin
    d. Allethrin

93. Methoprene and fenoxycarb are ingredients found increasingly in flea and other insect products. What are they?
    a. Insecticides
    b. Repellents
    c. Insect growth regulators
    d. Synergists

Questions 94 through 97

The following information was provided for a prescription written by a veterinarian:

Dr. Pete Bill—Veterinary Associates, Inc.
    325 Sentry Highway
    West Lafayette, IN 47907
    Indiana License Number #4xxx
    (317) 555-8636
For: Mr. R.K. Jones
    111 Melrose Place
    Loomisville, IN 47905
Canine patient *SIG:* Amoxicillin 100 mg
    1 tab q8h PO prn
    2 refills Date:1/5/96
    Signature: *Pete Bill*

94. What vital information is missing from this prescription that must be present for it to be filled?
    a. Veterinarian's Drug Enforcement Administration (DEA) license number
    b. Pet's name
    c. Owner's telephone number
    d. Number of tablets

95. In the prescription what does *PO* mean?
    a. Administer every other day
    b. Administer by mouth
    c. Administer as needed
    d. Administer on an empty stomach

96. How many times a day is this medication to be given?
    a. Once
    b. Twice
    c. Three times
    d. Four times

97. What does *prn* mean?
    a. Administer every other day
    b. Administer by mouth
    c. Administer as needed
    d. Administer on an empty stomach

98. The abbreviations *OD* and *OS* on a prescription refer to
    a. Administer by mouth and by rectum
    b. Administer every other day and every 3 days
    c. Right eye and left eye
    d. Administer with food and without food

99. What do 15 gr and 10 g mean on a prescription?
    a. 15 grains and 10 grams
    b. 15 grains and 10 grains
    c. 15 grams and 10 grams
    d. 15 grams and 10 grains

100. Most pharmaceutical agents that are measured in grains have how many milligrams per grain?
    a. 30
    b. 60
    c. 100
    d. 120

101. Which of the following is a concentration of a drug solution?
    a. 15 mg/kg
    b. 1,000 U/ml
    c. 20 gr/mg
    d. 250 g/lb 251

102. How many milliliters are in a teaspoon?
    a. 1
    b. 3
    c. 5
    d. 10

103. How many cubic centimeters are in a tablespoon?
    a. 5
    b. 15
    c. 25
    d. 30

104. Which equivalent is correct?
    a. q12h = QD
    b. q6h = QID
    c. q4h = TID
    d. q8h = BID

105. A 10-kg animal weighs how many pounds?
    a. 2
    b. 15
    c. 18
    d. 22

106. Which dosage form must be shaken before administration to an animal?
    a. Solution
    b. Ointment
    c. Gel
    d. Suspension

107. When a drug is used by a route, in a species, or for another indication than that specified by the manufacturer, this use is
    a. A felony offense
    b. An extra-label use
    c. Prohibited by the AVMA
    d. An implied consent from the manufacturer

108. Use of antibiotics and other drugs in food-producing animals has raised a concern over residues in the food that people eat. To avoid this problem, each drug is provided with a timetable that establishes the period between the last dose and when the animal can be slaughtered for food or when the milk can be used. What is this period called?
    a. Elimination half-life
    b. Secretion period
    c. Refractory period
    d. Withdrawal time

109. Sometimes drugs are first administered in a large dose and then given as a series of smaller doses. What is the first dose called?
    a. Initial dose
    b. Loading dose
    c. Distribution dose
    d. Bolus dose

110. Many drugs do not have X mg/ml listed on their labels but instead have their concentrations listed as a percent (e.g., 24% solution). When figuring a dose, however, you must know how many milligrams of drug are in each milliliter of solution. Which of the following most accurately reflects the percentage of a solution?
    a. X g/ml
    b. X g/10 ml
    c. X g/100 ml
    d. X mg/10 ml

111. How many milligrams are in each milliliter of a 24% solution?
    a. 24
    b. 2.4
    c. 240
    d. 0.24

112. Which class of drugs generally poses the greatest potential health threat to those handling the medication?
    a. Antibiotics
    b. Antineoplastics
    c. Antinematodals
    d. Antiprotozoals

113. What effect does renal failure or compromised liver function have on the pharmacokinetics of most drugs?
    a. Decreased absorption of drugs given orally
    b. Increased elimination rate of drugs from the body
    c. Decreased volume of distribution of drugs
    d. Increased half-life of drugs

Correct answers are on pages 254–262.

114. Controlled substances are drugs that
    a. Cannot be used in any animal intended for use as human food
    b. Have a high potential for abuse
    c. Are very hazardous to personnel handling them
    d. Are environmentally hazardous

115. Drugs that are administered intraarticularly are injected into
    a. The abdominal cavity
    b. The globe of the eye
    c. The ear canal
    d. A joint

116. If a drug that is very irritating to tissues is accidentally given outside of the cephalic vein (perivascularly), you should immediately
    a. Apply a tourniquet to prevent movement of the drug up the leg
    b. Infiltrate the area with sterile saline or other sterile isotonic fluid
    c. Aspirate the area with a needle and syringe to remove as much drug as possible
    d. Inject epinephrine into the area to constrict the capillaries and decrease drug absorption

117. Generally 1 fluid ounce is equal to approximately how many milliliters of liquid?
    a. 1
    b. 15
    c. 30
    d. 60

Answers

1. **c** *Giardia* and *Eimeria* are protozoa. The *-static* suffix means that the drug inhibits growth but does not kill the organism outright, as the *-cidal* drugs do.

2. **c** The minimum inhibitory concentration (MIC) for each pathologic organism can give an idea as to how effective the antibiotic will be. If antibiotic A has a high MIC for a particular bacterium as compared with antibiotic B, *more* antibiotic A must be present *at the site of infection* for it to be effective against the microorganism.

3. **d** Aminoglycosides are a diverse and commonly used group of antimicrobial drugs. They are powerful and have potentially severe side effects. It is therefore important to know which drugs are aminoglycosides so that precautions can be taken to decrease the risk of serious side effects.

4. **d** Aminoglycosides are *nephrotoxic* (kidney) and *ototoxic* (ear).

5. **a** High dosages may increase the risk of toxicity, but they usually are sufficient to kill bacteria and prevent the *survival of the fittest* selection process that occurs when low dosages or ineffective antibiotics are used.

6. **c** Penicillins interfere with formation of the bacterial cell wall, which occurs only just after bacteria have divided. Once the bacterial cell wall is formed, penicillin is ineffective against it.

7. **a** Antifungal agents (e.g., griseofulvin) can cause birth defects if given to pregnant animals. While quinolines (enrofloxacin—Baytril) work against bacterial DNA, they are selective for bacterial DNA and do *not* affect mammalian DNA. Some antiviral agents can alter mammalian DNA, but most of the agents used in veterinary medicine kill certain viruses by destroying the envelope that surrounds them.

8. **b** Penicillin G is readily destroyed by the acidic environment in the stomach.

9. **b** Allergic reaction and anaphylaxis are the most common side effects seen with penicillin. Fortunately these occur in a very small percentage of animals treated with this otherwise safe drug. It is important, however, that technicians be aware of the signs of this reaction in animals they are monitoring.

10. **b** Cloxacillin, dicloxacillin, and oxacillin are types of penicillin used in veterinary medicine that are effective against β-lactamase–producing bacteria. These penicillins, however, are not *super penicillins*. Their effectiveness against β-lactamase–producing bacteria must be balanced against their decreased effectiveness against other bacteria that penicillin G or amoxicillin is more likely to eliminate.

11. **b** All of these are *synergists*, meaning that they increase the killing power of another compound. Trimethoprim and ormetoprim are added to sulfa drugs, and piperonyl butoxide is added to pyrethrin flea and bug sprays to increase insecticidal activity.

12. **b** Procaine penicillin G must be given only every 1 to 2 days (as opposed to plain penicillin G, which must be given 2 to 3 times a day). Benzathine penicillin G must be given only every 5 days because of delayed absorption of the drug from the site of injection. Whereas procaine is indeed a weak local anesthetic, its addition to penicillin G is for the *repository* effect and not for its anesthetic quality.

13. **b** The latter generations tended to shift their spectrum of activity to a greater extent against Gram-negative bacteria and slightly away from Gram-positive bacteria. In severe infections with Gram-negative bacteria, the concept of generation when selecting a cephalosporin becomes very important.

14. **a** It is important to remember that aminoglycosides are largely ineffective against anaerobic bacteria. Thus, a closed abscess provides an environment in which this otherwise very effective antibiotic will not work. Aminoglycosides are effective against many Gram-positive bacteria; they act by disrupting protein production, not by destroying bacterial DNA.

15. **b** Aminoglycoside molecules are very *hydrophilic*, which means they do not effectively penetrate intact cellular membranes (such as that lining the gastrointestinal tract). Thus, neomycin, for the most part, remains in the bowel lumen and does not reach the kidneys.

16. **b** Aminoglycosides tend to accumulate in the fluid of the inner ear. If these concentrations rise high enough, they can damage the cells involved with hearing and balance and produce deafness and difficulty with maintaining balance.

17. **c** The risk of nephrotoxicity is diminished by ensuring that during the time between doses, the concentration of aminoglycoside in the body *decreases* below a certain critical level. This decrease in concentration slows accumulation of aminoglycosides in the kidney tissue and inner ear and decreases the risk of nephrotoxicity or ototoxicity. A continuous intravenous infusion (drip) would not allow the concentrations to drop below this critical level.

18. **d** Casts and protein appear in the urine during the early stages of kidney insult. BUN and creatinine levels do not increase until 66% to 75% of the kidney has already been severely damaged.

19. **c** Aminoglycosides work by binding to ribosomes (made from ribonucleic acid or RNA). If there are lysed white blood cells (WBCs) present, the nucleic acid from the cellular debris binds to the aminoglycosides and prevents them from acting against the bacteria.

20. **b** Enrofloxacin is more commonly used in veterinary medicine as Baytril (trade name).

21. **a** The prostate has a blood-tissue barrier that blocks entrance of many antibiotics in a way similar to the way in which the blood-brain barrier prevents many substances from entering the brain.

22. **b** Enrofloxacin adversely affects developing joint cartilage in dogs. Thus, enrofloxacin should not be used in small and medium-sized dogs between the ages of 2 and 8 months and even later in large-breed dogs. It should not be used in horses for the same reason.

23. **c** Tetracyclines are effective against the spirochetes (*Borrelia*) that cause Lyme disease. Penicillins are also effective against this organism.

24. **c** Calcium in the gastrointestinal tract chelates (combines with) tetracycline in such a way that the drug cannot be absorbed and is rendered ineffective. This is the reason oral tetracycline should not be given with milk products (cheese, cottage cheese). The same is true for magnesium-containing foods or products (e.g., antacids).

25. **b** The same attraction that chelates calcium to tetracycline binds tetracycline to bone and enamel. The yellow mottling of otherwise white dental enamel can be quite unsightly.

26. **b** Penicillins and cephalosporins require actively dividing bacteria to disrupt the forming bacterial cell wall and subsequently destroy the bacterium. Bacteriostatic drugs prevent bacteria from dividing; thus, penicillins and cephalosporins do not have an opportunity to disrupt the bacterial cell wall.

27. **d** Chloramphenicol exists largely in a non-ionized (lipophilic) form that can readily cross membranes. Most other antibiotics exist in an ionized (hydrophilic) form at normal body pH. Thus, they are prevented from readily crossing lipid membranes.

28. **a** Barbiturates rely heavily on the liver for their removal from the body. Any alteration in liver enzyme function is likely to affect barbiturate elimination and duration of action (e.g., prolongation of barbiturate anesthesia).

29. **b** The neonatal liver is not fully capable of functioning for several weeks. Thus, the neonate is unable to metabolize chloramphenicol very readily. The same is true for cats of any age.

30. **b** Chloramphenicol attaches to mitochondrial ribosomes in the bone marrow and can result in suppression of marrow blood cell formation. The result is severe anemia.

31. **c** The Food and Drug Administration (FDA) has banned use of chloramphenicol in any animal to be used for food production.

32. **b** When an animal is dehydrated, there is less water passing through the kidneys, resulting in possible precipitation of sulfate crystals that, in turn, can damage the kidneys.

33. **b** By themselves, most sulfonamides are largely bacteriostatic. With addition of ormetroprim or trimethoprim, the combined drugs are bactericidal.

34. **c** Irreversible and reversible keratoconjunctivitis sicca, or *dry eye,* has been reported several times. Excessive ocular discharge or behavior that indicates pain or discomfort associated with the eye in an animal receiving sulfa drugs should be seen by a veterinary professional.

35. **c** Metronidiazole is commonly prescribed as a therapeutic trial for suspected giardiasis even if the organism cannot be demonstrated on fecal examinations.

36. **d** These drugs are used to treat dermatophyte infections like ringworm but often have potentially severe side effects (including birth defects) if used inappropriately. The veterinary professional should be familiar with possible adverse reactions before using them.

37. **d** Primidone is still used, but it has enough side effects that it is no longer the drug of choice for controlling seizures. Phenytoin (Dilantin) is poorly absorbed in dogs and blood levels are difficult to control. Diazepam (Valium) is not very effective when given PO (although it is excellent when given IV) because little of the drug reaches systemic circulation because of the liver's *first-pass* effect.

38. **b** Approximately 85% of primidone is converted to phenobarbital, which in turn constitutes the major drug controlling seizure activity.

39. **b** This was the first anticonvulsant used in the late 1800s in people. Much of its mechanism of action is still unknown.

40. **d** Doxapram stimulates the brainstem respiratory centers.

41. **c**

42. **a**

43. **b**

44. **c** Butorphanol is also used as an analgesic in preanesthesia protocols.

45. **d** β_2-Receptors relax the smooth muscles that encircle the bronchioles.

46. **a** These drugs quickly reverse the bronchoconstriction caused by allergic insult, such as asthma. β_2-Receptors are also found on the arterioles, where stimulation can cause vasodilatation and a resulting drop in blood pressure. Therefore, these drugs should be used with caution or not at all in shock patients. Productive coughs should not be suppressed, as they are the most effective mechanism for removing large amounts of fluid and mucus from the respiratory tree.

47. **a** Aminophylline is actually made of 80% theophylline and 20% salt to decrease the gastrointestinal irritation when given PO.

48. **d** This is a very important consideration if the animal has an irregular heartbeat *and* a weak heart; the drug that controls the irregular heartbeat further weakens the strength of the contraction.

49. **b** Propranolol and procainamide are also antiarrhythmics but are not used as much as lidocaine.

50. **b** Propranolol is a rather nonspecific beta blocker (it blocks both β_1- and β_2-receptors). Blocking the receptors prevents the sympathetic nervous system from stimulating the heart and allows the parasympathetic system to naturally slow the heart rate.

51. **c** The therapeutic index measures how close toxic concentrations are to minimal therapeutic concentrations. *a* and *b* are incorrect because the terms *high* and *low* are meaningless by themselves. A toxic concentration may be *low,* but if the amount of drug needed to produce the beneficial effect is significantly *lower* than the toxic concentrations, the drug has a fairly wide or large therapeutic index. If, on the other hand, it takes *high* concentrations to produce toxicity but also *high* concentrations to have any beneficial effect, there is not much difference between the toxic dose and the beneficial dose; consequently, the therapeutic index is narrow or small.

52. **c** The gastrointestinal tract usually shows the first signs of digoxin toxicity.

53. **d** Hypokalemia, often caused by some diuretics used in patients with cardiovascular disease, increases the risk of digoxin toxicity. Low magnesium concentrations also do this. Sometimes patients receiving diuretics plus digoxin are given potassium supplementation to reduce the risk of digoxin toxicity.

54. **d** Because digoxin is excreted largely through the kidneys, any decrease in renal function (including old age changes) may require decreasing the digoxin dose.

55. **b** ACE inhibitors block the *a*ngiotensin-*c*onverting *e*nzyme, which is an enzyme that normally produces angiotensin II, a very potent vasoconstrictor. By blocking formation of vasoconstrictor, the ACE inhibitor allows vasodilatation. The α_1-receptors on arterioles cause vasoconstriction when they are stimulated. Blocking α_1-receptors allows the vessels to dilate.

56. **d** Hydralazine dilates arterioles; prazosin and captopril dilate both arterioles and venules.

57. **b** Nitroglycerin is a venodilator, and, perhaps more importantly, it also dilates cardiac arterioles, providing improved blood supply to the cardiac muscle.

58. **a** These three diuretics work on different parts of the renal nephron to promote diuresis (increased urine production).

59. **b** Aspirin is also used in heartworm disease to decrease clot formation and proliferation of the pulmonary arterial lining, both of which can significantly narrow the pulmonary arteries in dogs with heartworm disease.

60. **b** C-II are drugs with the highest potential for abuse that can be prescribed without special permission. C-I drugs have no proven or accepted medical application (heroin, marijuana, cocaine). C-V drugs have the lowest potential for abuse.

61. **c** Apomorphine is a potent emetic (stimulator of vomiting). It is usually administered via drops (crushed tablet in saline or water) or by placing the tablet directly into the conjunctival sac of the eye.

62. **d** Dimenhydrinate (Dramamine) and diphenhydramine (Benadryl) are antihistamines. Because histamine release is involved with vestibular stimulation of vomiting (vestibular function controls balance, sense of motion), blocking histamine receptors decreases vomiting caused by *motion sickness*. Acepromazine and other phenothiazine tranquilizers are also prescribed. Not one of these drugs is very effective in preventing vomiting associated with gastrointestinal irritation or causes other than motion.

63. **b** Syrup of ipecac is an emetic. It is important to remember that syrup of ipecac takes up to 20 minutes to work because it has to move into the duodenum to stimulate the gastrointestinal tract and be absorbed. Once absorbed it stimulates the chemoreceptor-trigger zone.

64. **b** Syrup of ipecac tends to coat the charcoal, preventing the toxicant from being absorbed by the charcoal. The charcoal tends to keep the syrup of ipecac away from the gastrointestinal wall, thus preventing it from irritating the gastrointestinal tract and inducing the desired emetic effect.

65. **d** These drugs are anticholinergic; that is, they work against acetylcholine. Acetylcholine is the neurotransmitter heavily involved with the parasympathetic nervous system. Blocking acetylcholine impairs the parasympathetic nervous system. The parasympathetic nervous system normally stimulates gastrointestinal movement, secretion, and blood flow. Therefore, anything that decreases the effect of the parasympathetic nervous system decreases gastrointestinal movement, secretion, and blood flow to the gut.

66. **c** Opioid drugs (narcotics) are used to treat diarrhea by increasing segmental contractions of the bowel, thus increasing the resistance to feces flow.

67. **c** Pepto-Bismol contains this ingredient. The salicylate blocks prostaglandin formation in the gastrointestinal tract. Prostaglandins normally stimulate fluid secretions; therefore, blocking prostaglandin formation decreases the fluid consistency of the feces.

68. **c** Naturally occurring prostaglandins have a protective effect on the gastrointestinal tract. They increase intestinal secretions (including gastric mucus) and maintain normal perfusion of tissues. Thus, the wall of the stomach and intestine is normally well protected and, if injured, repairs itself readily. Nonsteroidal antiinflammatory drugs (NSAIDs) block prostaglandin formation. And, as a side effect, they also block formation of the *good* prostaglandins that normally protect the stomach and intestinal tract.

69. **d** H$_2$ receptors are located on the cells that secrete hydrochloric acid into the stomach. When these receptors are blocked, the amount of acid dumped into the stomach is reduced. This is important for animals (and people) who have ulcers associated with gastric hyperacidity.

70. **a** This drug forms a sticky paste when exposed to the acidic pH of the stomach. The paste adheres to ulcer sites and covers them like a Band-Aid, protecting the ulcer from the acidic environment of the stomach.

71. **c** TSH is available only in injectable form. Thyroid extract is made from pulverized thyroid glands and its potency is somewhat inconsistent from dose to dose. T$_3$ is the active hormone, but using it as a supplement bypasses the normal regulatory mechanism that tissues have for converting just enough T$_4$ to T$_3$ to meet their metabolic needs. Therefore, T$_4$ is the best drug to use.

72. **c** These drugs prevent formation of new thyroid hormone, thus allowing concentrations of T$_3$ and T$_4$ to drop to normal levels. However, they do *not* *kill* the thyroid tumor cells, which are producing the increased T$_3$ and T$_4$, although they keep them from producing excess hormone. If use of the drugs is stopped, the levels of T$_3$ and T$_4$ quickly become elevated again.

73. **c**

74. **d**

75. **b** Progesterone increases uterine secretions and causes the endometrium to become a wonderful incubation site for bacteria, which can lead to pyometra.

76. **a** Pet owners must be aware of the risk before these drugs are used in their animals. Pyometra occurs because high levels of estrogens (e.g., ECP) cause the uterine cells to produce more receptors to progesterone, essentially making the uterus more susceptible to pyometra. Thus, when progesterone starts to be produced by the body, the uterus responds more strongly than normal as far as creating an *ideal* environment for a fetus or for bacteria.

77. **b** This is known by the trade name Ovaban.

78. **c** Acetaminophen, commonly marketed as Tylenol and other products, does not block prostaglandin formation as the NSAIDs do. It is this blockage of prostaglandins that leads to decreased mucus formation in the stomach, decreased perfusion of gastric tissues, and subsequently increased risk for gastritis and ulcer formation.

79. **d** Hydrocortisone is considered short acting (less than 12 hours). Prednisone, prednisolone, and triamcinolone are considered intermediate acting (12 to 36 hours). Dexamethasone exerts an effect on the body for 48 hours or longer.

80. **a** Increased water consumption necessitates that the owner make accommodations for greater urinary frequency if the pet is an indoor animal.

81. **c** Glucocorticoids cause eosinophils and lymphocytes to be sequestered (taken up or *hidden*) from the general circulation; as a result, their numbers in the CBC decrease. Neutrophils, by contrast, come off the walls of the blood vessels and reenter the general circulation, causing neutrophilia.

82. **c** Iatrogenic means caused by the treatment itself. Cushing's disease is hyperadrenocorticism, or the condition caused by excessive glucocorticoids.

83. **a**

84. **b** NSAIDs block prostaglandins. Prostaglandins maintain normal health of the gastrointestinal tract by increasing protective secretions and maintaining normal blood flow to the stomach; they also maintain normal blood supply to the kidneys in situations where renal blood flow is normally decreased (e.g., dehydration, shock, drop in blood pressure). Thus blocked prostaglandin formation predisposes an animal to gastritis, potential ulcer formation, and renal damage from inadequate blood and oxygen supplies.

85. **a** Phenylbutazone injection outside the vein can cause severe skin sloughing in horses.

86. **b** DMSO is also known for its potent *garlic* or *raw oyster* odor.

87. **b** Chlorpyrifos (Dursban) is an organophosphate, as is cythioate. Organophosphate insecticides (including malathion, diazinon, and dichlorvos) work by a similar mechanism to carbamate insecticides, such as carbaril (Sevin) and methocarbamate.

88. **b** Anticestodals are also sometimes referred to as *taeniacides.* Always check to see which tapeworms an anticestodal is effective against, as some important species of tapeworm may not be killed by all *anticestodal* medications.

89. **b** Even the once-a-month heartworm preventives have a cautionary statement, although they appear to be safe in collies when used according to label directions.

90. **c** Although not officially approved for this use, ivermectin is the drug of choice for clearing *Dirofilaria* microfilariae from the blood of dogs.

91. **d** Organophosphates stimulate the parasympathetic nervous system and therefore produce gastrointestinal hyperactivity (vomiting, diarrhea), bronchoconstriction, increased urination, and constricted pupils. Atropine blocks the parasympathetic nervous system receptor sites and therefore blocks the parasympathetic effects.

92. **b** Amitraz (Mitaban) was developed to treat demodectic mange, a traditionally difficult condition to manage. Fenoxycarb is an insect growth regulator. Pyrethrin and allethrin are pyrethroid insecticides.

93. **c** Insect growth regulators prevent growth of the insect, which results in death of the insect. Synergists (piperonyl butoxide) are compounds added to insecticides (like pyrethrins) to improve their insecticidal activity. Repellents used in veterinary products include butoxypolypropylene glycol (Butox PPG) and diethyltoluamide (DEET).

94. **d** The pharmacist is not likely to know how many tablets must be dispensed. The DEA number is not required except for prescriptions for controlled substances (barbiturates, tranquilizers), in which case some states require that a different prescription form be submitted.

95. **b**

96. **c** q8h = every 8 hours or three times daily (tid).

97. **c**

98. **c** OD = oculus dexter *(dexter* means right) and OS = oculus sinister *(sinister* means left).

99. **a** (*gr* means grain, but *g* means gram.)

100. **b** Although traditionally 65 mg = 1 grain, many products (phenobarbital, aspirin) that are measured in grains use the conversion 60 mg = 1 grain.

101. **b** The concentration of a solution is a weight (mg, kg, g, gr, IU, u) per volume (ml, L, cc); *units per ml* (sometimes expressed as IU/ml) is commonly used for penicillin and insulin.

102. **c**

103. **b** 1 cc = 1 ml, so there are 15 milliliters in a tablespoon.

104. **b** Every 6 hours = 4 times daily (or per 24 hr); the abbreviation for *4 times daily* (QID) should not be confused with the abbreviation for *every day* (QD).

105. **d** There are 2.2 lb for each kg (10 × 2.2 = 22).

106. **d** A suspension must be stirred up or shaken before dispensing to ensure uniform distribution of the drug throughout the liquid (or oil, in the case of emulsions) vehicle.

107. **b** Any manner of use other than that specified on the drug label is termed *extra-label*. This is quite common in veterinary medicine. However, it should be done only when there is an established veterinarian-client-patient relationship, when no other drug is available that will accomplish the goal, and when safety precautions are taken to prevent contamination of meat and milk in food-producing animals.

108. **d** Any time a medication is administered to food animals, the withdrawal time *must* be clearly indicated to the livestock owner.

109. **b** The loading dose establishes adequate concentrations of the drug in the body. The smaller maintenance doses are then designed to keep the concentrations within that acceptable range.

110. **c** A 5% solution contains 5 g/100 ml.

111. **c** Careful here! There are 24 *grams* per 100 milliliters, which is 0.24 *gram* per milliliter; 0.24 g = 240 mg.

112. **b** Antineoplastic drugs are cancer-fighting agents. They are potent and lethal to rapidly dividing cells, regardless of what animal (including the technician) they contact.

113. **d** Because most drugs leave the body through the kidneys and liver, a decrease in the function of these organs *decreases* the rate at which the drugs leave the body. Elimination rate is decreased, and half-life (the time it takes for half of the drug to leave the body) is prolonged or increased.

114. **b** Drugs are rated from C-I (most potential for abuse) to C-V (least potential for abuse).

115. **d**

116. **b** Diluting the agent is most important. Sometimes lidocaine is added to the infiltrate. Massaging the area and applying heat are also sometimes suggested.

117. **c** 16 fluid ounces = 473 ml; therefore, 1 fluid ounce (oz) = 29.6 ml, which is approximately 30 ml.

Radiography

Connie Han, RVT   *Cheryl Hurd, RVT*
Blaine R. Russell, DVM

Recommended Reading

Barber DL, Lewis RE: *Guide for radiology service in veterinary medicine,* Athens, 1982, University of Georgia.
Lavin LM: *Radiography in veterinary technology,* Philadelphia, 1994, WB Saunders.
McCurnin DM: *Clinical textbook for veterinary technicians,* ed 3, Philadelphia, 1994, WB Saunders.

Questions

General

1. The milliamp (mA) selector
   a. Controls the number of electrons produced by the filament
   b. Controls the duration of exposure
   c. Determines the penetrability of the x-ray beam
   d. Determines the energy of the x-ray beam

2. Which ratio grid requires the highest milliamperes (mAs) to obtain the desired density on a finished radiographic film?
   a. 8:1
   b. 12:1
   c. 10:1
   d. 5:1

3. Which ratio grid is most efficient?
   a. 8:1 with 102 lines/inch
   b. 5:1 with 80 lines/inch
   c. 10:1 with 103 lines/inch
   d. 12:1with 113 lines/inch

Practice answer sheet is on page 341.

Correct answers are on pages 277–283.

4. How does milliamperage affect the electrons in an x-ray beam?
   a. Increasing the milliamperage increases the number of electrons produced and increases the number of x-rays produced
   b. Increasing the milliamperage increases the speed at which the electrons hit the anode, which increases the penetrating power of the x-ray beam
   c. Decreasing the milliamperage increases the number of electrons generated and decreases the number of x-rays produced
   d. Decreasing the milliamperage decreases the speed at which the electrons hit the anode, which decreases the number of x-rays available

5. Which type of x-ray machine allows for faster time and more output?
   a. Half-wave rectified, single phase
   b. Full-wave rectified, single phase
   c. Full-wave rectified, three phase
   d. Self-rectified

6. Which of the following controls radiographic contrast?
   a. kVp
   b. mAs
   c. Focal film distance
   d. Object film distance

7. Which of the following does *not* affect radiographic density?
   a. kVp
   b. mAs
   c. Focal-film distance
   d. Object-film distance

8. The focusing cup of an x-ray machine is a
   a. Small depression where the filament is placed
   b. Negative electrode
   c. Tungsten coil that emits electrons when heated
   d. Positive electrode

9. The target of an x-ray machine is
   a. A tungsten coil that emits electrons when heated
   b. A small depression where the filament is placed
   c. An area of the anode struck by electrons during an exposure
   d. A positive electrode

10. The filament of an x-ray tube is the
    a. Negative electrode
    b. Positive electrode
    c. Area of the anode struck by electrons during an exposure
    d. Tungsten coil that emits electrons when heated

11. When a spin top test is performed on a full-wave rectified machine, how many dots should you see in $\frac{1}{60}$ second?
    a. 6
    b. 2
    c. 1
    d. 12

12. If you suspect that your machine is *not* producing x-radiation, what test can you perform?
    a. Spin top
    b. Film/screen contact
    c. Step wedge
    d. Screen fluorescence

13. Tube saturation can occur with a
    a. Too-high kVp reading
    b. Too-high mA reading
    c. Too-low kVp reading
    d. Too-low mA reading

14. Which of the following absorbs the most x-rays?
    a. Fat
    b. Air
    c. Metal
    d. Bone

15. Which direction should a grid move in relation to the grid lines in order to blur lines?
    a. Same direction as the grid lines
    b. Perpendicular to the grid lines
    c. Always stationary
    d. Moves in both directions

16. If the focal-film distance is increased by a factor of 2, how must the milliamps be adjusted to maintain density?
    a. Increased by a factor or 4
    b. Increased by a factor of 2
    c. Decreased by a factor of 4
    d. Decreased by a factor of 2

17. If a radiographic film appears overexposed, is it too light or too dark? Would you *increase* or *decrease* the exposure to improve the quality?
    a. Too dark; exposure should be increased
    b. Too light; exposure should be increased
    c. Too dark; exposure should be decreased
    d. Too light; exposure should be decreased

18. How does kVp affect the electrons and the x-ray beam?
    a. Increasing it increases the number of electrons produced and also increases the penetrating power of the x-ray beam
    b. Decreasing it decreases the number of electrons produced and also decreases the number of x-rays produced
    c. Increasing it increases the speed at which electrons are pulled across to the anode and also increases the penetrating power of the x-ray beam
    d. Increasing it increases the speed at which electrons are pulled across to the anode and lengthens the wavelength of the x-rays produced, making them more penetrating

19. A radiographic film is underexposed. It does not appear to be properly penetrated. The technique used to make the film was 5 mA and 60 kVp. Which technique might be chosen to *increase* the density and penetration of the radiographic film?
    a. 10 mA and 60 kVp
    b. 5 mA and 70 kVp
    c. 2.5 mA and 70 kVp
    d. 10 mA and 50 kVp

20. An abdominal radiographic film is made at 12 mA and 68 kVp. It is now necessary to *halve* the radiographic density. What techniques would you use?
    a. 6 mA and 82 kVp
    b. 12 mA and 82 kVp
    c. 6 mA and 68 kVp
    d. 10 mA and 68 kVp

21. Tube overload occurs with:
    a. Too-high kVp and mAs
    b. Too-low kVp and mAs
    c. Too-high kVp
    d. Too-low mAs

22. What effect does doubling the mAs have on radiographic density?
    a. Doubles it
    b. Halves it
    c. Density is the same
    d. Radiographic film is blackened

23. The electron cloud is generated at the
    a. Anode
    b. Cathode
    c. Focal spot
    d. Effective focal spot

24. Which technique produces the image with the most radiographic density?
    a. 100 mA, $\frac{1}{10}$ sec
    b. 150 mA, $\frac{1}{30}$ sec
    c. 200 mA, $\frac{1}{20}$ sec
    d. 200 mA, $\frac{1}{10}$ sec

Correct answers are on pages 277–283.

25. Which contrast study best demonstrates a diaphragmatic hernia?
    a. Pneumocystography
    b. Pneumoperitoneography
    c. Double-contrast cystography
    d. Celiography

26. Which contrast medium is considered negative contrast?
    a. Water-soluble organic iodide
    b. Barium sulfate
    c. Air
    d. Organic iodide

27. Which contrast procedure generally uses both positive and negative contrast media?
    a. Barium enema
    b. Urethrography
    c. Excretory urogram
    d. Myelography

28. Which contrast medium is *contraindicated* if a rupture or perforation of the bowel is suspected?
    a. Diatrizoate
    b. Barium sulfate
    c. Water-soluble organic iodide
    d. Air

29. Which contrast study requires the patient's head to be elevated after injection of contrast medium?
    a. Arthrography
    b. Fistulography
    c. Myelography
    d. Pneumoperitonography

30. Which contrast medium is be considered positive contrast?
    a. Nitrous oxide
    b. Air
    c. Barium sulfate
    d. Oxygen

31. Which contrast study is used to evaluate the kidneys, ureters, and urinary bladder?
    a. Urethrography
    b. Positive-contrast cystography
    c. Double-contrast cystography
    d. Excretory urography

32. Which contrast medium appears radiolucent on the finished radiographic film?
    a. Barium sulfate
    b. Metrizamide
    c. Air
    d. Water-soluble organic iodide

33. Which contrast study of the gastrointestinal tract is monitored until contrast medium reaches the colon?
    a. Gastrography
    b. Upper gastrointestinal series
    c. Barium enema
    d. Esophagography

34. Which of the following is *not* a reason why survey radiographic films should always be made before administering contrast medium?
    a. To establish proper exposure technique
    b. To establish proper patient preparation
    c. To make a diagnosis
    d. To help determine the dosage of contrast medium

35. Which contrast medium appears radiopaque on a radiographic film?
    a. Air
    b. Nitrous oxide
    c. Oxygen
    d. Barium sulfate

36. Which contrast study is indicated if a draining tract is present?
    a. Arthrography
    b. Celiography
    c. Fistulography
    d. Myelography

37. Which contrast study is used to detect ectopic ureters?
    a. Excretory urogram
    b. Urethrography
    c. Vaginography
    d. Positive-contrast cystography

38. With the heel effect, the x-ray beam intensity is greater toward the
    a. Anode
    b. Collimator
    c. Cathode
    d. Tube window

39. Which factor does *not* affect the amount of penumbra on a radiographic film and does *not* contribute to the penumbra?
    a. Object-film distance
    b. kVp
    c. Focal-film distance
    d. Focal spot size

40. The spin top test is performed when you suspect a problem with the
    a. mA stations
    b. X-ray tube
    c. Timer
    d. kVp

DARKROOM

A good layout of a darkroom should include dry bench and wet bench areas, separate from one another. For Questions 41 through 44, select the area where each task should be performed from the two choices below.

    a. Wet bench
    b. Dry bench

41. Loading and unloading cassettes.

42. Drying washed films.

43. Film storage.

44. Film processing.

45. How do low-grade light leaks in the darkroom affect film quality?
    a. They have no effect on the film quality
    b. They increase film quality by decreasing scatter radiation
    c. They decrease film quality by increasing overall fog of the film
    d. They decrease film quality by decreasing radiographic density

46. When must radiographs be labeled for certification organizations and for legal purposes?
    a. Before exposure and after processing
    b. During or after exposure but before processing
    c. After exposure and after processing
    d. Before filing or mailing

47. What is the total time the film should be placed in the fixer?
    a. Two times the developing time
    b. Three times the developing time
    c. The same as the developing time
    d. 30 seconds

48. A radiographic film of a dog's thorax is made. What occurs when the film is placed in the developer?
    a. The sensitized silver halide crystals are changed into black metallic silver
    b. The potassium bromide crystals are changed into black metallic silver
    c. The silver halide crystals are cleared from the film
    d. All the silver halide crystals are changed into black metallic silver

When manually processing films, there are two methods for maintaining the tanks: the exhausted method and the replenishing method. Answer Questions 49 through 51 by matching the two methods with the statements.

    a. Exhausted method
    b. Replenishing method

49. Allows chemicals to drain from the film back into their respective tanks.

50. Allows chemicals to drain only into the wash tank.

51. Periodically, chemicals are added to bring chemical levels back up to the top of the tanks.

Correct answers are on pages 277–283.

52. How often should the manual processing tanks be drained and cleaned and old chemicals replaced with fresh chemicals?
    a. Once a day
    b. Once a week
    c. At least every 3 months
    d. Once a year

53. What would happen if exposed film were accidentally placed in the fixer before being placed in the developer?
    a. The radiographic film turns black
    b. The radiographic film becomes clear
    c. If the mistake is detected soon enough, the image can be spared
    d. The radiographic film appears underexposed

54. The pH of the developer chemicals is
    a. Strongly acidic
    b. Neutral
    c. Alkaline
    d. Slightly acidic

55. When reconstituting the powder form of processing chemicals, what is one important factor to remember?
    a. Always reconstitute the chemicals in the darkroom
    b. Always reconstitute the chemicals under bright lights
    c. Always use sterile saline to reconstitute the chemicals
    d. Never reconstitute the chemicals in the darkroom

56. A radiographic film of a cat's thorax is made. When viewing the film, you note a decrease in radiographic density and a gray swirly appearance of the background. What caused this problem?
    a. Processing chemicals were too hot
    b. Film was not left in the fixer long enough
    c. Processing chemicals were too cold
    d. Film was not washed for 30 minutes after processing

57. Radiographic films made 5 years earlier have turned brown. What was the cause?
    a. Too long in the developer
    b. Too long in the fixer
    c. Incomplete development
    d. Incomplete final wash

58. When using a direct safelight system, the distance from the workbench should be at least
    a. 20 inches
    b. 30 inches
    c. 48 inches
    d. 72 inches

59. Lateral and ventrodorsal projections of a dog's abdomen are made and manually processed at the same time. However, both radiographic films have identical areas of decreased radiographic density. What could have caused this artifact on both films?
    a. They stuck together in the fixer
    b. They stuck together in the developer
    c. They stuck together in the wash tank
    d. They were overexposed

FILM

60. What is a latent image?
    a. An image on the film after processing
    b. Calcium tungstate crystals in the film's emulsion that have been exposed to radiant energy before processing
    c. Silver halide crystals in the film's emulsion that have been exposed to radiant energy before processing
    d. An image on the film before exposure

61. Screen-type film
    a. Is most sensitive to light produced by the intensifying screen
    b. Is most sensitive to direct x-ray beams
    c. Requires a longer exposure time than direct-exposure film
    d. Can be processed only manually

Answers

General

1. **a** The mA selector controls the number of electrons produced at the filament.

2. **b** With a 12:1 ratio grid, more x-rays are absorbed, requiring more x-rays to be produced or a higher mAs.

3. **d** A 12:1 ratio grid with 113 lines per inch absorbs more scatter, producing an image with better contrast and less fogging on the finished radiographic film.

4. **a**

5. **c** A full-wave rectified, three phase allows for more positive potential across the terminals of the tube, producing a higher energy of electrons and a more constant energy x-ray beam.

6. **a** kVp controls radiographic contrast by increasing or decreasing the shades of gray. The higher the kVp, the longer the scale of contrast. (More grays can be seen.)

7. **d** The object-film distance does not influence radiographic density.

8. **a** The focusing cup focuses the beam of electrons on the focal spot of the anode.

9. **c** The target of an x-ray machine is the area of the anode struck by electrons during an exposure.

10. **d**

11. **b** Two dots are seen when a spin top test is performed on a full-wave rectified machine in $1/60$ second. The spin top is the number of dots = pulsation frequency × exposure time.

12. **d** A screen can be placed open under the x-ray beam and a low exposure made. If x-radiation is being produced, the screen will fluoresce.

13. **c** Tube saturation occurs when there is not enough positive potential (voltage) between the cathode and anode to pull all the electrons across the tube. The extra electrons accumulate on the glass envelope and can crack the tube.

14. **c** Metal has the highest x-ray absorption because it is the most dense.

15. **b** A grid moves in the opposite direction from the grid lines. This erases the lines so they are not visible on the radiographic film.

16. **a** The Inverse Square Law states that the intensity of the x-ray beam is inversely proportional to the square of the distance from the source of the x-rays. The same number of x-rays must diverge, covering an area that is four times as large.

17. **c**

18. **c**

19. **b** Increasing the kVp 20% doubles the radiographic density and increases the penetration.

20. **c** Because mAs controls the number of x-rays produced, reducing the mAs reduces radiographic density.

21. **a** When kVp and mAs are too high for the machine, too much heat is created, causing the anode to crack.

22. **a** mAs controls the number of x-rays produced. If the mAs is doubled, this doubles the density on the radiographic film.

23. **b** The cathode holds the filament. When current is applied to the filament, electrons *boil off*, producing an electron cloud.

24. **d** 200 mA, $^1/_{10}$ second = 20 mAs. This is the highest mAs, which produces more x-rays.

25. **d** Celiography is useful when studying the abdominal cavity and the integrity of the diaphragm.

26. **c** Air appears black on a radiographic film.

27. **a** A barium enema generally uses both positive- and negative-contrast media to evaluate the colon.

28. **b** Barium sulfate can be toxic to the peritoneum.

29. **c** The head is elevated after injection for a myelogram to decrease the chance of seizure.

30. **c** Barium sulfate has a high atomic number and appears white on a radiographic film.

31. **d** Excretory urography provides information relative to renal function and the structure of the kidneys, ureters, and bladder.

32. **c** Air appears radiolucent (black) on a radiographic film.

33. **b** This contrast study is used to evaluate the stomach and small intestines. The contrast medium is administered orally, and films are made during transit of the contrast medium through the stomach and small bowel into the colon.

34. **d** The dose of contrast medium is calculated using the weight of the animal.

35. **d** Barium sulfate appears radiopaque (white) on a radiographic film.

36. **c** Fistulography is a contrast study that delineates the extent and possibly the origin of fistulous tracts.

37. **a** An excretory urogram identifies the size, shape, location, and margination of the kidneys and ureters.

38. **c** The cathode has the higher x-ray beam intensity because x-rays are absorbed by the target and anode.

39. **b** kVp controls the penetration power and scale of contrast on the film; it has no effect on penumbra. Penumbra causes a loss of detail. There are three main factors in the amount of penumbra on a radiographic film; these are focal-film distance, object-film distance, and focal-spot size.

40. **c** The spin top is number of dots = pulsation frequency × exposure time. If the number of dots is incorrect, there is a problem with the timer.

DARKROOM

41. **b**

42. **a**

43. **b**

44. **a**

45. **c** When film is exposed to low-grade light leaks, a base fog decreases the overall quality of the finished radiographic film, decreasing contrast and detail.

46. **b** For radiographic films to be legal in court and for the certification organizations to accept them, they must be permanently identified. This can be done during the exposure with lead letters or radiopaque tape or after the exposure, but the film should be identified before the film is processed with manual or photo labelers.

47. **a** The total time the film must be in the fixer is double the time it was in the developer. The film can be viewed on a view box after the film has been in the fixer for only 30 seconds; however, it must be placed back into the fixer for the remaining time to complete the process.

48. **a**

49. **a**

50. **b**

51. **b**

52. **c** The fluids in manual processing tanks should be changed at least every 3 months. In busy practices the frequency may need to be increased to maintain the quality of the radiographic film.

53. **b** The radiographic film is clear because the fixer removes all the silver halide crystals that remain after being in the developer. If the film has not been placed in the developer, the sensitized silver halide crystals have not yet been changed into black metallic silver. The fixer then removes all the silver halide crystals, clearing the film of any image.

54. **c** Developer chemicals are kept at an alkaline pH, usually 9.8 to 11.4. Developer chemicals cannot function in a neutral or acid solution.

55. **d** The chemicals should be mixed in a bucket outside the darkroom to prevent the chemical dust from contaminating unprotected films, thus causing artifacts.

56. **c** Most manufacturers recommend the processing chemicals be at least 68° F for the chemicals to be efficient.

57. **d** If the films were not completely washed, the fixer that remained in the emulsion would oxidize, turning them a brownish color.

58. **c** A direct system shines the safelight directly toward the workbench. To prevent possible fogging of the film, the safelight should be placed at least 48 inches from the workbench.

59. **b** Because both had identical areas of decreased density, this means the films were stuck together in the developer. The density is decreased because the developer was not able to change the sensitized silver halide crystals into black metallic silver; consequently, the fixer clears the remaining silver halide crystals. This leaves an area of decreased density.

FILM

60. **c** A latent image is the silver halide crystals in the film's emulsion that have been exposed to radiant energy, causing them to become susceptible to chemical change.

61. **a** Screen-type film is more sensitive to the light from intensifying screens than it is to direct x-ray exposure.

62. **b** The emulsion is too thick for some types of direct-exposure film to be automatically processed. The processing chemicals cannot reach all of the silver halide crystals in the time it takes to automatically process.

63. **b** Direct-exposure film requires that more x-rays be generated to expose it, as it does not use the intensifying effect of the screens.

64. **c** Film is most sensitive after it has been exposed, but before it is processed. Care must be taken when handling the film after it has been exposed.

65. **b** The crystal size in high-speed film is larger, allowing a decrease in mAs; however, the detail is decreased as compared with that of slow-speed film.

66. **b** Long-latitude film can produce a long scale of contrast.

67. **d** Film should be stored away from strong chemical fumes to prevent a base fog on the film.

68. **d** When identifying films, the label should include the clinic's name; the date; the owner's and patient's names; and the species, sex, and age of the patient.

ANIMAL POSITIONING

69. **a** An oblique projection is used to delineate an area that would normally be superimposed over another (e.g., the right and left sides of the mandible on a lateral projection of the skull).

70. **b** To include the entire thorax on a radiographic film, the cranial landmark is the manubrium sterni and the caudal landmark is halfway between the xiphoid and the last rib.

71. **c** To include the entire abdomen on a radiographic film, the cranial landmark is three rib spaces cranial to the xiphoid and the caudal landmark is the greater trochanter.

72. **b**

73. **c** The endotracheal tube is removed to prevent superimposition over the main bony structures.

74. **a** Foreshortening occurs when the long bone is not parallel to the cassette, causing the bone to appear shorter than it actually is.

75. **c** Centering the beam on the joint maximizes the size of the joint space and minimize the amount of false narrowing that can occur as the center of the primary beam is moved away from the joint.

76. **b** Extending the head caudodorsally moves the trachea off the shoulder joint; extending the contralateral limb farther caudally moves the manubrium away from the shoulder joint.

77. **a**

78. **b**

79. **b**

80. **a**

81. **c**

82. **a**

83. **b** With a dorsolateral-palmaromedial oblique projection, the lateral sesamoid is imaged without superimposition of any other bones.

84. **b**

85. **b** With a left 20-degree ventral/right dorsal oblique projection of the skull, the right tympanic bulla is delineated from the left.

IMAGE PRODUCTION

86. **b** Placing the thick part of the patient toward the cathode of the x-ray tube produces a more uniform density on the radiographic film.

87. **a** Radiographic films are legal medical records and must contain all the information found in answer *a*.

88. **c** L4 is midway between the pubis and the xyphoid cartilage in a dog lying in the ventrodorsal position.

89. **c** T7 is approximately midway between the 1st and 13th rib.

90. **d** To reduce the divergent x-ray energy beam, a restriction device can focus the column of energy on the cassette.

91. **b** mA × time (in seconds) = mAs

92. **c** The larger the crystal size, the more light is produced. High-speed screens have larger crystals, even bigger than the rare-earth crystals.

93. **b** Change in kVp changes the energy level of the x-ray beam.

94. **a** The distance between the source of an x-ray (focal spot) and the image receptor (x-ray film) is called the focal-film distance.

95. **b** If the object being x-rayed is farther from the receptor, the image formed on the film is magnified because the x-ray beam strikes the object farther from the projected shadow.

96. **b** A less penetrating x-ray beam produces less scatter. A focused beam also produces less scatter, and a grid reduces the scatter. All three of these features increase detail by reducing the effect of scatter radiation.

97. **c** X-rays are more visibly converted to light by rare-earth phosphorus than by calcium tungstate, a major factor in reducing exposure time. All the other items have no effect on exposure time reduction.

98. **a**

99. **d** The area of contrast is dependent upon the density and mass of the tissue or subject.

100. **c** Scatter radiation originates from the patient as the primary beam strikes the first solid object and produces secondary radiation.

101. **a** Increasing kVp causes increased scatter radiation. As a result of the increase in energy, more x-rays penetrate farther into the patient and increase the opportunity for scatter radiation.

102. **b** If a grid is used outside the specified range, grid cutoff may occur. This produces a progressive decrease in transmitted x-ray intensity near the edge of the grid.

103. **b** Calcium tungstate emits light in the blue and ultraviolet regions of the spectrum when struck by an x-ray beam.

104. **d** The larger the crystals, the faster the screen, the less the detail, and the more grainy the appearance of the image.

105. **d** Increased film speed leads to a radiographic artifact known as quantum mottle. This occurs because the faster screens are sensitive to radiation; as a result, the reduced energy levels of the settings do not produce the desired uniformity of density.

106. **c** The crystals of a fluoroscopy unit emit green light, to which the human eye is sensitive. Motion radiographic films can be seen because conventional film is substituted for the fluoroscopy screen.

107. **a** Silver halide is a compound of silver and bromine, chlorine, or iodine that forms a latent image when ionized by light or radiation.

108. **b** Ionizing radiation causes latent images to be formed on nonscreen film without intensifying screens.

109. **a** Radiographs made with nonscreen film have greater detail compared with other speed film because there is no loss of detail from intensifying screens.

110. **c** The very small silver halide crystals in the emulsion of slow x-ray film produce less change in radiographic density with changes in exposure factors.

111. **b** A processing system must be compatible with the film speed and the type of cassette to produce quality radiographic films.

112. **b** Light exposes the radiographic film unevenly, and the image on the film appears darkened, commonly known as *fogged.*

113. **b** The light bulb is commonly filtered with brown- or blue-light–sensitive film.

114. **b** The filter commonly used for the safelight when using green-light–sensitive film is dark red.

115. **a** If a lateral view of the tarsus was exposed with the toes of the patient facing to the right side of the cassette, the craniocaudal view should have the toes facing the same side of the cassette.

116. **b** If the fixer is exhausted or time in the fixer is limited, the film does not harden properly and the gelatin turns yellow.

117. **b** The 8:1 grid ratio is adequate for the average patient.

118. **c** Static electricity causes dark images as a result of the light produced over the unexposed film.

119. **b** Because x-ray film is more sensitive to light than to radiation, the use of fluorescent intensifying screens dramatically decreases the amount of radiation needed; therefore, much lower mAs settings and shorter exposure times can be used.

120. **d** Scatter radiation increases with an increase in the thickness of the body part; therefore, a better image results if scatter is reduced by absorbing the nonparallel x-rays with a grid. Body parts thicker than 10 cm scatter enough radiation to cause distortion of the image.

121. **c** Crystals in the screens fluoresce or emit light during exposure to x-rays.

122. **d** Light leakage in a darkroom, from any source, adds to the overall darkness of the image, fogging the radiographic film.

123. **d** Cross-over roller dirt is the most common cause of streaks and stains on automatically processed film.

RADIATION SAFETY

124. **a** Radiation absorbed dose (rad) is the quantity of energy imparted to matter by ionizing radiation.

125. **c** Roentgen equivalent man (rem) measures ionizing radiation absorbed by tissue.

126. **b** The dosimeter measures the actual amount of ionizing radiation, whereas the other monitoring devices indicate exposure.

127. **b** For people over 18 years of age, the upper limit is 5 rem.

128. **c** 7.5 rems × 1,000 millirems/rem = 7,500 millirems

129. **d** Wear the monitor badge in the area where exposure is most likely to occur.

130. **c** All states have one safety code in common. It requires that at least 2.5 mm of aluminum filtration of the primary beam be used in any diagnostic machine with a capacity over 70 kVp.

131. **b** The filter eliminates the less penetrating or "soft" x-rays, which have low energy.

132. **d** At no time should any part of your body even when shielded with protective covering, be exposed to the primary beam.

133. **d** Regulations in veterinary radiography require 0.5 mm of lead equivalent in the aprons and gloves because the restrainer is often very close to the primary beam.

134. **c** The intensity of the primary x-ray beam is inversely proportional to the source-image distance. At twice the distance, the beam intensity is 1/4 of the original intensity.

135. **d** The reduced radiation needed for diagnostic x-rays with rare-earth intensifying screens considerably reduces the exposure risk to the technician.

136. **d** Rare-earth screens are sensitive to green light and reduce the exposure settings necessary for image production; they therefore reduce possible radiation exposure.

137. **b** When more radiographs are made, there is more chance of exposure to ionizing radiation.

138. **b** Careful collimation reduces the amount of secondary scatter and therefore reduces exposure of the operator.

139. **d** Good technique results in less exposure because of fewer repeats.

140. **a** Chemical restraint should be used when possible so the technician does not have to be in the room with the animal during the exposure.

141. **b** Film badge reports are usually submitted monthly.

142. **a** Radiation protection is regulated by the National Committee on Radiation Protection and Measurements. Their recommendation is to supply monitoring badges at a potential level of 1/4 MPD.

143. **c** The monitor does not protect from radiation but detects radiation.

144. **c** Exposure units are physical amounts of radiation known as roentgens. Absorbed units are rads and the measurement of biological effect is a rem measurement. Radon is a radioactive gas.

145. **d** Increased distance from the primary beam greatly reduces the risk of exposure as compared with that provided by any of the devices positioned next to the primary beam.

146. **b** Nonoccupationally exposed persons can receive 10% of the adult dose. The maximum permissible dose (MPD) for the general public is set at a much lower level because the public is not monitored and is untrained to recognize and avoid exposure.

Notes

Notes

Surgical Nursing

Marta M. Bates, CAHT

Thomas Colville, DVM, MSc

Kimberly S. Cullen, CAHT

Shannon M. Dowie, CAHT

Anne D. Hope, CAHT

Marilyn L. Meyers, RVT

Mary K. Walsh, RN

Recommended Reading

Kagan KG: Aseptic technique, *Vet Tech* 13:205–211, 1992.

Knecht CD, Allen AR, Williams DJ, Johnson JH: *Fundamental techniques in veterinary surgery,* ed 3, Philadelphia, 1987, WB Saunders.

McCurnin DM: *Clinical textbook for veterinary technicians,* ed 3, Philadelphia, 1994, WB Saunders.

Slatter DH: *Textbook of small animal surgery,* Philadelphia, 1994, WB Saunders, vol 1.

Tracy DL, editor: *Small animal surgical nursing,* St Louis, 1983, Mosby.

Turner A, Simon BV, McIlwraith WC: *Techniques in large animal surgery,* ed 2, Philadelphia, 1989, Lea & Febiger.

Questions

GENERAL

1. Healing of a properly sutured surgical wound is most appropriately termed
   a. First-intention healing
   b. Granulation
   c. Secondary union
   d. Second-intention healing

2. Which of the following has the poorest potential for healing and return to normal function after damage and effective surgical repair?
   a. Bone
   b. Gastrointestinal tract
   c. Liver
   d. Nervous tissue

Practice answer sheet is on page 343.

Correct answers are on pages 305–311.

3. Which of the following best describes the location of an incision extending from the xiphoid process to the umbilicus of an animal?
   a. Flank
   b. Paracostal
   c. Paramedian
   d. Ventral midline

Questions 4 through 6

   a. Autoclave
   b. Dry heat
   c. Ethylene oxide gas
   d. Liquid chemical disinfectant

4. Agent, method, or device most appropriate for sterilizing an electric drill to be used in an orthopedic surgical procedure.

5. Agent, method, or device most appropriate for sterilizing a needle holder to be used in a surgical procedure.

6. Agent, method, or device most appropriate for sterilizing a pair of dissecting scissors to be used in a surgical procedure.

7. Which of the following describes the *minimum* exposure time and temperature to which all parts of an autoclaved surgical pack should be exposed?
   a. 121° C for 15 minutes
   b. 121° F for 15 minutes
   c. 250° C for 20 minutes
   d. 250° F for 20 minutes

8. Which of the following is the most effective and timely indicator that sterilization conditions have been met in an autoclaved surgery pack?
   a. Autoclave tape
   b. Chemical indicator
   c. Culture test
   d. Melting pellet

9. What is the proper term for microorganisms that gain entrance into an incision during a surgical procedure?
   a. Contamination
   b. Debridement
   c. Infection
   d. Septicemia

10. Which of the following does *not* have to be sterile during a surgical procedure to maintain aseptic technique?
    a. Drapes
    b. Gloves
    c. Gown
    d. Mask

11. Which of the following is the agent for autoclave sterilization?
    a. Chemical disinfectant solution
    b. Dry heat
    c. Ethylene oxide gas
    d. Steam

12. Which size of electrical clipper blade is most commonly used for removing the hair from a surgical site?
    a. #10
    b. #20
    c. #30
    d. #40

13. Which of the following is *not* an effective form of surgical hemostasis?
    a. Crushing
    b. Curettage
    c. Ligation
    d. Pressure

14. Which of the following is *not* a likely cause of dehiscence of an abdominal incision?
    a. Excessive physical activity
    b. Stormy recovery from anesthesia
    c. Surgical wound infection
    d. Suture material larger than needed

15. Which of the following is *not* an effective aseptic surgical technique?
    a. Consider a sterile item to be nonsterile if it touches a nonsterile item
    b. If the sterility of an item is in doubt, consider it sterile
    c. Nonscrubbed personnel can touch only nonsterile items
    d. Only sterile items can touch other sterile items

16. Which of the following does *not* enhance the healing of an open wound?
    a. Debridement
    b. Exuberant granulation tissue
    c. Granulation tissue
    d. Wound flushing

17. Which of the following is *not* a characteristic of first-intention wound healing?
    a. Minimal contamination
    b. Minimal tissue damage
    c. No continuous movement of wound edges from body movement
    d. Wound edges not approximated

18. Which incision is most appropriate for exploratory surgery of the abdomen of a dog in which the precise location of the problem is not known?
    a. Flank
    b. Paracostal
    c. Paramedian
    d. Ventral midline

19. Which of the following is *not* an early sign of wound dehiscence during the first 24 hours after abdominal surgery?
    a. Body temperature elevation of 1° to 2°
    b. Serosanguineous discharge from the incision
    c. Swollen incision
    d. Very warm incision

20. The main goal of aseptic surgical technique is to prevent contamination of the
    a. Sterile fields
    b. Sterile zones
    c. Surgical instruments
    d. Surgical wound

21. Which factor relating to infection of a surgical wound can aseptic technique reasonably expect to significantly influence?
    a. Number of microorganisms entering the wound
    b. Pathogenicity of microorganisms entering the wound
    c. Route of exposure to infectious microorganisms
    d. Susceptibility of the patient

22. The effectiveness of a surgical scrub of the hands and arms with a bactericidal soap depends on the
    a. Combination of contact time and scrubbing action
    b. Time the soap is in contact with the skin
    c. Scrubbing action of the brush
    d. Temperature of the water

23. Which of the following is a surgical scrub soap that forms a bacteriostatic film over the skin when it is used exclusively?
    a. Chlorhexidine
    b. Chlorpheniramine
    c. Hexachlorophene
    d. Povidone-iodine

24. Which of the following does *not* normally need to be sterilized as a part of good aseptic surgical technique?
    a. Cap
    b. Drapes
    c. Gown
    d. Scrub brush

Correct answers are on pages 305–311.

25. Liquid chemical sterilization is used primarily for
    a. Electrical equipment
    b. Instruments with sharp edges
    c. Orthopedic equipment
    d. Surgical drapes

26. The time necessary to disinfect surgical instruments with liquid chemicals can be shortened by
    a. Cooling the solution
    b. Making the solution less concentrated than recommended
    c. Making the solution more concentrated than recommended
    d. Warming the solution

27. Which surgical drape material prevents bacteria from penetrating the drape by capillary action when the top surface of the drape becomes wet?
    a. Cloth
    b. Muslin
    c. Paper
    d. Plastic

28. Which surgical instrument should *not* be routinely steam sterilized?
    a. Backhaus towel clamp
    b. Halstead mosquito forceps
    c. Mayo-Hegar needle holder
    d. Metzenbaum scissors

29. What is the most appropriate wound flushing solution?
    a. Hydrogen peroxide
    b. Isotonic saline
    c. Povidone-iodine solution
    d. Tap water

30. Which incision is most appropriate for rumenotomy in a standing cow?
    a. Left flank
    b. Right ventral paramedian
    c. Left ventral paramedian
    d. Ventral midline

31. Which, if any, operating room personnel should always face *away* from sterile fields during a surgical procedure?
    a. Nonscrubbed personnel only
    b. Scrubbed personnel only
    c. Both nonscrubbed and scrubbed personnel
    d. Neither nonscrubbed nor scrubbed personnel

32. What is the significance of ventral midline surgical wound dehiscence of the muscle, subcutaneous tissue, and skin layers?
    a. Emergency
    b. Cosmetic only
    c. Minor significance
    d. Serious, but not an emergency

33. Why is a recent surgical wound usually slightly warmer than surrounding normal tissues?
    a. Contamination
    b. Debridement
    c. Infection
    d. Inflammation

34. When does a sutured surgical wound begin to gain significant strength from production of collagen strands so that the wound edges are held together by not only the sutures?
    a. Immediately
    b. 5 days
    c. 14 days
    d. 35 days

35. Wound contraction is produced by
    a. Movement of the dermis only
    b. Movement of the epidermis only
    c. Movement of the whole thickness of skin
    d. Reproduction of epidermal cells

36. As a part of effective aseptic technique, surgical gowns
    a. Are commonly made of cloth or paper
    b. Are put on by touching only the outside
    c. Are routinely sterilized by ethylene oxide gas
    d. Do not need to be sterile, only clean

37. Which of the following is *not* a sign of hemorrhagic shock in a postsurgical patient?
    a. Deep, slow breathing
    b. Slow capillary refill
    c. Tachycardia
    d. Weakness

38. The usual significance of a seroma beneath a skin suture line is
    a. Emergency
    b. Cosmetic only
    c. Minor significance
    d. Serious, but not an emergency

39. The healing potential for a fractured bone that is properly aligned and kept immobile is
    a. Excellent
    b. Fair
    c. Good
    d. Poor

40. Which coloration indicates the best blood supply to the edges of a wound in unpigmented skin?
    a. Bluish-purple
    b. Gray
    c. Pink
    d. White

41. Which abdominal incision is most appropriate for a standing cesarean section on a heifer?
    a. Ventral midline
    b. Flank
    c. Paracostal
    d. Ventral paramedian

42. What portion of a surgical gown is considered sterile during surgery?
    a. Front and sides, from the neck to the bottom, including the arms
    b. Front, from the neck to the bottom, including the arms
    c. Front and sides, from the waist to the neck
    d. Front, from the waist up, including the arms

43. Which bacterial form is most easily destroyed by common sterilization methods?
    a. Spores of aerobes
    b. Spores of anaerobes
    c. Dormant form
    d. Vegetative form

44. The first phase of the wound healing process is the
    a. Epithelial
    b. Fibroblast
    c. Inflammatory
    d. Maturation

45. In the first 24 hours of primary union wound healing, most of the resistance to opening of the wound is provided by
    a. Collagen strands
    b. Fibrin strands
    c. Granulation tissue
    d. Sutures

46. In which type of abdominal incision can the muscle wall be most effectively closed with one layer of sutures?
    a. Flank
    b. Paracostal
    c. Paramedian
    d. Ventral midline

Correct answers are on pages 305–311.

47. Scrubbed surgical personnel become contaminated if they touch
    a. Objects in sterile fields
    b. Objects outside the sterile zone
    c. Properly sterilized surgical instruments
    d. Freshly exposed tissues of the patient

48. Nonscrubbed surgical personnel may properly touch anything that is
    a. Contaminated
    b. Inside the patient's body
    c. Inside the sterile zone
    d. Part of a sterile field

49. How should scrubbed personnel pass each other in the operating room?
    a. Back to back
    b. Back to front
    c. Front to back
    d. Front to front

50. When not otherwise occupied, scrubbed surgical personnel should stand with their
    a. Arms folded
    b. Hands above shoulder level
    c. Hands clasped between waist and shoulder level
    d. Hands down at their sides

51. When is it permissible for nonscrubbed surgical personnel to pass between scrubbed personnel and the patient during surgery?
    a. Never
    b. When opening suture material
    c. When adjusting the anesthesia machine
    d. When adjusting the intravenous drip

52. When aseptically opening a sterile surgical pack on an instrument stand, it is *not* proper for nonscrubbed surgical personnel to touch the
    a. Autoclave tape
    b. Contents of the pack
    c. Corners of the wrap
    d. Instrument stand

53. Which characteristic is *true* of ethylene oxide gas?
    a. Flammable
    b. Exposure is not considered a health hazard
    c. Noncombustible
    d. Nontoxic to tissues

54. Which of the following is *not* a likely contributor to postoperative wound dehiscence?
    a. Chronic postoperative vomiting
    b. Internal suture ends cut too short
    c. Infection
    d. Skin sutures left in too long

55. Which type of dressing best helps debride a wound with extensive tissue damage?
    a. Dry gauze
    b. Gauze dressing with an oily antiseptic
    c. Gauze dressing with a water-soluble antiseptic
    d. Wet saline dressing

56. Most of the clinical signs seen in an animal in shock from excessive blood loss are attributable to
    a. Acidosis
    b. Alkalosis
    c. Cell death
    d. Redistribution of blood flow

57. The main goal of surgery to remove a pus-filled uterus (pyometra) is
    a. As a prophylactic measure
    b. To make a diagnosis
    c. To restore the animal to a normal reproductive state
    d. To return the animal to health without restoring normal reproductive function

58. What tissue must form in a wound that is healing by second intention before wound contraction or epithelial regeneration can occur?
    a. Collagen fibers
    b. Fibrin clot
    c. Granulation tissue
    d. Scar tissue

59. When gloving for surgery, which of the following is *not* permitted?
    a. One gloved thumb touches the other gloved thumb
    b. The outside of the glove is touched by the scrubbed fingers
    c. The outside of the gown cuff is touched by inside of the glove cuff
    d. The scrubbed fingers touch the inside of the glove cuff

60. How should a pack be placed in an autoclave for sterilization?
    a. Diagonally
    b. Horizontally
    c. Tightly packed
    d. Vertically

COMMON SURGICAL INSTRUMENTS

61. Metzenbaum scissors are used for
    a. Cutting sutures
    b. Soft tissue dissection
    c. Cutting the linea alba
    d. Cutting skin

62. Which retractors are *not* hand held?
    a. Deaver
    b. Senns
    c. Rake
    d. Gelpi

63. Which instrument is commonly used in a fetlock arthrotomy?
    a. Scanlon Fernoer elevator
    b. Periosteum elevator
    c. Sharp obturator
    d. Hohmann retractor

64. What is the appropriate time to soak an instrument for *cold sterilization*?
    a. 30 min
    b. 15 min
    c. 45 min
    d. 10 min

65. How long does an instrument that is wrapped in paper remain sterile?
    a. 6 months
    b. 1 week
    c. 1 month
    d. 1 year

66. A dust cover extends the sterility time of an instrument from 1 month to
    a. 6 months
    b. 2 months
    c. 12 months
    d. 2 years

67. Instrument milk is used for all of the following *except*
    a. Lubrication
    b. Rust inhibition
    c. Extending the life of the instrument
    d. Cleaning the instrument

68. For which bovine surgical procedure are obstetric (OB) chains used?
    a. Rumenotomy
    b. Abomasopexy
    c. Cesarean section
    d. Uterine torsion correction

69. To flash sterilize an instrument, the autoclave settings should be
    a. 250°F, 20 lb pressure, 30 min, fast exhaust and dry
    b. 270°F, 20 lb pressure, 30 min, fast exhaust and dry
    c. 250°F, 30 lb pressure, 4 min, fast exhaust
    d. 270°F, 30 lb pressure, 4 min, fast exhaust

70. Which of the following does *not* have to be gas sterilized?
    a. Arthroscope
    b. Simplex
    c. Polyethylene tubing
    d. Plastic spray bottles

71. Ultrasonic cleaners are used for
    a. Removing small particles of blood and tissue
    b. Removing rust
    c. Disinfecting instruments
    d. Lubricating instruments

72. A laryngeal bur is used in
    a. Arthroscopy
    b. Abomasopexy
    c. Staphylectomy
    d. Sacculectomy

Correct answers are on pages 305–311.

73. Which of the following is *not* a consideration when evaluating a surgical pack for sterility?
    a. Sterilization date
    b. Indicator color change
    c. Holes or moisture damage
    d. Incorrect labeling

74. Mayo-Hegar scissors are used in all of the following situations *except* for cutting
    a. Sutures
    b. Delicate tissue
    c. Paper drapes
    d. Skin or muscle

75. When steam autoclaving bottles of solution, what two preparations should be made to prevent explosion of the bottles?
    a. Vent the bottles and set the autoclave to slow exhaust
    b. Cap the bottles and set the autoclave to slow exhaust
    c. Vent the bottles and set the autoclave to fast exhaust and dry
    d. Cap the bottles and set the autoclave to flash

76. How long must instruments be aerated after ethelene oxide gas sterilization?
    a. 12 hours
    b. 1 to 7 days
    c. 7 to 14 days
    d. 1 hour

77. What size scalpel blade is used in an arthroscopy for making the stab incision into the joint?
    a. #10
    b. #11
    c. # 12
    d. # 15

78. What size scalpel blade is used for making an abdominal skin incision?
    a. #10
    b. #11
    c. #12
    d. #15

79. Which type of sterilization technique is *not* acceptable for instruments used in a laryngoplasty?
    a. Gas sterilization
    b. Autoclaving
    c. Chemical sterilization
    d. Boiling

80. All of the following are objectives of the surgical hand scrub *except*
    a. To remove gross dirt and oil from the hands
    b. To sterilize the hands
    c. To reduce the microorganism count on the hands to as close to zero as possible
    d. To have a prolonged depressant effect on numbers of microflora on the hands and forearms

81. What type of surgical scrub solution is most effective in reducing numbers of bacteria on the skin?
    a. Hexaclorophene
    b. Povidone-iodine
    c. Chlorhexidine gluconate
    d. Polypropylene

82. When a surgeon encounters bleeding, all of the following can be used to control it *except*
    a. Electrocautery
    b. A hemostat
    c. Suction
    d. Rat tooth forceps

83. How long does a sealed item remain sterilized by gamma radiation?
    a. 1 year
    b. 6 months
    c. Until it is opened
    d. 1 month

84. Which item would be considered sterile on August 19, 1996?
    a. An item wrapped in double-layered muslin, with moisture on the outer layer
    b. An item sterlized with blood still on it
    c. An item wrapped in a peel pouch dated August 20, 1995
    d. An item wrapped in paper and a dust cover dated August 20, 1995

85. Which retractor is *not* self-retaining?
    a. Weitlaner
    b. Alms
    c. Sauerbruch
    d. Balfour

86. Sterilization is the process of killing microorganisms by physical or chemical means. What is the most reliable form of sterilization?
    a. Steam under pressure
    b. Gas
    c. Dry heat
    d. Radiation

87. Instruments wrapped in a single linen wrap can become contaminated with microbes within 2 to 3 days. How long does double wrapping an instrument extend the sterility period?
    a. 6 months
    b. 4 weeks
    c. 4 to 6 days
    d. 1 year

88. What is the best type of cleaner to use when hand-washing surgical instruments?
    a. Ordinary hand soap
    b. Abrasive compounds
    c. Low-sudsing detergents
    d. Plain hot water

Suturing

89. Which of the following are *nonabsorbable* sutures?
    a. Chromic gut and Prolene
    b. Dermalon and Mersilene
    c. Polydioxanone (PDS) and surgical steel
    d. Vicryl (polyglactin 910) and silk

90. All of the following are considered benefits of using skin staples except
    a. Skin is more resistant to abscess formation than when sutures are used
    b. Staples provide excellent wound healing
    c. Staples are more cost effective
    d. Staples save time

91. If skin edges are under extreme tension (e.g., in a large skin wound), what is the suture pattern of choice?
    a. Simple continuous
    b. Simple interrupted
    c. Interrupted horizontal mattress
    d. Continuous horizontal mattress

92. Which suture pattern is most commonly used in large animal surgery?
    a. Simple continous
    b. Simple interrupted
    c. Interrupted horizontal mattress
    d. Continuous horizontal mattress

93. Which suture is *not* recommended for skin closure?
    a. Polydioxanone
    b. Nylon
    c. Chromic gut
    d. Stainless steel

Correct answers are on pages 305–311.

94. What is the purpose of using a subcuticular suture pattern for final closure?
    a. To keep tissues apposed for quick healing
    b. To eliminate small scars produced around suture holes of the more common patterns
    c. To eliminate infection
    d. To be more cost effective

95. Which suture patterns are used for closure of hollow organs?
    a. Lembert, Cushing, pursestring
    b. Pursestring, Ford interlocking, cruciate
    c. Lembert, cruciate, Cushing
    d. Halsted, Ford interlocking, Lembert

96. After deflating gas-distended bowel with a hypodermic needle, which suture pattern is used to close the small hole?
    a. Simple interrupted
    b. Cruciate (cross mattress)
    c. Near-far-far-near
    d. Vertical mattress

97. In what way is a surgeon's knot different from a square knot?
    a. A surgeon's knot is less likely to stay locked in place
    b. A surgeon's knot has two throws on the first suture
    c. A square knot has two throws on the first suture
    d. A square knot is stronger than a surgeon's knot

98. Why is it better to ligate many small vessels rather than one mass ligation of tissues?
    a. Mass ligation of tissues is unsightly
    b. Mass ligation of tissue may result in an infected area
    c. Mass ligation of tissue is more likely to fail
    d. Tissues included in a mass ligation may be too difficult for the body to resorb

99. What is the purpose of a transfixation ligature?
    a. To make the ligature stronger
    b. To close a hollow organ
    c. To prevent breakage of the suture
    d. To prevent slippage of the suture

100. All of the following are good reasons for using an instrument tie (with the use of a needleholder) *except*
    a. It is economical; small pieces of suture can be used and therefore suture material not wasted
    b. It saves time
    c. It is more accurate than a one- or two-handed tie
    d. It is readily adaptable to any type of wound closure

101. Which of the following is *not* a consideration when choosing a needle for use in a surgical procedure?
    a. Type of tissue to be sutured
    b. Location of the tissue to be sutured
    c. Size of suture material
    d. Strength of suture material

102. When suturing skin, the needle of choice is .
    a. Special K
    b. Trocar
    c. Cutting
    d. Taper

103. What is the most significant advantage of using a swaged-on needle as opposed to a closed-eye needle?
    a. There is little chance of the needle's separating from the suture
    b. The suture and needle are approximately the same diameter
    c. Tissues are subjected to less trauma because a single strand is pulled through the tissue
    d. It saves time

169. Ethyl and isopropyl alcohols
    a. Have characteristics that make them ideal for sterilizing instruments
    b. At lower concentrations are bacteriostatic rather than bactericidal, and therefore are not very effective
    c. Have an excellent residual effect because of their rapid evaporation
    d. Have no place in veterinary surgery

170. An effective disinfectant to clean a cage after an animal that has had a *Pseudomonas*-contaminated wound is
    a. Chlorhexidine
    b. Isopropyl alcohol
    c. Quaternary ammonium
    d. Povidone-iodine

171. A good solution to instill in the conjunctival sac before surgery is
    a. 10% chlorhexidine gluconate
    b. 1:25 povidone-iodine solution
    c. 5% isopropyl alcohol
    d. Dilute soapy water

172. *Clean-contaminated* surgery refers to
    a. All surgeries
    b. Incisions in sterile areas that become contaminated during surgery
    c. Incisions made in contaminated areas
    d. Incisions in a previously contaminated area that has been rendered sterile

173. In terms of surgical contamination, endogenous organisms are those that
    a. Originate from the patient's own body
    b. Come from the external surgical environment
    c. Rarely cause any problem in surgical wounds
    d. Come from the surgeon's cutting his finger and bleeding into the wound

174. When a break in aseptic technique occurs,
    a. The surgery must be called off immediately
    b. The break can be ignored and surgery can continue
    c. The patient is unlikely to recover from the surgery
    d. Steps must be taken to immediately remedy the situation to the best of everyone's ability

175. A good time to clean the surgery room is
    a. On the night before surgery to allow air-borne dust to settle before surgery
    b. Immediately before the surgery so things can be as clean as possible
    c. Once a week
    d. Once a month

176. If during surgery you notice an item close to the edge of the sterile field, you should
    a. Ask others to find out if it was contaminated
    b. Consider it unsterile if you are not absolutely certain
    c. Consider it sterile
    d. Move it farther into the sterile field

177. Preparing a patient's skin for surgery
    a. Renders the skin completely sterile
    b. Does nothing to affect the outcome of the surgery
    c. Reduces the bacterial flora to a level that can be controlled by the patient's defense mechanisms
    d. Is not necessary if antibiotics are given

Correct answers are on pages 305–311.

178. Lavaging (flushing) a body cavity with warm, sterile saline after a surgical procedure is completed and before closing the incision
   a. Is of no value
   b. Decreases the amount of bacteria left behind and, additionally, warms the patient
   c. Serves only as a medium for bacteria to multiply
   d. Is necessary only if there has been a break in aseptic technique

SURGICAL TERMINOLOGY

179. An example of an elective procedure is
   a. Ovariohysterectomy
   b. Nephrotomy
   c. Exploratory laparotomy
   d. Thyroidectomy

180. A tapered suture needle is
   a. Best to use in skin
   b. The least traumatic and most often used in deep tissue layers
   c. Not used very often because of its relative inability to penetrate tissue
   d. Too expensive for routine surgical use

181. A thoracotomy is an incision into the
   a. Abdomen
   b. Chest
   c. Skull
   d. Ear canal

182. The suffix -ectomy refers to
   a. Surgical removal
   b. Reduction
   c. Drainage
   d. Incision into

183. Which orthopedic fixation consists of pins that penetrate fractured bones and are held in place externally by bolts?
   a. Rush pinning
   b. Steinmann fixation
   c. Stack pinning
   d. Kirschner-Ehmer fixation

184. The term *arthrotomy* refers to an incision into
   a. An artery
   b. A joint
   c. A muscle
   d. A long bone

185. Arresting the flow of blood from a vessel or to a part is called
   a. Aspiration
   b. Fibrinolysis
   c. Hemostasis
   d. Hemolysis

186. *Peritonitis* refers to
   a. Inflammation of the pericardial space
   b. Inflammation of the lining of the abdominal cavity
   c. Inflammation caused by parasite infection
   d. Incision into the peritoneum

187. Cryptorchidectomy is performed on male dogs
   a. With one or both testicles that have not descended into the scrotal sac
   b. When no other treatment for cryptosporidiosis is available
   c. And is similar to the vasectomy procedure done in people
   d. When complications from routine castration arise

188. *Fenestration* refers to
   a. Cutting a part exactly in half
   b. Creating a window in tissue
   c. The draping procedure
   d. Folding back the top skin layer

189. Ovariohysterectomy is routinely performed
   a. In excitable dogs that need immediate calming
   b. In young female dogs that the owners wish rendered sterile
   c. In male dogs with female characteristics
   d. Exclusively in female dogs who have already had litters of puppies

190. *Hepatic* refers to
    a. Heparin preparations
    b. Liver
    c. Hemoglobin
    d. Stomach

191. Blood vessels are ligated
    a. To remove them completely from the body
    b. When they are larger than 1.5 mm and blood flow needs to be stopped
    c. With as much trauma as possible to coagulate the blood
    d. Rarely and only in emergency situations

192. Chemical cauterization
    a. Is an excellent method of stopping blood flow
    b. Is rarely used in veterinary medicine
    c. Is traumatic to adjacent tissues and, therefore, not used in surgical cases
    d. Is a misnomer; chemicals cannot stop bleeding

193. Keeping tissues moist during a surgical procedure
    a. Is important because dry tissues are less resistant to bacterial infection
    b. Is undesirable because wet tissue is an ideal medium for bacterial regeneration
    c. Is of little value
    d. Should be accomplished with 70% isopropyl alcohol

194. Plating a fractured bone
    a. Refers to coating it with a rigid metallic substance to induce healing
    b. Is impractical in veterinary patients
    c. Is an internal method of fracture fixation involving stainless-steel plates and screws
    d. Can be done without skin incision

195. The distal portion of a long bone is
    a. The one closest to the trunk of the body
    b. The one farthest away from the trunk of the body
    c. Exactly in the middle of the long bone
    d. The outer layer of the bone

196. Perineal urethrostomies are performed only on
    a. Pregnant cats
    b. Male cats with urethral obstruction
    c. Large-breed dogs with gastric torsion
    d. Small dogs with pyometra

197. *Torsion* of an organ or part refers to
    a. Swelling or expansion
    b. Inflation with fluid
    c. Inflation with gas
    d. Twisting or rotation

198. Which surgical procedure is *least* likely to combat canine hip dysplasia's debilitating complications?
    a. Triple pelvic osteotomy
    b. Total hip replacement
    c. Intramedullary pinning
    d. Pectineal myotomy

199. Ear canal *ablation* refers to
    a. Irrigation of the ear canal
    b. Instilling antibiotics to correct otitis media
    c. Surgical removal and closure of the external ear canal
    d. Enlarging the external ear canal

200. *Perioperatively* refers to
    a. Before surgery
    b. After surgery
    c. Around the time of surgery
    d. During surgery

Correct answers are on pages 305–311.

201. A *proptosed* eye is one that is
    a. Normally positioned
    b. Displaced rostrally from the socket
    c. Shrunken and shrivelled
    d. Deviated in any direction other than normal

202. Onychectomy
    a. Is the procedure used to remove a cat's testicles
    b. Is the common practice of removing a cat's claws and associated phalanges
    c. Can be done without anesthesia
    d. Should be performed only on cats living outdoors

203. Postoperative complications
    a. Do not occur if the surgeon is skilled
    b. Should never be discussed with a client
    c. Can occur even if the surgery went well
    d. Are almost always attributable to poor assistance in surgery

204. Fracture reduction
    a. Involves trimming the areas of bone adjacent to the fracture site
    b. Involves apposing (pulling together) the fractured bone ends
    c. Is rarely necessary for good healing
    d. Can usually be done without anesthesia

205. A diaphragmatic hernia
    a. Is a diaphragm that is spastic
    b. Is displacement of the heart into the abdomen
    c. Cannot be corrected
    d. Is a common finding in car trauma patients and should be suspected if the animal is dyspneic

206. When an animal is sent home after surgery,
    a. The wound should already be completely healed
    b. The client should be given written detailed home care instructions
    c. The animal is no longer legally your patient and no longer your concern
    d. The technician should make daily visits to ensure the patient is given the same care as in the hospital

207. Absorbable gelatin sponges
    a. Are typically soaked or sutured into a bleeding site
    b. Should never be left in the body after surgery
    c. Are radiopaque
    d. Are impractical for veterinary surgery

208. Exteriorizing a body part or organ during surgery
    a. Is a routine practice when the part or organ contains contaminants
    b. Is very hazardous to the patient and not routinely done
    c. Precludes the need for lavaging
    d. Is done only if that part or organ is to be rejected (surgically removed)

Answers

GENERAL

1. **a** The basic requirements for *first-intention healing* are minimal tissue damage and apposition of the wound edges, usually with sutures.

2. **d** The basic functional unit of the nervous system, the neuron, is incapable of reproduction; consequently, damage to the nervous system is often repaired by scar tissue. The other organs and tissues listed have excellent healing potential.

3. **d** The xiphoid process and umbilicus are both on the animal's ventral midline.

4. **c** An electric drill would be damaged or inadequately sterilized by any of the other methods.

5. **a** Steam sterilization in an autoclave is used most often for instruments and equipment that would not be damaged by moisture or heat.

6. **d** The sharp edges of scissors are dulled by steam in an autoclave; boiling and dry heat are not sufficiently effective; and the expense and danger of ethylene oxide use are not warranted.

7. **a** The minimum standard for sterilization of surgical instruments in an autoclave is 121° C (250° F) for at least 15 minutes.

8. **b** Chemical autoclave indicators are the only type listed that can give immediate information on all three of the basic criteria for autoclave sterilization—(1) the presence of steam at the proper combination, (2) exposure time, and (3) temperature.

9. **a** Microorganisms in a wound during surgery are considered contaminants until, or unless, they multiply and cause damage.

10. **d** A surgical mask does not come in contact with anything sterile during a surgical procedure, so it has only to be clean.

11. **d** An autoclave sterilizes by exposing packs to high-temperature steam under pressure.

12. **d** A #40 clipper blade is a *surgical* blade. It clips the hair off at the skin surface.

13. **b** Curettage involves scraping of a tissue or cavity.

14. **d** Using overly large suture material would not cause a wound to break down. It would actually have greater holding power than a smaller size of suture material.

15. **b** Contaminated items look identical to sterile items; if there is any doubt about the sterility of an item, it must be considered contaminated.

16. **b** Exuberant granulation tissue (proud flesh) inhibits wound healing and epithelial regeneration. The other choices would likely enhance wound healing.

17. **d** One of the most important characteristics of wound healing by first intention is approximation of the wound edges.

18. **d** The ventral midline approach gives the most extensive access to the abdominal cavity.

19. **a** A slight elevation of body temperature that lasts for a day or two is normal after major surgery. The other choices are all early indicators of wound dehiscence.

20. **d** Prevention of surgical wound contamination is the whole purpose of aseptic technique in the operating room.

21. **a** This is the only choice that can be influenced by aseptic technique. The others are inherent in the patient, the surgical procedure being performed, or the microorganisms in the environment.

22. **a** The antimicrobial effect of a surgical scrub is dependent on sufficient exposure of the skin to the soap, as well as the scrubbing action that loosens dead skin and debris and works the soap into the cracks and crevices of the skin.

23. **c** Hexachlorophene forms a bacteriostatic film on the skin if used exclusively to wash the hands and arms. Other soaps remove the protective film.

24. **a** The surgical cap does not come in contact with the tissues of the patient, either directly or indirectly. It therefore needs to be clean, not sterile.

25. **b** Liquid chemical sterilization does not dull sharp edges.

26. **d** Warming the solution speeds up the chemical reactions necessary to kill microorganisms.

27. **d** Cloth and paper drapes are subject to capillary action; plastic drapes are not.

28. **d** Steam dulls the sharp edges of scissors.

29. **b** The other solutions listed are either irritating to the tissues or not isotonic with the patient's tissue fluids.

30. **a** None of the other approaches can be used in a standing cow, nor do they provide good access to the rumen.

31. **d** All personnel in the operating room should face toward sterile fields so they are aware of their relationship to them.

32. **a** Dehiscence of all layers of the body wall exposes abdominal viscera. Repair must be immediate to prevent serious damage to the abdominal organs and structures.

33. **d** Inflammation results from any injury to the body whether intentional (surgical) or unintentional (traumatic). The increased blood supply to an area of inflammation results in increased warmth to the area. Good surgical technique minimizes inflammation but does not eliminate it.

34. **b** It takes 4 to 6 days for production of collagen strands in a wound to reach a significant level. Until that time, the sutures are the main thing holding the suture line together.

35. **c** Wound contraction represents movement of the whole thickness of the skin toward the center of the wound.

36. **a**

37. **a** A patient in shock would be expected to show rapid, shallow breathing in an effort to oxygenate the blood as rapidly as possible.

38. **b** Unless very large or ruptured, postoperative seromas are unsightly but of little importance to the animal's health.

39. **a** Bones have excellent healing capacities, provided the fragments are properly aligned and movement is minimized.

40. **a** Bluish-purple wound edges indicate that the blood vessels of and under the skin are congested with blood.

41. **b** None of the other approaches would be appropriate for a standing animal.

42. **d** This is the only portion of a surgical gown that is considered sterile during surgery.

43. **d** The vegetative form of bacteria is the actively feeding, growing, reproducing form, and is most easily destroyed by common sterilization and disinfection methods.

44. **c** Inflammation is the first step in wound healing.

45. **d** Other than the sutures, a surgical wound has no appreciable strength until significant numbers of collagen fibers are produced in about 4 to 6 days.

46. **d** The linea alba, on the ventral midline of the abdominal wall, is the tendinous attachment of all of the ventral abdominal muscles. One layer of sutures in this area effectively closes the abdominal wall.

47. **b** Anything outside the sterile zone in an operating room is considered contaminated.

48. **a** Nonscrubbed personnel should touch only items that are not sterile.

49. **a** Passing back to back prevents accidental contamination.

50. **c** The hands of scrubbed personnel should always be held between waist level and shoulder level to help prevent inadvertent contamination. Clasping the hands when not otherwise occupied helps prevent fatigue from compromising the position of the hands and arms.

51. **a** Nonscrubbed personnel should never violate the sterile zone in which scrubbed personnel are working.

52. **b** Sterility is destroyed if pack contents are touched by a nonscrubbed person.

53. **a** Ethylene oxide gas is very flammable.

54. **d** Leaving skin sutures in too long increases scarring but does not directly contribute to breakdown of the surgical wound.

55. **d** Wet saline dressings are useful to help debride wounds with extensive tissue damage. They absorb and remove inflammatory products from the wound.

56. **d** Redistribution of blood flow results in the pale mucous membranes, poor capillary refill, and cold extremities seen in an animal in shock.

57. **d** Removal of the uterus would restore the animal to health, but absence of the uterus would preclude future breeding.

58. **c** Once the dead and damaged tissue has been removed from a wound by inflammation, a bed of granulation tissue, consisting primarily of collagen fibers and capillaries, must form on the floor of the wound before wound contraction can begin.

59. **b** If the outside of the glove is touched by anything that is not sterile, including the freshly scrubbed fingers, it becomes contaminated and must not be used for surgery.

60. **d** A pack placed vertically in the autoclave receives the best circulation of steam around its contents.

Common Surgical Instruments

61. **b** These scissors are made only for delicate tissue dissection. They become dull or spring open if used on heavier material.

62. **d** These retractors have a ratchet device to hold them in place during use.

63. **a**

64. **d**

65. **d**

66. **a**

67. **d** There are no cleansing agents in instrument milk.

68. **c** A cesarean section is the surgical removal of the calf from the cow, and OB chains are used to slip over the calf's hocks to help pull it out.

69. **d**

70. **b** A simplex, made of heavy rubber, can be sterilized effectively in an autoclave, whereas all of the others would be damaged by the high heat or moisture.

71. **a** All of the other answers are features of instrument milk, not ultrasonic cleaners.

72. **d** A laryngeal bur is used to remove the laryngeal saccule.

73. **d**

74. **b** These scissors are heavy and can cut thicker things. If used on delicate tissue, they might crush the tissue instead of cleanly cutting it.

75. **a** Bottles must be vented to prevent pressure from building up. Slow exhaust is necessary to avoid evacuation of solution from the bottles.

76. **b**

77. **b** A #11 blade has a sharp point for making a small incision just large enough for the arthroscope or canula to enter the joint.

78. **a** A #10 blade is a broad blade with the proper shape for a skin incision.

79. **d** Boiling does not sterilize instruments but is only a disinfectant. It is acceptable only for contaminated or clean-contaminated surgery. A laryngoplasty is sterile surgery.

80. **b** It is impossible to sterilize a surgeon's hands.

81. **c** Of those listed, chlorhexidene gluconate produces the greatest initial reduction of bacterial numbers.

82. **d** A rat tooth forceps is used for grasping tissue; it cannot control bleeding.

83. **c** As long as an item remains sealed, it remains sterile indefinitely when subjected to gamma radiation.

84. **c** *a*—any moisture on a cloth-wrapped item constitutes contamination; *b*—blood constitutes contamination; *d*—a dust cover only extends the sterility time to 6 months, so this item is out of date.

85. **c** A Sauerbruch retractor has no ratchet and must be held in the hand to be functional.

86. **a** Steam under pressure can permeate rapidly and then condense; this kills the microorganisms most effectively.

87. **b**

88. **c** *a*—ordinary hand soaps can leave behind insoluble alkaline residue; *b*—abrasive compounds can damage the surface of the instruments; *d*—plain water is too slow and less thorough than a low-sudsing detergent.

SUTURING

89. **b**

90. **c** Skin staples are more expensive than skin sutures.

91. **c** The interrupted horizontal mattress provides more strength than any of the other suture patterns. It also is the one most easily used with rubber tubing for tension reduction.

92. **b** This is a fast and efficient way of closing most incisions.

93. **c** Gut is an absorbable suture that breaks down rapidly.

94. **b** *a*—is true of many patterns; *c*—does not apply; *d*—does not apply.

95. a

96. b

97. b Both have the ability for locking into place. *c*—is incorrect because a square knot has only one throw on the first suture; *d*—is incorrect because both knots have the same strength.

98. c With mass ligation, the blood supply to the area may still be great enough to cause the suture to break.

99. d

100. c

101. d The strength of the suture is not affected by the type of needle and vice versa.

102. c A cutting needle penetrates the skin with the least amount of trauma. Also, it is the strongest for skin closure.

103. c All of the answers are true; however, trauma to the tissues is the most important factor to consider.

104. c Tendons and nerves should be sutured with tension sutures whereas viscera should be closed with inverting sutures; therefore, the skin should be closed with appositional sutures.

105. c

106. c The #2 suture is the largest of these answers, and a cow's uterus, being large and heavy, requires larger suture material.

107. c

108. c

109. d

110. b A good suture material would *not* constitute a favorable environment for bacterial growth.

111. a

112. b

113. c

114. d

115. b With each suture placed, the stress on the other sutures is decreased; thus, more sutures are better than fewer.

116. c

117. a This chemical reaction increases strength, decreases absorption, and reduces tissue reaction.

118. b The suture is coiled and more difficult to tighten down; none of the other answers are direct results of memory.

ASEPTIC TECHNIQUE

119. d

120. c If proper aseptic technique is used, antibiotics should not be given for short, routine, uncomplicated procedures.

121. c

122. a

123. b

124. d

125. b It does not stain and has a broader antimicrobial spectrum than iodophors.

126. b

127. b

128. b The anal sacs and ducts should be avoided to prevent postoperative problems.

129. d

130. c

131. b Finochietto retractors are used to hold the split sternum in thoracotomies; Gelpi retractors hold muscle layers apart.

132. b

133. a

134. d

135. c

136. c

137. a

138. a Metzenbaums are for cutting fine tissue *only*.

139. b

140. a

141. b Cold sterilization would work; but gas processing is more effective, and indicator strips can be used to ensure complete processing.

142. b

143. d

144. c

145. b

146. b

147. b It is not atraumatic and must be used judiciously.

148. b

149. c

150. b

151. b

152. d

153. c Good records should be kept of nosocomial outbreaks in your clinic so that effective disinfectants can be selected.

154. d

155. c

156. a

157. c

158. b Masks should be changed every few hours for this reason.

159. d

160. c Surgeons should pass each other in the surgery room either back to back or front to front.

161. c Hands should not drop below waist or instrument table level.

162. c

163. b

164. b Closed gloving provides the least chance for glove contamination.

165. b The dirtiest water is at the elbow; this should not be allowed to travel back down to the hands.

166. b

167. d

168. a

169. b

170. c

171. b Any of the others could severely damage the eye.

172. c Contaminated areas, such as the mouth and bladder, cannot be made sterile.

173. a Exogenous organisms are those from sources outside the patient's body.

174. d Breaks will occur; it is important to have plans to remedy the situation.

175. a

176. b

177. c

178. b

SURGICAL TERMINOLOGY

179. a Elective procedures are not necessary to the patients's immediate health.

180. b Cutting needles are used in skin and other tough tissues.

181. b

182. a

183. d Often shortened to "K-E" apparatus.

184. b

185. c

186. b

187. a

188. **b** Fenestrated drapes have a small window for the incision site; the surgeon fenestrates an intervertebral disc to remove disc material.

189. **b**

190. **b**

191. **b**

192. **c**

193. **a** "Moist tissues are happy tissues."

194. **c**

195. **b** Proximal refers to the area of bone closest to the trunk.

196. **b**

197. **d**

198. **c** Intramedullary pinning is performed on fractured long bones, such as the femur.

199. **c**

200. **c**

201. **b**

202. **b**

203. **c** The client should be well informed of surgical risks and possible complications.

204. **b**

205. **d** Displacement of abdominal contents into the thorax constitutes an emergency situation.

206. **b**

207. **a**

208. **a** Care must be taken to keep the exteriorized part moist.

Notes

Anatomy and Physiology

Fill in a circled letter to indicate your answer choice.

CELLS AND TISSUES

1. (a) (b) (c) (d)
2. (a) (b) (c) (d)
3. (a) (b) (c) (d)
4. (a) (b) (c) (d)
5. (a) (b) (c) (d)
6. (a) (b) (c) (d)
7. (a) (b) (c) (d)
8. (a) (b) (c) (d)
9. (a) (b) (c) (d)
10. (a) (b) (c) (d)
11. (a) (b) (c) (d)
12. (a) (b) (c) (d)
13. (a) (b) (c) (d)
14. (a) (b) (c) (d)
15. (a) (b) (c) (d)

CIRCULATORY SYSTEM

16. (a) (b) (c) (d)
17. (a) (b) (c) (d)
18. (a) (b) (c) (d)
19. (a) (b) (c) (d)
20. (a) (b) (c) (d)
21. (a) (b) (c) (d)
22. (a) (b) (c) (d)
23. (a) (b) (c) (d)
24. (a) (b) (c) (d)
25. (a) (b) (c) (d)
26. (a) (b) (c) (d)
27. (a) (b) (c) (d)
28. (a) (b) (c) (d)
29. (a) (b) (c) (d)
30. (a) (b) (c) (d)
31. (a) (b) (c) (d)
32. (a) (b) (c) (d)
33. (a) (b) (c) (d)
34. (a) (b) (c) (d)
35. (a) (b) (c) (d)
36. (a) (b) (c) (d)
37. (a) (b) (c) (d)
38. (a) (b) (c) (d)
39. (a) (b) (c) (d)

40. (a) (b) (c) (d)
41. (a) (b) (c) (d)
42. (a) (b) (c) (d)
43. (a) (b) (c) (d)
44. (a) (b) (c) (d)
45. (a) (b) (c) (d)
46. (a) (b) (c) (d)
47. (a) (b) (c) (d)
48. (a) (b) (c) (d)
49. (a) (b) (c) (d)
50. (a) (b) (c) (d)
51. (a) (b) (c) (d)
52. (a) (b) (c) (d)
53. (a) (b) (c) (d)
54. (a) (b) (c) (d)
55. (a) (b) (c) (d)
56. (a) (b) (c) (d)
57. (a) (b) (c) (d)
58. (a) (b) (c) (d)
59. (a) (b) (c) (d)
60. (a) (b) (c) (d)
61. (a) (b) (c) (d)
62. (a) (b) (c) (d)
63. (a) (b) (c) (d)
64. (a) (b) (c) (d)
65. (a) (b) (c) (d)
66. (a) (b) (c) (d)
67. (a) (b) (c) (d)
68. (a) (b) (c) (d)
69. (a) (b) (c) (d)
70. (a) (b) (c) (d)
71. (a) (b) (c) (d)

DIGESTIVE SYSTEM

72. (a) (b) (c) (d)
73. (a) (b) (c) (d)
74. (a) (b) (c) (d)
75. (a) (b) (c) (d)
76. (a) (b) (c) (d)
77. (a) (b) (c) (d)
78. (a) (b) (c) (d)
79. (a) (b) (c) (d)

80. (a) (b) (c) (d)
81. (a) (b) (c) (d)
82. (a) (b) (c) (d)
83. (a) (b) (c) (d)
84. (a) (b) (c) (d)
85. (a) (b) (c) (d)
86. (a) (b) (c) (d)
87. (a) (b) (c) (d)
88. (a) (b) (c) (d)
89. (a) (b) (c) (d)
90. (a) (b) (c) (d)
91. (a) (b) (c) (d)
92. (a) (b) (c) (d)
93. (a) (b) (c) (d)
94. (a) (b) (c) (d)
95. (a) (b) (c) (d)
96. (a) (b) (c) (d)
97. (a) (b) (c) (d)
98. (a) (b) (c) (d)
99. (a) (b) (c) (d)
100. (a) (b) (c) (d)
101. (a) (b) (c) (d)
102. (a) (b) (c) (d)
103. (a) (b) (c) (d)
104. (a) (b) (c) (d)
105. (a) (b) (c) (d)
106. (a) (b) (c) (d)
107. (a) (b) (c) (d)
108. (a) (b) (c) (d)
109. (a) (b) (c) (d)
110. (a) (b) (c) (d)
111. (a) (b) (c) (d)

ENDOCRINE SYSTEM

112. (a) (b) (c) (d)
113. (a) (b) (c) (d)
114. (a) (b) (c) (d)
115. (a) (b) (c) (d)
116. (a) (b) (c) (d)
117. (a) (b) (c) (d)
118. (a) (b) (c) (d)
119. (a) (b) (c) (d)

120. (a) (b) (c) (d)
121. (a) (b) (c) (d)
122. (a) (b) (c) (d)
123. (a) (b) (c) (d)
124. (a) (b) (c) (d)
125. (a) (b) (c) (d)
126. (a) (b) (c) (d)
127. (a) (b) (c) (d)
128. (a) (b) (c) (d)
129. (a) (b) (c) (d)
130. (a) (b) (c) (d)
131. (a) (b) (c) (d)
132. (a) (b) (c) (d)
133. (a) (b) (c) (d)
134. (a) (b) (c) (d)
135. (a) (b) (c) (d)
136. (a) (b) (c) (d)

INTEGUMENARY SYSTEM

137. (a) (b) (c) (d)
138. (a) (b) (c) (d)
139. (a) (b) (c) (d)
140. (a) (b) (c) (d)
141. (a) (b) (c) (d)
142. (a) (b) (c) (d)
143. (a) (b) (c) (d)
144. (a) (b) (c) (d)
145. (a) (b) (c) (d)
146. (a) (b) (c) (d)
147. (a) (b) (c) (d)
148. (a) (b) (c) (d)
149. (a) (b) (c) (d)
150. (a) (b) (c) (d)
151. (a) (b) (c) (d)
152. (a) (b) (c) (d)
153. (a) (b) (c) (d)
154. (a) (b) (c) (d)
155. (a) (b) (c) (d)
156. (a) (b) (c) (d)

Mammary Glands and Lactation

157. (a) (b) (c) (d)
158. (a) (b) (c) (d)
159. (a) (b) (c) (d)
160. (a) (b) (c) (d)
161. (a) (b) (c) (d)
162. (a) (b) (c) (d)
163. (a) (b) (c) (d)
164. (a) (b) (c) (d)
165. (a) (b) (c) (d)
166. (a) (b) (c) (d)
167. (a) (b) (c) (d)
168. (a) (b) (c) (d)
169. (a) (b) (c) (d)
170. (a) (b) (c) (d)
171. (a) (b) (c) (d)

Muscular System

172. (a) (b) (c) (d)
173. (a) (b) (c) (d)
174. (a) (b) (c) (d)
175. (a) (b) (c) (d)
176. (a) (b) (c) (d)
177. (a) (b) (c) (d)
178. (a) (b) (c) (d)
179. (a) (b) (c) (d)
180. (a) (b) (c) (d)
181. (a) (b) (c) (d)
182. (a) (b) (c) (d)
183. (a) (b) (c) (d)
184. (a) (b) (c) (d)
185. (a) (b) (c) (d)
186. (a) (b) (c) (d)
187. (a) (b) (c) (d)
188. (a) (b) (c) (d)
189. (a) (b) (c) (d)
190. (a) (b) (c) (d)
191. (a) (b) (c) (d)
192. (a) (b) (c) (d)
193. (a) (b) (c) (d)
194. (a) (b) (c) (d)
195. (a) (b) (c) (d)

Nervous System

196. (a) (b) (c) (d)
197. (a) (b) (c) (d)
198. (a) (b) (c) (d)
199. (a) (b) (c) (d)

200. (a) (b) (c) (d)
201. (a) (b) (c) (d)
202. (a) (b) (c) (d)
203. (a) (b) (c) (d)
204. (a) (b) (c) (d)
205. (a) (b) (c) (d)
206. (a) (b) (c) (d)
207. (a) (b) (c) (d)
208. (a) (b) (c) (d)
209. (a) (b) (c) (d)
210. (a) (b) (c) (d)
211. (a) (b) (c) (d)
212. (a) (b) (c) (d)
213. (a) (b) (c) (d)
214. (a) (b) (c) (d)
215. (a) (b) (c) (d)
216. (a) (b) (c) (d)
217. (a) (b) (c) (d)
218. (a) (b) (c) (d)
219. (a) (b) (c) (d)
220. (a) (b) (c) (d)
221. (a) (b) (c) (d)
222. (a) (b) (c) (d)
223. (a) (b) (c) (d)
224. (a) (b) (c) (d)
225. (a) (b) (c) (d)
226. (a) (b) (c) (d)
227. (a) (b) (c) (d)
228. (a) (b) (c) (d)
229. (a) (b) (c) (d)
230. (a) (b) (c) (d)

Reproductive System

231. (a) (b) (c) (d)
232. (a) (b) (c) (d)
233. (a) (b) (c) (d)
234. (a) (b) (c) (d)
235. (a) (b) (c) (d)
236. (a) (b) (c) (d)
237. (a) (b) (c) (d)
238. (a) (b) (c) (d)
239. (a) (b) (c) (d)
240. (a) (b) (c) (d)
241. (a) (b) (c) (d)
242. (a) (b) (c) (d)
243. (a) (b) (c) (d)
244. (a) (b) (c) (d)
245. (a) (b) (c) (d)
246. (a) (b) (c) (d)
247. (a) (b) (c) (d)
248. (a) (b) (c) (d)

249. (a) (b) (c) (d)
250. (a) (b) (c) (d)
251. (a) (b) (c) (d)
252. (a) (b) (c) (d)
253. (a) (b) (c) (d)
254. (a) (b) (c) (d)
255. (a) (b) (c) (d)
256. (a) (b) (c) (d)
257. (a) (b) (c) (d)
258. (a) (b) (c) (d)
259. (a) (b) (c) (d)
260. (a) (b) (c) (d)
261. (a) (b) (c) (d)
262. (a) (b) (c) (d)
263. (a) (b) (c) (d)
264. (a) (b) (c) (d)
265. (a) (b) (c) (d)
266. (a) (b) (c) (d)
267. (a) (b) (c) (d)
268. (a) (b) (c) (d)
269. (a) (b) (c) (d)
270. (a) (b) (c) (d)
271. (a) (b) (c) (d)
272. (a) (b) (c) (d)
273. (a) (b) (c) (d)
274. (a) (b) (c) (d)
275. (a) (b) (c) (d)
276. (a) (b) (c) (d)
277. (a) (b) (c) (d)
278. (a) (b) (c) (d)
279. (a) (b) (c) (d)
280. (a) (b) (c) (d)
281. (a) (b) (c) (d)
282. (a) (b) (c) (d)
283. (a) (b) (c) (d)
284. (a) (b) (c) (d)
285. (a) (b) (c) (d)
286. (a) (b) (c) (d)
287. (a) (b) (c) (d)
288. (a) (b) (c) (d)
289. (a) (b) (c) (d)
290. (a) (b) (c) (d)
291. (a) (b) (c) (d)

Respiratory System

292. (a) (b) (c) (d)
293. (a) (b) (c) (d)
294. (a) (b) (c) (d)
295. (a) (b) (c) (d)
296. (a) (b) (c) (d)
297. (a) (b) (c) (d)

298. (a) (b) (c) (d)
299. (a) (b) (c) (d)
300. (a) (b) (c) (d)
301. (a) (b) (c) (d)
302. (a) (b) (c) (d)
303. (a) (b) (c) (d)
304. (a) (b) (c) (d)
305. (a) (b) (c) (d)
306. (a) (b) (c) (d)
307. (a) (b) (c) (d)
308. (a) (b) (c) (d)
309. (a) (b) (c) (d)
310. (a) (b) (c) (d)

Sensory System

311. (a) (b) (c) (d)
312. (a) (b) (c) (d)
313. (a) (b) (c) (d)
314. (a) (b) (c) (d)
315. (a) (b) (c) (d)
316. (a) (b) (c) (d)
317. (a) (b) (c) (d)
318. (a) (b) (c) (d)
319. (a) (b) (c) (d)
320. (a) (b) (c) (d)
321. (a) (b) (c) (d)
322. (a) (b) (c) (d)
323. (a) (b) (c) (d)
324. (a) (b) (c) (d)
325. (a) (b) (c) (d)
326. (a) (b) (c) (d)
327. (a) (b) (c) (d)
328. (a) (b) (c) (d)
329. (a) (b) (c) (d)
330. (a) (b) (c) (d)
331. (a) (b) (c) (d)
332. (a) (b) (c) (d)
333. (a) (b) (c) (d)
334. (a) (b) (c) (d)
335. (a) (b) (c) (d)
336. (a) (b) (c) (d)
337. (a) (b) (c) (d)
338. (a) (b) (c) (d)
339. (a) (b) (c) (d)
340. (a) (b) (c) (d)
341. (a) (b) (c) (d)
342. (a) (b) (c) (d)
343. (a) (b) (c) (d)
344. (a) (b) (c) (d)
345. (a) (b) (c) (d)

Skeletal System Including Joints

346. (a) (b) (c) (d)
347. (a) (b) (c) (d)
348. (a) (b) (c) (d)
349. (a) (b) (c) (d)
350. (a) (b) (c) (d)
351. (a) (b) (c) (d)
352. (a) (b) (c) (d)
353. (a) (b) (c) (d)
354. (a) (b) (c) (d)
355. (a) (b) (c) (d)
356. (a) (b) (c) (d)
357. (a) (b) (c) (d)
358. (a) (b) (c) (d)

359. (a) (b) (c) (d)
360. (a) (b) (c) (d)
361. (a) (b) (c) (d)
362. (a) (b) (c) (d)
363. (a) (b) (c) (d)
364. (a) (b) (c) (d)
365. (a) (b) (c) (d)
366. (a) (b) (c) (d)
367. (a) (b) (c) (d)
368. (a) (b) (c) (d)
369. (a) (b) (c) (d)
370. (a) (b) (c) (d)
371. (a) (b) (c) (d)
372. (a) (b) (c) (d)
373. (a) (b) (c) (d)
374. (a) (b) (c) (d)

375. (a) (b) (c) (d)
376. (a) (b) (c) (d)
377. (a) (b) (c) (d)
378. (a) (b) (c) (d)

Urinary System

379. (a) (b) (c) (d)
380. (a) (b) (c) (d)
381. (a) (b) (c) (d)
382. (a) (b) (c) (d)
383. (a) (b) (c) (d)
384. (a) (b) (c) (d)
385. (a) (b) (c) (d)
386. (a) (b) (c) (d)
387. (a) (b) (c) (d)

388. (a) (b) (c) (d)
389. (a) (b) (c) (d)
390. (a) (b) (c) (d)
391. (a) (b) (c) (d)
392. (a) (b) (c) (d)
393. (a) (b) (c) (d)
394. (a) (b) (c) (d)
395. (a) (b) (c) (d)
396. (a) (b) (c) (d)
397. (a) (b) (c) (d)
398. (a) (b) (c) (d)
399. (a) (b) (c) (d)
400. (a) (b) (c) (d)
401. (a) (b) (c) (d)
402. (a) (b) (c) (d)

Corresponding questions are on pages 2-32.

Anesthesiology

Fill in a circled letter to indicate your answer choice.

TYPES OF ANESTHETICS/DRUGS

1. ⓐ ⓑ ⓒ ⓓ
2. ⓐ ⓑ ⓒ ⓓ
3. ⓐ ⓑ ⓒ ⓓ
4. ⓐ ⓑ ⓒ ⓓ
5. ⓐ ⓑ ⓒ ⓓ
6. ⓐ ⓑ ⓒ ⓓ
7. ⓐ ⓑ ⓒ ⓓ
8. ⓐ ⓑ ⓒ ⓓ
9. ⓐ ⓑ ⓒ ⓓ
10. ⓐ ⓑ ⓒ ⓓ
11. ⓐ ⓑ ⓒ ⓓ
12. ⓐ ⓑ ⓒ ⓓ
13. ⓐ ⓑ ⓒ ⓓ
14. ⓐ ⓑ ⓒ ⓓ
15. ⓐ ⓑ ⓒ ⓓ
16. ⓐ ⓑ ⓒ ⓓ
17. ⓐ ⓑ ⓒ ⓓ
18. ⓐ ⓑ ⓒ ⓓ
19. ⓐ ⓑ ⓒ ⓓ
20. ⓐ ⓑ ⓒ ⓓ
21. ⓐ ⓑ ⓒ ⓓ
22. ⓐ ⓑ ⓒ ⓓ
23. ⓐ ⓑ ⓒ ⓓ
24. ⓐ ⓑ ⓒ ⓓ
25. ⓐ ⓑ ⓒ ⓓ
26. ⓐ ⓑ ⓒ ⓓ
27. ⓐ ⓑ ⓒ ⓓ
28. ⓐ ⓑ ⓒ ⓓ
29. ⓐ ⓑ ⓒ ⓓ
30. ⓐ ⓑ ⓒ ⓓ
31. ⓐ ⓑ ⓒ ⓓ
32. ⓐ ⓑ ⓒ ⓓ
33. ⓐ ⓑ ⓒ ⓓ
34. ⓐ ⓑ ⓒ ⓓ
35. ⓐ ⓑ ⓒ ⓓ
36. ⓐ ⓑ ⓒ ⓓ
37. ⓐ ⓑ ⓒ ⓓ
38. ⓐ ⓑ ⓒ ⓓ
39. ⓐ ⓑ ⓒ ⓓ
40. ⓐ ⓑ ⓒ ⓓ
41. ⓐ ⓑ ⓒ ⓓ
42. ⓐ ⓑ ⓒ ⓓ
43. ⓐ ⓑ ⓒ ⓓ
44. ⓐ ⓑ ⓒ ⓓ
45. ⓐ ⓑ ⓒ ⓓ
46. ⓐ ⓑ ⓒ ⓓ
47. ⓐ ⓑ ⓒ ⓓ
48. ⓐ ⓑ ⓒ ⓓ
49. ⓐ ⓑ ⓒ ⓓ
50. ⓐ ⓑ ⓒ ⓓ
51. ⓐ ⓑ ⓒ ⓓ
52. ⓐ ⓑ ⓒ ⓓ
53. ⓐ ⓑ ⓒ ⓓ
54. ⓐ ⓑ ⓒ ⓓ

MACHINES AND EQUIPMENT

55. ⓐ ⓑ ⓒ ⓓ
56. ⓐ ⓑ ⓒ ⓓ
57. ⓐ ⓑ ⓒ ⓓ
58. ⓐ ⓑ ⓒ ⓓ
59. ⓐ ⓑ ⓒ ⓓ
60. ⓐ ⓑ ⓒ ⓓ
61. ⓐ ⓑ ⓒ ⓓ
62. ⓐ ⓑ ⓒ ⓓ
63. ⓐ ⓑ ⓒ ⓓ
64. ⓐ ⓑ ⓒ ⓓ
65. ⓐ ⓑ ⓒ ⓓ
66. ⓐ ⓑ ⓒ ⓓ
67. ⓐ ⓑ ⓒ ⓓ
68. ⓐ ⓑ ⓒ ⓓ
69. ⓐ ⓑ ⓒ ⓓ
70. ⓐ ⓑ ⓒ ⓓ
71. ⓐ ⓑ ⓒ ⓓ
72. ⓐ ⓑ ⓒ ⓓ
73. ⓐ ⓑ ⓒ ⓓ
74. ⓐ ⓑ ⓒ ⓓ
75. ⓐ ⓑ ⓒ ⓓ
76. ⓐ ⓑ ⓒ ⓓ
77. ⓐ ⓑ ⓒ ⓓ
78. ⓐ ⓑ ⓒ ⓓ
79. ⓐ ⓑ ⓒ ⓓ
80. ⓐ ⓑ ⓒ ⓓ
81. ⓐ ⓑ ⓒ ⓓ

INTUBATION

82. ⓐ ⓑ ⓒ ⓓ
83. ⓐ ⓑ ⓒ ⓓ
84. ⓐ ⓑ ⓒ ⓓ
85. ⓐ ⓑ ⓒ ⓓ
86. ⓐ ⓑ ⓒ ⓓ
87. ⓐ ⓑ ⓒ ⓓ
88. ⓐ ⓑ ⓒ ⓓ
89. ⓐ ⓑ ⓒ ⓓ
90. ⓐ ⓑ ⓒ ⓓ
91. ⓐ ⓑ ⓒ ⓓ
92. ⓐ ⓑ ⓒ ⓓ
93. ⓐ ⓑ ⓒ ⓓ
94. ⓐ ⓑ ⓒ ⓓ
95. ⓐ ⓑ ⓒ ⓓ

MONITORING THE ANESTHETIZED PATIENT

96. ⓐ ⓑ ⓒ ⓓ
97. ⓐ ⓑ ⓒ ⓓ
98. ⓐ ⓑ ⓒ ⓓ
99. ⓐ ⓑ ⓒ ⓓ
100. ⓐ ⓑ ⓒ ⓓ
101. ⓐ ⓑ ⓒ ⓓ
102. ⓐ ⓑ ⓒ ⓓ
103. ⓐ ⓑ ⓒ ⓓ
104. ⓐ ⓑ ⓒ ⓓ
105. ⓐ ⓑ ⓒ ⓓ
106. ⓐ ⓑ ⓒ ⓓ
107. ⓐ ⓑ ⓒ ⓓ
108. ⓐ ⓑ ⓒ ⓓ
109. ⓐ ⓑ ⓒ ⓓ
110. ⓐ ⓑ ⓒ ⓓ
111. ⓐ ⓑ ⓒ ⓓ
112. ⓐ ⓑ ⓒ ⓓ

113. ⓐ ⓑ ⓒ ⓓ
114. ⓐ ⓑ ⓒ ⓓ
115. ⓐ ⓑ ⓒ ⓓ
116. ⓐ ⓑ ⓒ ⓓ
117. ⓐ ⓑ ⓒ ⓓ
118. ⓐ ⓑ ⓒ ⓓ
119. ⓐ ⓑ ⓒ ⓓ
120. ⓐ ⓑ ⓒ ⓓ
121. ⓐ ⓑ ⓒ ⓓ
122. ⓐ ⓑ ⓒ ⓓ
123. ⓐ ⓑ ⓒ ⓓ
124. ⓐ ⓑ ⓒ ⓓ
125. ⓐ ⓑ ⓒ ⓓ
126. ⓐ ⓑ ⓒ ⓓ
127. ⓐ ⓑ ⓒ ⓓ
128. ⓐ ⓑ ⓒ ⓓ

ANESTHETIC EMERGENCIES

129. ⓐ ⓑ ⓒ ⓓ
130. ⓐ ⓑ ⓒ ⓓ
131. ⓐ ⓑ ⓒ ⓓ
132. ⓐ ⓑ ⓒ ⓓ
133. ⓐ ⓑ ⓒ ⓓ
134. ⓐ ⓑ ⓒ ⓓ
135. ⓐ ⓑ ⓒ ⓓ
136. ⓐ ⓑ ⓒ ⓓ
137. ⓐ ⓑ ⓒ ⓓ
138. ⓐ ⓑ ⓒ ⓓ
139. ⓐ ⓑ ⓒ ⓓ
140. ⓐ ⓑ ⓒ ⓓ
141. ⓐ ⓑ ⓒ ⓓ
142. ⓐ ⓑ ⓒ ⓓ
143. ⓐ ⓑ ⓒ ⓓ
144. ⓐ ⓑ ⓒ ⓓ
145. ⓐ ⓑ ⓒ ⓓ
146. ⓐ ⓑ ⓒ ⓓ
147. ⓐ ⓑ ⓒ ⓓ
148. ⓐ ⓑ ⓒ ⓓ
149. ⓐ ⓑ ⓒ ⓓ
150. ⓐ ⓑ ⓒ ⓓ

151.	ⓐ	ⓑ	ⓒ	ⓓ	155.	ⓐ	ⓑ	ⓒ	ⓓ	159.	ⓐ	ⓑ	ⓒ	ⓓ	163.	ⓐ	ⓑ	ⓒ	ⓓ
152.	ⓐ	ⓑ	ⓒ	ⓓ	156.	ⓐ	ⓑ	ⓒ	ⓓ	160.	ⓐ	ⓑ	ⓒ	ⓓ	164.	ⓐ	ⓑ	ⓒ	ⓓ
153.	ⓐ	ⓑ	ⓒ	ⓓ	157.	ⓐ	ⓑ	ⓒ	ⓓ	161.	ⓐ	ⓑ	ⓒ	ⓓ					
154.	ⓐ	ⓑ	ⓒ	ⓓ	158.	ⓐ	ⓑ	ⓒ	ⓓ	162.	ⓐ	ⓑ	ⓒ	ⓓ					

Animal Care

Fill in a circled letter to indicate your answer choice.

HOUSING
General

1. (a) (b) (c) (d)
2. (a) (b) (c) (d)
3. (a) (b) (c) (d)
4. (a) (b) (c) (d)
5. (a) (b) (c) (d)
6. (a) (b) (c) (d)
7. (a) (b) (c) (d)
8. (a) (b) (c) (d)
9. (a) (b) (c) (d)
10. (a) (b) (c) (d)
11. (a) (b) (c) (d)
12. (a) (b) (c) (d)
13. (a) (b) (c) (d)
14. (a) (b) (c) (d)
15. (a) (b) (c) (d)
16. (a) (b) (c) (d)
17. (a) (b) (c) (d)
18. (a) (b) (c) (d)
19. (a) (b) (c) (d)
20. (a) (b) (c) (d)
21. (a) (b) (c) (d)
22. (a) (b) (c) (d)
23. (a) (b) (c) (d)
24. (a) (b) (c) (d)
25. (a) (b) (c) (d)
26. (a) (b) (c) (d)

SWINE

27. (a) (b) (c) (d)
28. (a) (b) (c) (d)
29. (a) (b) (c) (d)
30. (a) (b) (c) (d)
31. (a) (b) (c) (d)
32. (a) (b) (c) (d)
33. (a) (b) (c) (d)
34. (a) (b) (c) (d)
35. (a) (b) (c) (d)
36. (a) (b) (c) (d)
37. (a) (b) (c) (d)

38. (a) (b) (c) (d)
39. (a) (b) (c) (d)
40. (a) (b) (c) (d)
41. (a) (b) (c) (d)

NUTRITION
General

42. (a) (b) (c) (d)
43. (a) (b) (c) (d)
44. (a) (b) (c) (d)
45. (a) (b) (c) (d)
46. (a) (b) (c) (d)
47. (a) (b) (c) (d)
48. (a) (b) (c) (d)
49. (a) (b) (c) (d)
50. (a) (b) (c) (d)
51. (a) (b) (c) (d)
52. (a) (b) (c) (d)
53. (a) (b) (c) (d)
54. (a) (b) (c) (d)
55. (a) (b) (c) (d)
56. (a) (b) (c) (d)
57. (a) (b) (c) (d)
58. (a) (b) (c) (d)
59. (a) (b) (c) (d)
60. (a) (b) (c) (d)
61. (a) (b) (c) (d)
62. (a) (b) (c) (d)
63. (a) (b) (c) (d)
64. (a) (b) (c) (d)
65. (a) (b) (c) (d)
66. (a) (b) (c) (d)
67. (a) (b) (c) (d)
68. (a) (b) (c) (d)
69. (a) (b) (c) (d)
70. (a) (b) (c) (d)
71. (a) (b) (c) (d)
72. (a) (b) (c) (d)
73. (a) (b) (c) (d)
74. (a) (b) (c) (d)
75. (a) (b) (c) (d)
76. (a) (b) (c) (d)

77. (a) (b) (c) (d)
78. (a) (b) (c) (d)
79. (a) (b) (c) (d)
80. (a) (b) (c) (d)
81. (a) (b) (c) (d)
82. (a) (b) (c) (d)
83. (a) (b) (c) (d)
84. (a) (b) (c) (d)
85. (a) (b) (c) (d)
86. (a) (b) (c) (d)
87. (a) (b) (c) (d)
88. (a) (b) (c) (d)
89. (a) (b) (c) (d)
90. (a) (b) (c) (d)
91. (a) (b) (c) (d)
92. (a) (b) (c) (d)
93. (a) (b) (c) (d)
94. (a) (b) (c) (d)
95. (a) (b) (c) (d)
96. (a) (b) (c) (d)
97. (a) (b) (c) (d)
98. (a) (b) (c) (d)
99. (a) (b) (c) (d)
100. (a) (b) (c) (d)
101. (a) (b) (c) (d)
102. (a) (b) (c) (d)
103. (a) (b) (c) (d)
104. (a) (b) (c) (d)
105. (a) (b) (c) (d)

SWINE

106. (a) (b) (c) (d)
107. (a) (b) (c) (d)
108. (a) (b) (c) (d)
109. (a) (b) (c) (d)
110. (a) (b) (c) (d)
111. (a) (b) (c) (d)
112. (a) (b) (c) (d)
113. (a) (b) (c) (d)
114. (a) (b) (c) (d)
115. (a) (b) (c) (d)
116. (a) (b) (c) (d)

117. (a) (b) (c) (d)
118. (a) (b) (c) (d)
119. (a) (b) (c) (d)
120. (a) (b) (c) (d)

PHYSICAL RESTRAINT
General

121. (a) (b) (c) (d)
122. (a) (b) (c) (d)
123. (a) (b) (c) (d)
124. (a) (b) (c) (d)
125. (a) (b) (c) (d)
126. (a) (b) (c) (d)
127. (a) (b) (c) (d)
128. (a) (b) (c) (d)
129. (a) (b) (c) (d)
130. (a) (b) (c) (d)
131. (a) (b) (c) (d)
132. (a) (b) (c) (d)
133. (a) (b) (c) (d)
134. (a) (b) (c) (d)
135. (a) (b) (c) (d)
136. (a) (b) (c) (d)
137. (a) (b) (c) (d)
138. (a) (b) (c) (d)
139. (a) (b) (c) (d)
140. (a) (b) (c) (d)
141. (a) (b) (c) (d)
142. (a) (b) (c) (d)
143. (a) (b) (c) (d)
144. (a) (b) (c) (d)
145. (a) (b) (c) (d)
146. (a) (b) (c) (d)
147. (a) (b) (c) (d)
148. (a) (b) (c) (d)
149. (a) (b) (c) (d)
150. (a) (b) (c) (d)
151. (a) (b) (c) (d)
152. (a) (b) (c) (d)
153. (a) (b) (c) (d)
154. (a) (b) (c) (d)
155. (a) (b) (c) (d)

156.	(a)	(b)	(c)	(d)
157.	(a)	(b)	(c)	(d)
158.	(a)	(b)	(c)	(d)
159.	(a)	(b)	(c)	(d)
160.	(a)	(b)	(c)	(d)
161.	(a)	(b)	(c)	(d)
162.	(a)	(b)	(c)	(d)
163.	(a)	(b)	(c)	(d)
164.	(a)	(b)	(c)	(d)
165.	(a)	(b)	(c)	(d)
166.	(a)	(b)	(c)	(d)
167.	(a)	(b)	(c)	(d)
168.	(a)	(b)	(c)	(d)
169.	(a)	(b)	(c)	(d)
170.	(a)	(b)	(c)	(d)
171.	(a)	(b)	(c)	(d)
172.	(a)	(b)	(c)	(d)
173.	(a)	(b)	(c)	(d)
174.	(a)	(b)	(c)	(d)
175.	(a)	(b)	(c)	(d)

176.	(a)	(b)	(c)	(d)
177.	(a)	(b)	(c)	(d)
178.	(a)	(b)	(c)	(d)
179.	(a)	(b)	(c)	(d)
180.	(a)	(b)	(c)	(d)

SWINE

Restraint and Behavior

181.	(a)	(b)	(c)	(d)
182.	(a)	(b)	(c)	(d)
183.	(a)	(b)	(c)	(d)
184.	(a)	(b)	(c)	(d)
185.	(a)	(b)	(c)	(d)
186.	(a)	(b)	(c)	(d)
187.	(a)	(b)	(c)	(d)
188.	(a)	(b)	(c)	(d)
189.	(a)	(b)	(c)	(d)
190.	(a)	(b)	(c)	(d)

191.	(a)	(b)	(c)	(d)
192.	(a)	(b)	(c)	(d)
193.	(a)	(b)	(c)	(d)
194.	(a)	(b)	(c)	(d)
195.	(a)	(b)	(c)	(d)

SANITATION

196.	(a)	(b)	(c)	(d)
197.	(a)	(b)	(c)	(d)
198.	(a)	(b)	(c)	(d)
199.	(a)	(b)	(c)	(d)
200.	(a)	(b)	(c)	(d)
201.	(a)	(b)	(c)	(d)
202.	(a)	(b)	(c)	(d)
203.	(a)	(b)	(c)	(d)
204.	(a)	(b)	(c)	(d)
205.	(a)	(b)	(c)	(d)
206.	(a)	(b)	(c)	(d)
207.	(a)	(b)	(c)	(d)

208.	(a)	(b)	(c)	(d)
209.	(a)	(b)	(c)	(d)
210.	(a)	(b)	(c)	(d)
211.	(a)	(b)	(c)	(d)
212.	(a)	(b)	(c)	(d)
213.	(a)	(b)	(c)	(d)
214.	(a)	(b)	(c)	(d)
215.	(a)	(b)	(c)	(d)
216.	(a)	(b)	(c)	(d)
217.	(a)	(b)	(c)	(d)
218.	(a)	(b)	(c)	(d)
219.	(a)	(b)	(c)	(d)
220.	(a)	(b)	(c)	(d)
221.	(a)	(b)	(c)	(d)
222.	(a)	(b)	(c)	(d)
223.	(a)	(b)	(c)	(d)
224.	(a)	(b)	(c)	(d)
225.	(a)	(b)	(c)	(d)

Dentistry

Fill in a circled letter to indicate your answer choice.

1. (a) (b) (c) (d)
2. (a) (b) (c) (d)
3. (a) (b) (c) (d)
4. (a) (b) (c) (d)
5. (a) (b) (c) (d)
6. (a) (b) (c) (d)
7. (a) (b) (c) (d)
8. (a) (b) (c) (d)
9. (a) (b) (c) (d)
10. (a) (b) (c) (d)
11. (a) (b) (c) (d)
12. (a) (b) (c) (d)
13. (a) (b) (c) (d)
14. (a) (b) (c) (d)

MATCHING

15. (a) (b) (c) (d)
16. (a) (b) (c) (d)
17. (a) (b) (c) (d)
18. (a) (b) (c) (d)
19. (a) (b) (c) (d)
20. (a) (b) (c) (d)
21. (a) (b) (c) (d)
22. (a) (b) (c) (d)
23. (a) (b) (c) (d)
24. (a) (b) (c) (d)
25. (a) (b) (c) (d)
26. (a) (b) (c) (d)
27. (a) (b) (c) (d)

28. (a) (b) (c) (d)
29. (a) (b) (c) (d)
30. (a) (b) (c) (d)
31. (a) (b) (c) (d)
32. (a) (b) (c) (d)
33. (a) (b) (c) (d)
34. (a) (b) (c) (d)
35. (a) (b) (c) (d)
36. (a) (b) (c) (d)
37. (a) (b) (c) (d)
38. (a) (b) (c) (d)
39. (a) (b) (c) (d)
40. (a) (b) (c) (d)
41. (a) (b) (c) (d)
42. (a) (b) (c) (d)

43. (a) (b) (c) (d)
44. (a) (b) (c) (d)
45. (a) (b) (c) (d)
46. (a) (b) (c) (d)
47. (a) (b) (c) (d)
48. (a) (b) (c) (d)
49. (a) (b) (c) (d)
50. (a) (b) (c) (d)
51. (a) (b) (c) (d)
52. (a) (b) (c) (d)
53. (a) (b) (c) (d)
54. (a) (b) (c) (d)
55. (a) (b) (c) (d)
56. (a) (b) (c) (d)
57. (a) (b) (c) (d)

Emergency Care

Fill in a circled letter to indicate your answer choice.

EMERGENCY ASSESSMENT

1. (a) (b) (c) (d)
2. (a) (b) (c) (d)
3. (a) (b) (c) (d)
4. (a) (b) (c) (d)
5. (a) (b) (c) (d)
6. (a) (b) (c) (d)
7. (a) (b) (c) (d)
8. (a) (b) (c) (d)
9. (a) (b) (c) (d)
10. (a) (b) (c) (d)
11. (a) (b) (c) (d)
12. (a) (b) (c) (d)
13. (a) (b) (c) (d)
14. (a) (b) (c) (d)
15. (a) (b) (c) (d)
16. (a) (b) (c) (d)
17. (a) (b) (c) (d)
18. (a) (b) (c) (d)
19. (a) (b) (c) (d)
20. (a) (b) (c) (d)
21. (a) (b) (c) (d)
22. (a) (b) (c) (d)

FIRST AID

23. (a) (b) (c) (d)
24. (a) (b) (c) (d)
25. (a) (b) (c) (d)
26. (a) (b) (c) (d)
27. (a) (b) (c) (d)
28. (a) (b) (c) (d)
29. (a) (b) (c) (d)
30. (a) (b) (c) (d)
31. (a) (b) (c) (d)
32. (a) (b) (c) (d)
33. (a) (b) (c) (d)
34. (a) (b) (c) (d)
35. (a) (b) (c) (d)
36. (a) (b) (c) (d)
37. (a) (b) (c) (d)
38. (a) (b) (c) (d)
39. (a) (b) (c) (d)
40. (a) (b) (c) (d)
41. (a) (b) (c) (d)
42. (a) (b) (c) (d)
43. (a) (b) (c) (d)
44. (a) (b) (c) (d)
45. (a) (b) (c) (d)
46. (a) (b) (c) (d)
47. (a) (b) (c) (d)

48. (a) (b) (c) (d)
49. (a) (b) (c) (d)
50. (a) (b) (c) (d)
51. (a) (b) (c) (d)
52. (a) (b) (c) (d)
53. (a) (b) (c) (d)
54. (a) (b) (c) (d)
55. (a) (b) (c) (d)
56. (a) (b) (c) (d)
57. (a) (b) (c) (d)

CRITICAL CARE

58. (a) (b) (c) (d)
59. (a) (b) (c) (d)
60. (a) (b) (c) (d)
61. (a) (b) (c) (d)
62. (a) (b) (c) (d)
63. (a) (b) (c) (d)
64. (a) (b) (c) (d)
65. (a) (b) (c) (d)
66. (a) (b) (c) (d)
67. (a) (b) (c) (d)
68. (a) (b) (c) (d)
69. (a) (b) (c) (d)
70. (a) (b) (c) (d)
71. (a) (b) (c) (d)

72. (a) (b) (c) (d)
73. (a) (b) (c) (d)
74. (a) (b) (c) (d)
75. (a) (b) (c) (d)
76. (a) (b) (c) (d)
77. (a) (b) (c) (d)
78. (a) (b) (c) (d)
79. (a) (b) (c) (d)
80. (a) (b) (c) (d)
81. (a) (b) (c) (d)
82. (a) (b) (c) (d)
83. (a) (b) (c) (d)
84. (a) (b) (c) (d)
85. (a) (b) (c) (d)
86. (a) (b) (c) (d)
87. (a) (b) (c) (d)
88. (a) (b) (c) (d)
89. (a) (b) (c) (d)
90. (a) (b) (c) (d)
91. (a) (b) (c) (d)
92. (a) (b) (c) (d)
93. (a) (b) (c) (d)
94. (a) (b) (c) (d)
95. (a) (b) (c) (d)
96. (a) (b) (c) (d)

Hospital Management

Fill in a circled letter to indicate your answer choice.

RECORD KEEPING

1. (a) (b) (c) (d)
2. (a) (b) (c) (d)
3. (a) (b) (c) (d)
4. (a) (b) (c) (d)
5. (a) (b) (c) (d)
6. (a) (b) (c) (d)
7. (a) (b) (c) (d)
8. (a) (b) (c) (d)
9. (a) (b) (c) (d)
10. (a) (b) (c) (d)
11. (a) (b) (c) (d)
12. (a) (b) (c) (d)
13. (a) (b) (c) (d)
14. (a) (b) (c) (d)
15. (a) (b) (c) (d)
16. (a) (b) (c) (d)

17. (a) (b) (c) (d)
18. (a) (b) (c) (d)
19. (a) (b) (c) (d)
20. (a) (b) (c) (d)
21. (a) (b) (c) (d)
22. (a) (b) (c) (d)
23. (a) (b) (c) (d)
24. (a) (b) (c) (d)
25. (a) (b) (c) (d)

ETHICS AND JURISPRUDENCE

26. (a) (b) (c) (d)
27. (a) (b) (c) (d)
28. (a) (b) (c) (d)
29. (a) (b) (c) (d)
30. (a) (b) (c) (d)

31. (a) (b) (c) (d)
32. (a) (b) (c) (d)
33. (a) (b) (c) (d)
34. (a) (b) (c) (d)
35. (a) (b) (c) (d)
36. (a) (b) (c) (d)
37. (a) (b) (c) (d)
38. (a) (b) (c) (d)
39. (a) (b) (c) (d)
40. (a) (b) (c) (d)
41. (a) (b) (c) (d)
42. (a) (b) (c) (d)
43. (a) (b) (c) (d)
44. (a) (b) (c) (d)
45. (a) (b) (c) (d)
46. (a) (b) (c) (d)
47. (a) (b) (c) (d)
48. (a) (b) (c) (d)

49. (a) (b) (c) (d)
50. (a) (b) (c) (d)
51. (a) (b) (c) (d)
52. (a) (b) (c) (d)
53. (a) (b) (c) (d)
54. (a) (b) (c) (d)
55. (a) (b) (c) (d)
56. (a) (b) (c) (d)
57. (a) (b) (c) (d)
58. (a) (b) (c) (d)
59. (a) (b) (c) (d)
60. (a) (b) (c) (d)
61. (a) (b) (c) (d)
62. (a) (b) (c) (d)
63. (a) (b) (c) (d)
64. (a) (b) (c) (d)

Laboratory Animals

Fill in a circled letter to indicate your answer choice.

1. ⓐ ⓑ ⓒ ⓓ	16. ⓐ ⓑ ⓒ ⓓ	31. ⓐ ⓑ ⓒ ⓓ	46. ⓐ ⓑ ⓒ ⓓ
2. ⓐ ⓑ ⓒ ⓓ	17. ⓐ ⓑ ⓒ ⓓ	32. ⓐ ⓑ ⓒ ⓓ	47. ⓐ ⓑ ⓒ ⓓ
3. ⓐ ⓑ ⓒ ⓓ	18. ⓐ ⓑ ⓒ ⓓ	33. ⓐ ⓑ ⓒ ⓓ	48. ⓐ ⓑ ⓒ ⓓ
4. ⓐ ⓑ ⓒ ⓓ	19. ⓐ ⓑ ⓒ ⓓ	34. ⓐ ⓑ ⓒ ⓓ	49. ⓐ ⓑ ⓒ ⓓ
5. ⓐ ⓑ ⓒ ⓓ	20. ⓐ ⓑ ⓒ ⓓ	35. ⓐ ⓑ ⓒ ⓓ	50. ⓐ ⓑ ⓒ ⓓ
6. ⓐ ⓑ ⓒ ⓓ	21. ⓐ ⓑ ⓒ ⓓ	36. ⓐ ⓑ ⓒ ⓓ	51. ⓐ ⓑ ⓒ ⓓ
7. ⓐ ⓑ ⓒ ⓓ	22. ⓐ ⓑ ⓒ ⓓ	37. ⓐ ⓑ ⓒ ⓓ	52. ⓐ ⓑ ⓒ ⓓ
8. ⓐ ⓑ ⓒ ⓓ	23. ⓐ ⓑ ⓒ ⓓ	38. ⓐ ⓑ ⓒ ⓓ	53. ⓐ ⓑ ⓒ ⓓ
9. ⓐ ⓑ ⓒ ⓓ	24. ⓐ ⓑ ⓒ ⓓ	39. ⓐ ⓑ ⓒ ⓓ	54. ⓐ ⓑ ⓒ ⓓ
10. ⓐ ⓑ ⓒ ⓓ	25. ⓐ ⓑ ⓒ ⓓ	40. ⓐ ⓑ ⓒ ⓓ	55. ⓐ ⓑ ⓒ ⓓ
11. ⓐ ⓑ ⓒ ⓓ	26. ⓐ ⓑ ⓒ ⓓ	41. ⓐ ⓑ ⓒ ⓓ	56. ⓐ ⓑ ⓒ ⓓ
12. ⓐ ⓑ ⓒ ⓓ	27. ⓐ ⓑ ⓒ ⓓ	42. ⓐ ⓑ ⓒ ⓓ	57. ⓐ ⓑ ⓒ ⓓ
13. ⓐ ⓑ ⓒ ⓓ	28. ⓐ ⓑ ⓒ ⓓ	43. ⓐ ⓑ ⓒ ⓓ	58. ⓐ ⓑ ⓒ ⓓ
14. ⓐ ⓑ ⓒ ⓓ	29. ⓐ ⓑ ⓒ ⓓ	44. ⓐ ⓑ ⓒ ⓓ	59. ⓐ ⓑ ⓒ ⓓ
15. ⓐ ⓑ ⓒ ⓓ	30. ⓐ ⓑ ⓒ ⓓ	45. ⓐ ⓑ ⓒ ⓓ	60. ⓐ ⓑ ⓒ ⓓ

Laboratory Procedures

Fill in a circled letter to indicate your answer choice.

QUALITY CONTROL

1. (a) (b) (c) (d)
2. (a) (b) (c) (d)
3. (a) (b) (c) (d)
4. (a) (b) (c) (d)
5. (a) (b) (c) (d)
6. (a) (b) (c) (d)
7. (a) (b) (c) (d)
8. (a) (b) (c) (d)
9. (a) (b) (c) (d)
10. (a) (b) (c) (d)
11. (a) (b) (c) (d)
12. (a) (b) (c) (d)
13. (a) (b) (c) (d)
14. (a) (b) (c) (d)
15. (a) (b) (c) (d)
16. (a) (b) (c) (d)
17. (a) (b) (c) (d)
18. (a) (b) (c) (d)
19. (a) (b) (c) (d)
20. (a) (b) (c) (d)

SAMPLE HANDLING, COLLECTION, AND STORAGE

21. (a) (b) (c) (d)
22. (a) (b) (c) (d)
23. (a) (b) (c) (d)
24. (a) (b) (c) (d)
25. (a) (b) (c) (d)
26. (a) (b) (c) (d)
27. (a) (b) (c) (d)
28. (a) (b) (c) (d)
29. (a) (b) (c) (d)
30. (a) (b) (c) (d)
31. (a) (b) (c) (d)
32. (a) (b) (c) (d)
33. (a) (b) (c) (d)
34. (a) (b) (c) (d)
35. (a) (b) (c) (d)
36. (a) (b) (c) (d)
37. (a) (b) (c) (d)

38. (a) (b) (c) (d)
39. (a) (b) (c) (d)
40. (a) (b) (c) (d)

BLOOD CHEMISTRY

41. (a) (b) (c) (d)
42. (a) (b) (c) (d)
43. (a) (b) (c) (d)
44. (a) (b) (c) (d)
45. (a) (b) (c) (d)
46. (a) (b) (c) (d)
47. (a) (b) (c) (d)
48. (a) (b) (c) (d)
49. (a) (b) (c) (d)
50. (a) (b) (c) (d)
51. (a) (b) (c) (d)
52. (a) (b) (c) (d)
53. (a) (b) (c) (d)
54. (a) (b) (c) (d)
55. (a) (b) (c) (d)
56. (a) (b) (c) (d)
57. (a) (b) (c) (d)
58. (a) (b) (c) (d)
59. (a) (b) (c) (d)
60. (a) (b) (c) (d)
61. (a) (b) (c) (d)
62. (a) (b) (c) (d)
63. (a) (b) (c) (d)
64. (a) (b) (c) (d)
65. (a) (b) (c) (d)
66. (a) (b) (c) (d)
67. (a) (b) (c) (d)
68. (a) (b) (c) (d)
69. (a) (b) (c) (d)
70. (a) (b) (c) (d)
71. (a) (b) (c) (d)
72. (a) (b) (c) (d)
73. (a) (b) (c) (d)
74. (a) (b) (c) (d)
75. (a) (b) (c) (d)
76. (a) (b) (c) (d)
77. (a) (b) (c) (d)
78. (a) (b) (c) (d)

79. (a) (b) (c) (d)
80. (a) (b) (c) (d)
81. (a) (b) (c) (d)
82. (a) (b) (c) (d)
83. (a) (b) (c) (d)
84. (a) (b) (c) (d)
85. (a) (b) (c) (d)
86. (a) (b) (c) (d)
87. (a) (b) (c) (d)
88. (a) (b) (c) (d)
89. (a) (b) (c) (d)
90. (a) (b) (c) (d)
91. (a) (b) (c) (d)
92. (a) (b) (c) (d)
93. (a) (b) (c) (d)
94. (a) (b) (c) (d)
95. (a) (b) (c) (d)
96. (a) (b) (c) (d)
97. (a) (b) (c) (d)
98. (a) (b) (c) (d)
99. (a) (b) (c) (d)
100. (a) (b) (c) (d)
101. (a) (b) (c) (d)
102. (a) (b) (c) (d)
103. (a) (b) (c) (d)
104. (a) (b) (c) (d)
105. (a) (b) (c) (d)
106. (a) (b) (c) (d)
107. (a) (b) (c) (d)
108. (a) (b) (c) (d)
109. (a) (b) (c) (d)
110. (a) (b) (c) (d)
111. (a) (b) (c) (d)
112. (a) (b) (c) (d)
113. (a) (b) (c) (d)
114. (a) (b) (c) (d)
115. (a) (b) (c) (d)
116. (a) (b) (c) (d)
117. (a) (b) (c) (d)
118. (a) (b) (c) (d)

CYTOLOGY

119. (a) (b) (c) (d)

120. (a) (b) (c) (d)
121. (a) (b) (c) (d)
122. (a) (b) (c) (d)
123. (a) (b) (c) (d)
124. (a) (b) (c) (d)
125. (a) (b) (c) (d)
126. (a) (b) (c) (d)
127. (a) (b) (c) (d)
128. (a) (b) (c) (d)
129. (a) (b) (c) (d)
130. (a) (b) (c) (d)
131. (a) (b) (c) (d)
132. (a) (b) (c) (d)
133. (a) (b) (c) (d)
134. (a) (b) (c) (d)
135. (a) (b) (c) (d)
136. (a) (b) (c) (d)
137. (a) (b) (c) (d)
138. (a) (b) (c) (d)
139. (a) (b) (c) (d)
140. (a) (b) (c) (d)
141. (a) (b) (c) (d)
142. (a) (b) (c) (d)
143. (a) (b) (c) (d)
144. (a) (b) (c) (d)
145. (a) (b) (c) (d)
146. (a) (b) (c) (d)
147. (a) (b) (c) (d)
148. (a) (b) (c) (d)
149. (a) (b) (c) (d)
150. (a) (b) (c) (d)

HEMATOLOGY

151. (a) (b) (c) (d)
152. (a) (b) (c) (d)
153. (a) (b) (c) (d)
154. (a) (b) (c) (d)
155. (a) (b) (c) (d)
156. (a) (b) (c) (d)
157. (a) (b) (c) (d)
158. (a) (b) (c) (d)
159. (a) (b) (c) (d)
160. (a) (b) (c) (d)

161.	ⓐ	ⓑ	ⓒ	ⓓ
162.	ⓐ	ⓑ	ⓒ	ⓓ
163.	ⓐ	ⓑ	ⓒ	ⓓ
164.	ⓐ	ⓑ	ⓒ	ⓓ
165.	ⓐ	ⓑ	ⓒ	ⓓ
166.	ⓐ	ⓑ	ⓒ	ⓓ
167.	ⓐ	ⓑ	ⓒ	ⓓ
168.	ⓐ	ⓑ	ⓒ	ⓓ
169.	ⓐ	ⓑ	ⓒ	ⓓ
170.	ⓐ	ⓑ	ⓒ	ⓓ
171.	ⓐ	ⓑ	ⓒ	ⓓ
172.	ⓐ	ⓑ	ⓒ	ⓓ
173.	ⓐ	ⓑ	ⓒ	ⓓ
174.	ⓐ	ⓑ	ⓒ	ⓓ
175.	ⓐ	ⓑ	ⓒ	ⓓ
176.	ⓐ	ⓑ	ⓒ	ⓓ
177.	ⓐ	ⓑ	ⓒ	ⓓ
178.	ⓐ	ⓑ	ⓒ	ⓓ
179.	ⓐ	ⓑ	ⓒ	ⓓ
180.	ⓐ	ⓑ	ⓒ	ⓓ
181.	ⓐ	ⓑ	ⓒ	ⓓ
182.	ⓐ	ⓑ	ⓒ	ⓓ
183.	ⓐ	ⓑ	ⓒ	ⓓ
184.	ⓐ	ⓑ	ⓒ	ⓓ
185.	ⓐ	ⓑ	ⓒ	ⓓ
186.	ⓐ	ⓑ	ⓒ	ⓓ
187.	ⓐ	ⓑ	ⓒ	ⓓ
188.	ⓐ	ⓑ	ⓒ	ⓓ
189.	ⓐ	ⓑ	ⓒ	ⓓ
190.	ⓐ	ⓑ	ⓒ	ⓓ
191.	ⓐ	ⓑ	ⓒ	ⓓ
192.	ⓐ	ⓑ	ⓒ	ⓓ
193.	ⓐ	ⓑ	ⓒ	ⓓ
194.	ⓐ	ⓑ	ⓒ	ⓓ
195.	ⓐ	ⓑ	ⓒ	ⓓ
196.	ⓐ	ⓑ	ⓒ	ⓓ
197.	ⓐ	ⓑ	ⓒ	ⓓ
198.	ⓐ	ⓑ	ⓒ	ⓓ
199.	ⓐ	ⓑ	ⓒ	ⓓ
200.	ⓐ	ⓑ	ⓒ	ⓓ
201.	ⓐ	ⓑ	ⓒ	ⓓ
202.	ⓐ	ⓑ	ⓒ	ⓓ
203.	ⓐ	ⓑ	ⓒ	ⓓ
204.	ⓐ	ⓑ	ⓒ	ⓓ
205.	ⓐ	ⓑ	ⓒ	ⓓ
206.	ⓐ	ⓑ	ⓒ	ⓓ
207.	ⓐ	ⓑ	ⓒ	ⓓ
208.	ⓐ	ⓑ	ⓒ	ⓓ
209.	ⓐ	ⓑ	ⓒ	ⓓ
210.	ⓐ	ⓑ	ⓒ	ⓓ
211.	ⓐ	ⓑ	ⓒ	ⓓ
212.	ⓐ	ⓑ	ⓒ	ⓓ
213.	ⓐ	ⓑ	ⓒ	ⓓ

214.	ⓐ	ⓑ	ⓒ	ⓓ
215.	ⓐ	ⓑ	ⓒ	ⓓ
216.	ⓐ	ⓑ	ⓒ	ⓓ
217.	ⓐ	ⓑ	ⓒ	ⓓ
218.	ⓐ	ⓑ	ⓒ	ⓓ
219.	ⓐ	ⓑ	ⓒ	ⓓ
220.	ⓐ	ⓑ	ⓒ	ⓓ
221.	ⓐ	ⓑ	ⓒ	ⓓ
222.	ⓐ	ⓑ	ⓒ	ⓓ
223.	ⓐ	ⓑ	ⓒ	ⓓ
224.	ⓐ	ⓑ	ⓒ	ⓓ
225.	ⓐ	ⓑ	ⓒ	ⓓ
226.	ⓐ	ⓑ	ⓒ	ⓓ
227.	ⓐ	ⓑ	ⓒ	ⓓ
228.	ⓐ	ⓑ	ⓒ	ⓓ
229.	ⓐ	ⓑ	ⓒ	ⓓ
230.	ⓐ	ⓑ	ⓒ	ⓓ
231.	ⓐ	ⓑ	ⓒ	ⓓ
232.	ⓐ	ⓑ	ⓒ	ⓓ
233.	ⓐ	ⓑ	ⓒ	ⓓ
234.	ⓐ	ⓑ	ⓒ	ⓓ
235.	ⓐ	ⓑ	ⓒ	ⓓ
236.	ⓐ	ⓑ	ⓒ	ⓓ
237.	ⓐ	ⓑ	ⓒ	ⓓ
238.	ⓐ	ⓑ	ⓒ	ⓓ
239.	ⓐ	ⓑ	ⓒ	ⓓ
240.	ⓐ	ⓑ	ⓒ	ⓓ

IMMUNOLOGY

241.	ⓐ	ⓑ	ⓒ	ⓓ
242.	ⓐ	ⓑ	ⓒ	ⓓ
243.	ⓐ	ⓑ	ⓒ	ⓓ
244.	ⓐ	ⓑ	ⓒ	ⓓ
245.	ⓐ	ⓑ	ⓒ	ⓓ
246.	ⓐ	ⓑ	ⓒ	ⓓ
247.	ⓐ	ⓑ	ⓒ	ⓓ
248.	ⓐ	ⓑ	ⓒ	ⓓ
249.	ⓐ	ⓑ	ⓒ	ⓓ
250.	ⓐ	ⓑ	ⓒ	ⓓ
251.	ⓐ	ⓑ	ⓒ	ⓓ
252.	ⓐ	ⓑ	ⓒ	ⓓ
253.	ⓐ	ⓑ	ⓒ	ⓓ
254.	ⓐ	ⓑ	ⓒ	ⓓ
255.	ⓐ	ⓑ	ⓒ	ⓓ
256.	ⓐ	ⓑ	ⓒ	ⓓ
257.	ⓐ	ⓑ	ⓒ	ⓓ
258.	ⓐ	ⓑ	ⓒ	ⓓ
259.	ⓐ	ⓑ	ⓒ	ⓓ
260.	ⓐ	ⓑ	ⓒ	ⓓ
261.	ⓐ	ⓑ	ⓒ	ⓓ
262.	ⓐ	ⓑ	ⓒ	ⓓ
263.	ⓐ	ⓑ	ⓒ	ⓓ

264.	ⓐ	ⓑ	ⓒ	ⓓ
265.	ⓐ	ⓑ	ⓒ	ⓓ
266.	ⓐ	ⓑ	ⓒ	ⓓ
267.	ⓐ	ⓑ	ⓒ	ⓓ
268.	ⓐ	ⓑ	ⓒ	ⓓ
269.	ⓐ	ⓑ	ⓒ	ⓓ
270.	ⓐ	ⓑ	ⓒ	ⓓ
271.	ⓐ	ⓑ	ⓒ	ⓓ
272.	ⓐ	ⓑ	ⓒ	ⓓ
273.	ⓐ	ⓑ	ⓒ	ⓓ
274.	ⓐ	ⓑ	ⓒ	ⓓ
275.	ⓐ	ⓑ	ⓒ	ⓓ
276.	ⓐ	ⓑ	ⓒ	ⓓ
277.	ⓐ	ⓑ	ⓒ	ⓓ
278.	ⓐ	ⓑ	ⓒ	ⓓ
279.	ⓐ	ⓑ	ⓒ	ⓓ
280.	ⓐ	ⓑ	ⓒ	ⓓ
281.	ⓐ	ⓑ	ⓒ	ⓓ
282.	ⓐ	ⓑ	ⓒ	ⓓ
283.	ⓐ	ⓑ	ⓒ	ⓓ
284.	ⓐ	ⓑ	ⓒ	ⓓ
285.	ⓐ	ⓑ	ⓒ	ⓓ
286.	ⓐ	ⓑ	ⓒ	ⓓ
287.	ⓐ	ⓑ	ⓒ	ⓓ
288.	ⓐ	ⓑ	ⓒ	ⓓ
289.	ⓐ	ⓑ	ⓒ	ⓓ
290.	ⓐ	ⓑ	ⓒ	ⓓ
291.	ⓐ	ⓑ	ⓒ	ⓓ
292.	ⓐ	ⓑ	ⓒ	ⓓ
293.	ⓐ	ⓑ	ⓒ	ⓓ
294.	ⓐ	ⓑ	ⓒ	ⓓ
295.	ⓐ	ⓑ	ⓒ	ⓓ

MICROBIOLOGY

296.	ⓐ	ⓑ	ⓒ	ⓓ
297.	ⓐ	ⓑ	ⓒ	ⓓ
298.	ⓐ	ⓑ	ⓒ	ⓓ
299.	ⓐ	ⓑ	ⓒ	ⓓ
300.	ⓐ	ⓑ	ⓒ	ⓓ
301.	ⓐ	ⓑ	ⓒ	ⓓ
302.	ⓐ	ⓑ	ⓒ	ⓓ
303.	ⓐ	ⓑ	ⓒ	ⓓ
304.	ⓐ	ⓑ	ⓒ	ⓓ
305.	ⓐ	ⓑ	ⓒ	ⓓ
306.	ⓐ	ⓑ	ⓒ	ⓓ
307.	ⓐ	ⓑ	ⓒ	ⓓ
308.	ⓐ	ⓑ	ⓒ	ⓓ
309.	ⓐ	ⓑ	ⓒ	ⓓ
310.	ⓐ	ⓑ	ⓒ	ⓓ
311.	ⓐ	ⓑ	ⓒ	ⓓ
312.	ⓐ	ⓑ	ⓒ	ⓓ
313.	ⓐ	ⓑ	ⓒ	ⓓ

314.	ⓐ	ⓑ	ⓒ	ⓓ
315.	ⓐ	ⓑ	ⓒ	ⓓ
316.	ⓐ	ⓑ	ⓒ	ⓓ
317.	ⓐ	ⓑ	ⓒ	ⓓ
318.	ⓐ	ⓑ	ⓒ	ⓓ
319.	ⓐ	ⓑ	ⓒ	ⓓ
320.	ⓐ	ⓑ	ⓒ	ⓓ
321.	ⓐ	ⓑ	ⓒ	ⓓ
322.	ⓐ	ⓑ	ⓒ	ⓓ
323.	ⓐ	ⓑ	ⓒ	ⓓ
324.	ⓐ	ⓑ	ⓒ	ⓓ
325.	ⓐ	ⓑ	ⓒ	ⓓ
326.	ⓐ	ⓑ	ⓒ	ⓓ
327.	ⓐ	ⓑ	ⓒ	ⓓ
328.	ⓐ	ⓑ	ⓒ	ⓓ
329.	ⓐ	ⓑ	ⓒ	ⓓ
330.	ⓐ	ⓑ	ⓒ	ⓓ
331.	ⓐ	ⓑ	ⓒ	ⓓ
332.	ⓐ	ⓑ	ⓒ	ⓓ
333.	ⓐ	ⓑ	ⓒ	ⓓ
334.	ⓐ	ⓑ	ⓒ	ⓓ
335.	ⓐ	ⓑ	ⓒ	ⓓ
336.	ⓐ	ⓑ	ⓒ	ⓓ
337.	ⓐ	ⓑ	ⓒ	ⓓ
338.	ⓐ	ⓑ	ⓒ	ⓓ
339.	ⓐ	ⓑ	ⓒ	ⓓ
340.	ⓐ	ⓑ	ⓒ	ⓓ
341.	ⓐ	ⓑ	ⓒ	ⓓ
342.	ⓐ	ⓑ	ⓒ	ⓓ
343.	ⓐ	ⓑ	ⓒ	ⓓ
344.	ⓐ	ⓑ	ⓒ	ⓓ
345.	ⓐ	ⓑ	ⓒ	ⓓ
346.	ⓐ	ⓑ	ⓒ	ⓓ
347.	ⓐ	ⓑ	ⓒ	ⓓ
348.	ⓐ	ⓑ	ⓒ	ⓓ
349.	ⓐ	ⓑ	ⓒ	ⓓ
350.	ⓐ	ⓑ	ⓒ	ⓓ
351.	ⓐ	ⓑ	ⓒ	ⓓ
352.	ⓐ	ⓑ	ⓒ	ⓓ
353.	ⓐ	ⓑ	ⓒ	ⓓ
354.	ⓐ	ⓑ	ⓒ	ⓓ
355.	ⓐ	ⓑ	ⓒ	ⓓ

PARASITOLOGY

356.	ⓐ	ⓑ	ⓒ	ⓓ
357.	ⓐ	ⓑ	ⓒ	ⓓ
358.	ⓐ	ⓑ	ⓒ	ⓓ
359.	ⓐ	ⓑ	ⓒ	ⓓ
360.	ⓐ	ⓑ	ⓒ	ⓓ
361.	ⓐ	ⓑ	ⓒ	ⓓ
362.	ⓐ	ⓑ	ⓒ	ⓓ
363.	ⓐ	ⓑ	ⓒ	ⓓ

364.	ⓐ	ⓑ	ⓒ	ⓓ	399.	ⓐ	ⓑ	ⓒ	ⓓ	434.	ⓐ	ⓑ	ⓒ	ⓓ	466.	ⓐ	ⓑ	ⓒ	ⓓ
365.	ⓐ	ⓑ	ⓒ	ⓓ	400.	ⓐ	ⓑ	ⓒ	ⓓ	435.	ⓐ	ⓑ	ⓒ	ⓓ	467.	ⓐ	ⓑ	ⓒ	ⓓ
366.	ⓐ	ⓑ	ⓒ	ⓓ	401.	ⓐ	ⓑ	ⓒ	ⓓ	436.	ⓐ	ⓑ	ⓒ	ⓓ	468.	ⓐ	ⓑ	ⓒ	ⓓ
367.	ⓐ	ⓑ	ⓒ	ⓓ	402.	ⓐ	ⓑ	ⓒ	ⓓ	437.	ⓐ	ⓑ	ⓒ	ⓓ	469.	ⓐ	ⓑ	ⓒ	ⓓ
368.	ⓐ	ⓑ	ⓒ	ⓓ	403.	ⓐ	ⓑ	ⓒ	ⓓ	438.	ⓐ	ⓑ	ⓒ	ⓓ	470.	ⓐ	ⓑ	ⓒ	ⓓ
369.	ⓐ	ⓑ	ⓒ	ⓓ	404.	ⓐ	ⓑ	ⓒ	ⓓ	439.	ⓐ	ⓑ	ⓒ	ⓓ	471.	ⓐ	ⓑ	ⓒ	ⓓ
370.	ⓐ	ⓑ	ⓒ	ⓓ	405.	ⓐ	ⓑ	ⓒ	ⓓ	440.	ⓐ	ⓑ	ⓒ	ⓓ	472.	ⓐ	ⓑ	ⓒ	ⓓ
371.	ⓐ	ⓑ	ⓒ	ⓓ	406.	ⓐ	ⓑ	ⓒ	ⓓ	441.	ⓐ	ⓑ	ⓒ	ⓓ	473.	ⓐ	ⓑ	ⓒ	ⓓ
372.	ⓐ	ⓑ	ⓒ	ⓓ	407.	ⓐ	ⓑ	ⓒ	ⓓ	442.	ⓐ	ⓑ	ⓒ	ⓓ	474.	ⓐ	ⓑ	ⓒ	ⓓ
373.	ⓐ	ⓑ	ⓒ	ⓓ	408.	ⓐ	ⓑ	ⓒ	ⓓ	443.	ⓐ	ⓑ	ⓒ	ⓓ	475.	ⓐ	ⓑ	ⓒ	ⓓ
374.	ⓐ	ⓑ	ⓒ	ⓓ	409.	ⓐ	ⓑ	ⓒ	ⓓ	444.	ⓐ	ⓑ	ⓒ	ⓓ	476.	ⓐ	ⓑ	ⓒ	ⓓ
375.	ⓐ	ⓑ	ⓒ	ⓓ	410.	ⓐ	ⓑ	ⓒ	ⓓ	445.	ⓐ	ⓑ	ⓒ	ⓓ	477.	ⓐ	ⓑ	ⓒ	ⓓ
376.	ⓐ	ⓑ	ⓒ	ⓓ	411.	ⓐ	ⓑ	ⓒ	ⓓ	446.	ⓐ	ⓑ	ⓒ	ⓓ	478.	ⓐ	ⓑ	ⓒ	ⓓ
377.	ⓐ	ⓑ	ⓒ	ⓓ	412.	ⓐ	ⓑ	ⓒ	ⓓ	447.	ⓐ	ⓑ	ⓒ	ⓓ	479.	ⓐ	ⓑ	ⓒ	ⓓ
378.	ⓐ	ⓑ	ⓒ	ⓓ	413.	ⓐ	ⓑ	ⓒ	ⓓ	448.	ⓐ	ⓑ	ⓒ	ⓓ	480.	ⓐ	ⓑ	ⓒ	ⓓ
379.	ⓐ	ⓑ	ⓒ	ⓓ	414.	ⓐ	ⓑ	ⓒ	ⓓ	449.	ⓐ	ⓑ	ⓒ	ⓓ	481.	ⓐ	ⓑ	ⓒ	ⓓ
380.	ⓐ	ⓑ	ⓒ	ⓓ	415.	ⓐ	ⓑ	ⓒ	ⓓ	450.	ⓐ	ⓑ	ⓒ	ⓓ	482.	ⓐ	ⓑ	ⓒ	ⓓ
381.	ⓐ	ⓑ	ⓒ	ⓓ	416.	ⓐ	ⓑ	ⓒ	ⓓ	451.	ⓐ	ⓑ	ⓒ	ⓓ	483.	ⓐ	ⓑ	ⓒ	ⓓ
382.	ⓐ	ⓑ	ⓒ	ⓓ	417.	ⓐ	ⓑ	ⓒ	ⓓ	452.	ⓐ	ⓑ	ⓒ	ⓓ	484.	ⓐ	ⓑ	ⓒ	ⓓ
383.	ⓐ	ⓑ	ⓒ	ⓓ	418.	ⓐ	ⓑ	ⓒ	ⓓ	453.	ⓐ	ⓑ	ⓒ	ⓓ	485.	ⓐ	ⓑ	ⓒ	ⓓ
384.	ⓐ	ⓑ	ⓒ	ⓓ	419.	ⓐ	ⓑ	ⓒ	ⓓ	454.	ⓐ	ⓑ	ⓒ	ⓓ	486.	ⓐ	ⓑ	ⓒ	ⓓ
385.	ⓐ	ⓑ	ⓒ	ⓓ	420.	ⓐ	ⓑ	ⓒ	ⓓ	455.	ⓐ	ⓑ	ⓒ	ⓓ	487.	ⓐ	ⓑ	ⓒ	ⓓ
386.	ⓐ	ⓑ	ⓒ	ⓓ	421.	ⓐ	ⓑ	ⓒ	ⓓ	456.	ⓐ	ⓑ	ⓒ	ⓓ	488.	ⓐ	ⓑ	ⓒ	ⓓ
387.	ⓐ	ⓑ	ⓒ	ⓓ	422.	ⓐ	ⓑ	ⓒ	ⓓ	457.	ⓐ	ⓑ	ⓒ	ⓓ	489.	ⓐ	ⓑ	ⓒ	ⓓ
388.	ⓐ	ⓑ	ⓒ	ⓓ	423.	ⓐ	ⓑ	ⓒ	ⓓ						490.	ⓐ	ⓑ	ⓒ	ⓓ
389.	ⓐ	ⓑ	ⓒ	ⓓ	424.	ⓐ	ⓑ	ⓒ	ⓓ	**URINALYSIS**					491.	ⓐ	ⓑ	ⓒ	ⓓ
390.	ⓐ	ⓑ	ⓒ	ⓓ	425.	ⓐ	ⓑ	ⓒ	ⓓ						492.	ⓐ	ⓑ	ⓒ	ⓓ
391.	ⓐ	ⓑ	ⓒ	ⓓ	426.	ⓐ	ⓑ	ⓒ	ⓓ	458.	ⓐ	ⓑ	ⓒ	ⓓ	493.	ⓐ	ⓑ	ⓒ	ⓓ
392.	ⓐ	ⓑ	ⓒ	ⓓ	427.	ⓐ	ⓑ	ⓒ	ⓓ	459.	ⓐ	ⓑ	ⓒ	ⓓ	494.	ⓐ	ⓑ	ⓒ	ⓓ
393.	ⓐ	ⓑ	ⓒ	ⓓ	428.	ⓐ	ⓑ	ⓒ	ⓓ	460.	ⓐ	ⓑ	ⓒ	ⓓ	495.	ⓐ	ⓑ	ⓒ	ⓓ
394.	ⓐ	ⓑ	ⓒ	ⓓ	429.	ⓐ	ⓑ	ⓒ	ⓓ	461.	ⓐ	ⓑ	ⓒ	ⓓ	496.	ⓐ	ⓑ	ⓒ	ⓓ
395.	ⓐ	ⓑ	ⓒ	ⓓ	430.	ⓐ	ⓑ	ⓒ	ⓓ	462.	ⓐ	ⓑ	ⓒ	ⓓ	497.	ⓐ	ⓑ	ⓒ	ⓓ
396.	ⓐ	ⓑ	ⓒ	ⓓ	431.	ⓐ	ⓑ	ⓒ	ⓓ	463.	ⓐ	ⓑ	ⓒ	ⓓ					
397.	ⓐ	ⓑ	ⓒ	ⓓ	432.	ⓐ	ⓑ	ⓒ	ⓓ	464.	ⓐ	ⓑ	ⓒ	ⓓ					
398.	ⓐ	ⓑ	ⓒ	ⓓ	433.	ⓐ	ⓑ	ⓒ	ⓓ	465.	ⓐ	ⓑ	ⓒ	ⓓ					

Corresponding questions are on pages 140-177.

Medical Calculations

Fill in a circled letter to indicate your answer choice.

1. ⓐ ⓑ ⓒ ⓓ	24. ⓐ ⓑ ⓒ ⓓ	47. ⓐ ⓑ ⓒ ⓓ	70. ⓐ ⓑ ⓒ ⓓ
2. ⓐ ⓑ ⓒ ⓓ	25. ⓐ ⓑ ⓒ ⓓ	48. ⓐ ⓑ ⓒ ⓓ	71. ⓐ ⓑ ⓒ ⓓ
3. ⓐ ⓑ ⓒ ⓓ	26. ⓐ ⓑ ⓒ ⓓ	49. ⓐ ⓑ ⓒ ⓓ	72. ⓐ ⓑ ⓒ ⓓ
4. ⓐ ⓑ ⓒ ⓓ	27. ⓐ ⓑ ⓒ ⓓ	50. ⓐ ⓑ ⓒ ⓓ	73. ⓐ ⓑ ⓒ ⓓ
5. ⓐ ⓑ ⓒ ⓓ	28. ⓐ ⓑ ⓒ ⓓ	51. ⓐ ⓑ ⓒ ⓓ	74. ⓐ ⓑ ⓒ ⓓ
6. ⓐ ⓑ ⓒ ⓓ	29. ⓐ ⓑ ⓒ ⓓ	52. ⓐ ⓑ ⓒ ⓓ	75. ⓐ ⓑ ⓒ ⓓ
7. ⓐ ⓑ ⓒ ⓓ	30. ⓐ ⓑ ⓒ ⓓ	53. ⓐ ⓑ ⓒ ⓓ	76. ⓐ ⓑ ⓒ ⓓ
8. ⓐ ⓑ ⓒ ⓓ	31. ⓐ ⓑ ⓒ ⓓ	54. ⓐ ⓑ ⓒ ⓓ	77. ⓐ ⓑ ⓒ ⓓ
9. ⓐ ⓑ ⓒ ⓓ	32. ⓐ ⓑ ⓒ ⓓ	55. ⓐ ⓑ ⓒ ⓓ	78. ⓐ ⓑ ⓒ ⓓ
10. ⓐ ⓑ ⓒ ⓓ	33. ⓐ ⓑ ⓒ ⓓ	56. ⓐ ⓑ ⓒ ⓓ	79. ⓐ ⓑ ⓒ ⓓ
11. ⓐ ⓑ ⓒ ⓓ	34. ⓐ ⓑ ⓒ ⓓ	57. ⓐ ⓑ ⓒ ⓓ	80. ⓐ ⓑ ⓒ ⓓ
12. ⓐ ⓑ ⓒ ⓓ	35. ⓐ ⓑ ⓒ ⓓ	58. ⓐ ⓑ ⓒ ⓓ	81. ⓐ ⓑ ⓒ ⓓ
13. ⓐ ⓑ ⓒ ⓓ	36. ⓐ ⓑ ⓒ ⓓ	59. ⓐ ⓑ ⓒ ⓓ	82. ⓐ ⓑ ⓒ ⓓ
14. ⓐ ⓑ ⓒ ⓓ	37. ⓐ ⓑ ⓒ ⓓ	60. ⓐ ⓑ ⓒ ⓓ	83. ⓐ ⓑ ⓒ ⓓ
15. ⓐ ⓑ ⓒ ⓓ	38. ⓐ ⓑ ⓒ ⓓ	61. ⓐ ⓑ ⓒ ⓓ	84. ⓐ ⓑ ⓒ ⓓ
16. ⓐ ⓑ ⓒ ⓓ	39. ⓐ ⓑ ⓒ ⓓ	62. ⓐ ⓑ ⓒ ⓓ	85. ⓐ ⓑ ⓒ ⓓ
17. ⓐ ⓑ ⓒ ⓓ	40. ⓐ ⓑ ⓒ ⓓ	63. ⓐ ⓑ ⓒ ⓓ	86. ⓐ ⓑ ⓒ ⓓ
18. ⓐ ⓑ ⓒ ⓓ	41. ⓐ ⓑ ⓒ ⓓ	64. ⓐ ⓑ ⓒ ⓓ	87. ⓐ ⓑ ⓒ ⓓ
19. ⓐ ⓑ ⓒ ⓓ	42. ⓐ ⓑ ⓒ ⓓ	65. ⓐ ⓑ ⓒ ⓓ	88. ⓐ ⓑ ⓒ ⓓ
20. ⓐ ⓑ ⓒ ⓓ	43. ⓐ ⓑ ⓒ ⓓ	66. ⓐ ⓑ ⓒ ⓓ	89. ⓐ ⓑ ⓒ ⓓ
21. ⓐ ⓑ ⓒ ⓓ	44. ⓐ ⓑ ⓒ ⓓ	67. ⓐ ⓑ ⓒ ⓓ	90. ⓐ ⓑ ⓒ ⓓ
22. ⓐ ⓑ ⓒ ⓓ	45. ⓐ ⓑ ⓒ ⓓ	68. ⓐ ⓑ ⓒ ⓓ	91. ⓐ ⓑ ⓒ ⓓ
23. ⓐ ⓑ ⓒ ⓓ	46. ⓐ ⓑ ⓒ ⓓ	69. ⓐ ⓑ ⓒ ⓓ	92. ⓐ ⓑ ⓒ ⓓ

Medical Nursing

Fill in a circled letter to indicate your answer choice.

PHYSICAL EXAMINATION

1. ⓐ ⓑ ⓒ ⓓ
2. ⓐ ⓑ ⓒ ⓓ
3. ⓐ ⓑ ⓒ ⓓ
4. ⓐ ⓑ ⓒ ⓓ
5. ⓐ ⓑ ⓒ ⓓ
6. ⓐ ⓑ ⓒ ⓓ
7. ⓐ ⓑ ⓒ ⓓ
8. ⓐ ⓑ ⓒ ⓓ
9. ⓐ ⓑ ⓒ ⓓ
10. ⓐ ⓑ ⓒ ⓓ
11. ⓐ ⓑ ⓒ ⓓ
12. ⓐ ⓑ ⓒ ⓓ
13. ⓐ ⓑ ⓒ ⓓ
14. ⓐ ⓑ ⓒ ⓓ
15. ⓐ ⓑ ⓒ ⓓ
16. ⓐ ⓑ ⓒ ⓓ
17. ⓐ ⓑ ⓒ ⓓ
18. ⓐ ⓑ ⓒ ⓓ
19. ⓐ ⓑ ⓒ ⓓ
20. ⓐ ⓑ ⓒ ⓓ
21. ⓐ ⓑ ⓒ ⓓ
22. ⓐ ⓑ ⓒ ⓓ
23. ⓐ ⓑ ⓒ ⓓ
24. ⓐ ⓑ ⓒ ⓓ
25. ⓐ ⓑ ⓒ ⓓ
26. ⓐ ⓑ ⓒ ⓓ
27. ⓐ ⓑ ⓒ ⓓ
28. ⓐ ⓑ ⓒ ⓓ
29. ⓐ ⓑ ⓒ ⓓ
30. ⓐ ⓑ ⓒ ⓓ
31. ⓐ ⓑ ⓒ ⓓ
32. ⓐ ⓑ ⓒ ⓓ
33. ⓐ ⓑ ⓒ ⓓ
34. ⓐ ⓑ ⓒ ⓓ
35. ⓐ ⓑ ⓒ ⓓ
36. ⓐ ⓑ ⓒ ⓓ
37. ⓐ ⓑ ⓒ ⓓ
38. ⓐ ⓑ ⓒ ⓓ
39. ⓐ ⓑ ⓒ ⓓ

NORMAL VALUES

40. ⓐ ⓑ ⓒ ⓓ
41. ⓐ ⓑ ⓒ ⓓ
42. ⓐ ⓑ ⓒ ⓓ
43. ⓐ ⓑ ⓒ ⓓ
44. ⓐ ⓑ ⓒ ⓓ
45. ⓐ ⓑ ⓒ ⓓ
46. ⓐ ⓑ ⓒ ⓓ
47. ⓐ ⓑ ⓒ ⓓ
48. ⓐ ⓑ ⓒ ⓓ
49. ⓐ ⓑ ⓒ ⓓ
50. ⓐ ⓑ ⓒ ⓓ
51. ⓐ ⓑ ⓒ ⓓ
52. ⓐ ⓑ ⓒ ⓓ
53. ⓐ ⓑ ⓒ ⓓ
54. ⓐ ⓑ ⓒ ⓓ
55. ⓐ ⓑ ⓒ ⓓ
56. ⓐ ⓑ ⓒ ⓓ
57. ⓐ ⓑ ⓒ ⓓ
58. ⓐ ⓑ ⓒ ⓓ
59. ⓐ ⓑ ⓒ ⓓ
60. ⓐ ⓑ ⓒ ⓓ

DRUG ADMINISTRATION

61. ⓐ ⓑ ⓒ ⓓ
62. ⓐ ⓑ ⓒ ⓓ
63. ⓐ ⓑ ⓒ ⓓ
64. ⓐ ⓑ ⓒ ⓓ
65. ⓐ ⓑ ⓒ ⓓ
66. ⓐ ⓑ ⓒ ⓓ
67. ⓐ ⓑ ⓒ ⓓ
68. ⓐ ⓑ ⓒ ⓓ
69. ⓐ ⓑ ⓒ ⓓ
70. ⓐ ⓑ ⓒ ⓓ
71. ⓐ ⓑ ⓒ ⓓ
72. ⓐ ⓑ ⓒ ⓓ
73. ⓐ ⓑ ⓒ ⓓ
74. ⓐ ⓑ ⓒ ⓓ
75. ⓐ ⓑ ⓒ ⓓ

76. ⓐ ⓑ ⓒ ⓓ
77. ⓐ ⓑ ⓒ ⓓ

FLUID THERAPY

78. ⓐ ⓑ ⓒ ⓓ
79. ⓐ ⓑ ⓒ ⓓ
80. ⓐ ⓑ ⓒ ⓓ
81. ⓐ ⓑ ⓒ ⓓ
82. ⓐ ⓑ ⓒ ⓓ
83. ⓐ ⓑ ⓒ ⓓ
84. ⓐ ⓑ ⓒ ⓓ
85. ⓐ ⓑ ⓒ ⓓ
86. ⓐ ⓑ ⓒ ⓓ
87. ⓐ ⓑ ⓒ ⓓ
88. ⓐ ⓑ ⓒ ⓓ
89. ⓐ ⓑ ⓒ ⓓ
90. ⓐ ⓑ ⓒ ⓓ

BANDAGING AND SPLINTS

91. ⓐ ⓑ ⓒ ⓓ
92. ⓐ ⓑ ⓒ ⓓ
93. ⓐ ⓑ ⓒ ⓓ
94. ⓐ ⓑ ⓒ ⓓ
95. ⓐ ⓑ ⓒ ⓓ
96. ⓐ ⓑ ⓒ ⓓ
97. ⓐ ⓑ ⓒ ⓓ
98. ⓐ ⓑ ⓒ ⓓ
99. ⓐ ⓑ ⓒ ⓓ
100. ⓐ ⓑ ⓒ ⓓ
101. ⓐ ⓑ ⓒ ⓓ
102. ⓐ ⓑ ⓒ ⓓ
103. ⓐ ⓑ ⓒ ⓓ
104. ⓐ ⓑ ⓒ ⓓ
105. ⓐ ⓑ ⓒ ⓓ

WOUND HEALING

106. ⓐ ⓑ ⓒ ⓓ
107. ⓐ ⓑ ⓒ ⓓ

108. ⓐ ⓑ ⓒ ⓓ
109. ⓐ ⓑ ⓒ ⓓ

BREED IDENTIFICATION

110. ⓐ ⓑ ⓒ ⓓ
111. ⓐ ⓑ ⓒ ⓓ
112. ⓐ ⓑ ⓒ ⓓ
113. ⓐ ⓑ ⓒ ⓓ
114. ⓐ ⓑ ⓒ ⓓ
115. ⓐ ⓑ ⓒ ⓓ
116. ⓐ ⓑ ⓒ ⓓ
117. ⓐ ⓑ ⓒ ⓓ
118. ⓐ ⓑ ⓒ ⓓ
119. ⓐ ⓑ ⓒ ⓓ
120. ⓐ ⓑ ⓒ ⓓ
121. ⓐ ⓑ ⓒ ⓓ
122. ⓐ ⓑ ⓒ ⓓ
123. ⓐ ⓑ ⓒ ⓓ
124. ⓐ ⓑ ⓒ ⓓ
125. ⓐ ⓑ ⓒ ⓓ
126. ⓐ ⓑ ⓒ ⓓ
127. ⓐ ⓑ ⓒ ⓓ
128. ⓐ ⓑ ⓒ ⓓ
129. ⓐ ⓑ ⓒ ⓓ
130. ⓐ ⓑ ⓒ ⓓ
131. ⓐ ⓑ ⓒ ⓓ
132. ⓐ ⓑ ⓒ ⓓ
133. ⓐ ⓑ ⓒ ⓓ
134. ⓐ ⓑ ⓒ ⓓ
135. ⓐ ⓑ ⓒ ⓓ
136. ⓐ ⓑ ⓒ ⓓ
137. ⓐ ⓑ ⓒ ⓓ
138. ⓐ ⓑ ⓒ ⓓ
139. ⓐ ⓑ ⓒ ⓓ
140. ⓐ ⓑ ⓒ ⓓ
141. ⓐ ⓑ ⓒ ⓓ
142. ⓐ ⓑ ⓒ ⓓ
143. ⓐ ⓑ ⓒ ⓓ
144. ⓐ ⓑ ⓒ ⓓ
145. ⓐ ⓑ ⓒ ⓓ
146. ⓐ ⓑ ⓒ ⓓ

147.	(a)	(b)	(c)	(d)
148.	(a)	(b)	(c)	(d)
149.	(a)	(b)	(c)	(d)
150.	(a)	(b)	(c)	(d)
151.	(a)	(b)	(c)	(d)
152.	(a)	(b)	(c)	(d)
153.	(a)	(b)	(c)	(d)
154.	(a)	(b)	(c)	(d)
155.	(a)	(b)	(c)	(d)
156.	(a)	(b)	(c)	(d)
157.	(a)	(b)	(c)	(d)
158.	(a)	(b)	(c)	(d)
159.	(a)	(b)	(c)	(d)

DISEASE CONTROL

160.	(a)	(b)	(c)	(d)
161.	(a)	(b)	(c)	(d)
162.	(a)	(b)	(c)	(d)
163.	(a)	(b)	(c)	(d)
164.	(a)	(b)	(c)	(d)
165.	(a)	(b)	(c)	(d)
166.	(a)	(b)	(c)	(d)
167.	(a)	(b)	(c)	(d)
168.	(a)	(b)	(c)	(d)

169.	(a)	(b)	(c)	(d)
170.	(a)	(b)	(c)	(d)
171.	(a)	(b)	(c)	(d)
172.	(a)	(b)	(c)	(d)
173.	(a)	(b)	(c)	(d)
174.	(a)	(b)	(c)	(d)
175.	(a)	(b)	(c)	(d)
176.	(a)	(b)	(c)	(d)
177.	(a)	(b)	(c)	(d)
178.	(a)	(b)	(c)	(d)
179.	(a)	(b)	(c)	(d)
180.	(a)	(b)	(c)	(d)
181.	(a)	(b)	(c)	(d)
182.	(a)	(b)	(c)	(d)
183.	(a)	(b)	(c)	(d)
184.	(a)	(b)	(c)	(d)
185.	(a)	(b)	(c)	(d)
186.	(a)	(b)	(c)	(d)
187.	(a)	(b)	(c)	(d)
188.	(a)	(b)	(c)	(d)
189.	(a)	(b)	(c)	(d)
190.	(a)	(b)	(c)	(d)
191.	(a)	(b)	(c)	(d)
192.	(a)	(b)	(c)	(d)
193.	(a)	(b)	(c)	(d)

194.	(a)	(b)	(c)	(d)
195.	(a)	(b)	(c)	(d)
196.	(a)	(b)	(c)	(d)
197.	(a)	(b)	(c)	(d)
198.	(a)	(b)	(c)	(d)

PUBLIC HEALTH AND ZOONOSES

199.	(a)	(b)	(c)	(d)
200.	(a)	(b)	(c)	(d)
201.	(a)	(b)	(c)	(d)
202.	(a)	(b)	(c)	(d)
203.	(a)	(b)	(c)	(d)
204.	(a)	(b)	(c)	(d)
205.	(a)	(b)	(c)	(d)
206.	(a)	(b)	(c)	(d)
207.	(a)	(b)	(c)	(d)
208.	(a)	(b)	(c)	(d)
209.	(a)	(b)	(c)	(d)
210.	(a)	(b)	(c)	(d)
211.	(a)	(b)	(c)	(d)
212.	(a)	(b)	(c)	(d)
213.	(a)	(b)	(c)	(d)
214.	(a)	(b)	(c)	(d)

215.	(a)	(b)	(c)	(d)
216.	(a)	(b)	(c)	(d)
217.	(a)	(b)	(c)	(d)
218.	(a)	(b)	(c)	(d)
219.	(a)	(b)	(c)	(d)
220.	(a)	(b)	(c)	(d)
221.	(a)	(b)	(c)	(d)
222.	(a)	(b)	(c)	(d)
223.	(a)	(b)	(c)	(d)
224.	(a)	(b)	(c)	(d)
225.	(a)	(b)	(c)	(d)
226.	(a)	(b)	(c)	(d)
227.	(a)	(b)	(c)	(d)
228.	(a)	(b)	(c)	(d)
229.	(a)	(b)	(c)	(d)
230.	(a)	(b)	(c)	(d)
231.	(a)	(b)	(c)	(d)
232.	(a)	(b)	(c)	(d)
233.	(a)	(b)	(c)	(d)
234.	(a)	(b)	(c)	(d)
235.	(a)	(b)	(c)	(d)
236.	(a)	(b)	(c)	(d)
237.	(a)	(b)	(c)	(d)
238.	(a)	(b)	(c)	(d)

Medical Terminology

Fill in a circled letter to indicate your answer choice.

1. ⓐ ⓑ ⓒ ⓓ
2. ⓐ ⓑ ⓒ ⓓ
3. ⓐ ⓑ ⓒ ⓓ
4. ⓐ ⓑ ⓒ ⓓ
5. ⓐ ⓑ ⓒ ⓓ
6. ⓐ ⓑ ⓒ ⓓ
7. ⓐ ⓑ ⓒ ⓓ
8. ⓐ ⓑ ⓒ ⓓ
9. ⓐ ⓑ ⓒ ⓓ
10. ⓐ ⓑ ⓒ ⓓ
11. ⓐ ⓑ ⓒ ⓓ
12. ⓐ ⓑ ⓒ ⓓ
13. ⓐ ⓑ ⓒ ⓓ
14. ⓐ ⓑ ⓒ ⓓ
15. ⓐ ⓑ ⓒ ⓓ
16. ⓐ ⓑ ⓒ ⓓ
17. ⓐ ⓑ ⓒ ⓓ
18. ⓐ ⓑ ⓒ ⓓ
19. ⓐ ⓑ ⓒ ⓓ
20. ⓐ ⓑ ⓒ ⓓ
21. ⓐ ⓑ ⓒ ⓓ
22. ⓐ ⓑ ⓒ ⓓ
23. ⓐ ⓑ ⓒ ⓓ

24. ⓐ ⓑ ⓒ ⓓ
25. ⓐ ⓑ ⓒ ⓓ
26. ⓐ ⓑ ⓒ ⓓ
27. ⓐ ⓑ ⓒ ⓓ
28. ⓐ ⓑ ⓒ ⓓ
29. ⓐ ⓑ ⓒ ⓓ
30. ⓐ ⓑ ⓒ ⓓ
31. ⓐ ⓑ ⓒ ⓓ
32. ⓐ ⓑ ⓒ ⓓ
33. ⓐ ⓑ ⓒ ⓓ
34. ⓐ ⓑ ⓒ ⓓ
35. ⓐ ⓑ ⓒ ⓓ
36. ⓐ ⓑ ⓒ ⓓ
37. ⓐ ⓑ ⓒ ⓓ
38. ⓐ ⓑ ⓒ ⓓ
39. ⓐ ⓑ ⓒ ⓓ
40. ⓐ ⓑ ⓒ ⓓ
41. ⓐ ⓑ ⓒ ⓓ
42. ⓐ ⓑ ⓒ ⓓ
43. ⓐ ⓑ ⓒ ⓓ
44. ⓐ ⓑ ⓒ ⓓ
45. ⓐ ⓑ ⓒ ⓓ
46. ⓐ ⓑ ⓒ ⓓ

47. ⓐ ⓑ ⓒ ⓓ
48. ⓐ ⓑ ⓒ ⓓ
49. ⓐ ⓑ ⓒ ⓓ
50. ⓐ ⓑ ⓒ ⓓ
51. ⓐ ⓑ ⓒ ⓓ
52. ⓐ ⓑ ⓒ ⓓ
53. ⓐ ⓑ ⓒ ⓓ
54. ⓐ ⓑ ⓒ ⓓ
55. ⓐ ⓑ ⓒ ⓓ
56. ⓐ ⓑ ⓒ ⓓ
57. ⓐ ⓑ ⓒ ⓓ
58. ⓐ ⓑ ⓒ ⓓ
59. ⓐ ⓑ ⓒ ⓓ
60. ⓐ ⓑ ⓒ ⓓ
61. ⓐ ⓑ ⓒ ⓓ
62. ⓐ ⓑ ⓒ ⓓ
63. ⓐ ⓑ ⓒ ⓓ
64. ⓐ ⓑ ⓒ ⓓ
65. ⓐ ⓑ ⓒ ⓓ
66. ⓐ ⓑ ⓒ ⓓ
67. ⓐ ⓑ ⓒ ⓓ
68. ⓐ ⓑ ⓒ ⓓ
69. ⓐ ⓑ ⓒ ⓓ

70. ⓐ ⓑ ⓒ ⓓ
71. ⓐ ⓑ ⓒ ⓓ
72. ⓐ ⓑ ⓒ ⓓ
73. ⓐ ⓑ ⓒ ⓓ
74. ⓐ ⓑ ⓒ ⓓ
75. ⓐ ⓑ ⓒ ⓓ
76. ⓐ ⓑ ⓒ ⓓ
77. ⓐ ⓑ ⓒ ⓓ
78. ⓐ ⓑ ⓒ ⓓ
79. ⓐ ⓑ ⓒ ⓓ
80. ⓐ ⓑ ⓒ ⓓ
81. ⓐ ⓑ ⓒ ⓓ
82. ⓐ ⓑ ⓒ ⓓ
83. ⓐ ⓑ ⓒ ⓓ
84. ⓐ ⓑ ⓒ ⓓ
85. ⓐ ⓑ ⓒ ⓓ
86. ⓐ ⓑ ⓒ ⓓ
87. ⓐ ⓑ ⓒ ⓓ
88. ⓐ ⓑ ⓒ ⓓ
89. ⓐ ⓑ ⓒ ⓓ
90. ⓐ ⓑ ⓒ ⓓ
91. ⓐ ⓑ ⓒ ⓓ

Pharmacology

Fill in a circled letter to indicate your answer choice.

1. ⓐ ⓑ ⓒ ⓓ	31. ⓐ ⓑ ⓒ ⓓ	61. ⓐ ⓑ ⓒ ⓓ	91. ⓐ ⓑ ⓒ ⓓ
2. ⓐ ⓑ ⓒ ⓓ	32. ⓐ ⓑ ⓒ ⓓ	62. ⓐ ⓑ ⓒ ⓓ	92. ⓐ ⓑ ⓒ ⓓ
3. ⓐ ⓑ ⓒ ⓓ	33. ⓐ ⓑ ⓒ ⓓ	63. ⓐ ⓑ ⓒ ⓓ	93. ⓐ ⓑ ⓒ ⓓ
4. ⓐ ⓑ ⓒ ⓓ	34. ⓐ ⓑ ⓒ ⓓ	64. ⓐ ⓑ ⓒ ⓓ	94. ⓐ ⓑ ⓒ ⓓ
5. ⓐ ⓑ ⓒ ⓓ	35. ⓐ ⓑ ⓒ ⓓ	65. ⓐ ⓑ ⓒ ⓓ	95. ⓐ ⓑ ⓒ ⓓ
6. ⓐ ⓑ ⓒ ⓓ	36. ⓐ ⓑ ⓒ ⓓ	66. ⓐ ⓑ ⓒ ⓓ	96. ⓐ ⓑ ⓒ ⓓ
7. ⓐ ⓑ ⓒ ⓓ	37. ⓐ ⓑ ⓒ ⓓ	67. ⓐ ⓑ ⓒ ⓓ	97. ⓐ ⓑ ⓒ ⓓ
8. ⓐ ⓑ ⓒ ⓓ	38. ⓐ ⓑ ⓒ ⓓ	68. ⓐ ⓑ ⓒ ⓓ	98. ⓐ ⓑ ⓒ ⓓ
9. ⓐ ⓑ ⓒ ⓓ	39. ⓐ ⓑ ⓒ ⓓ	69. ⓐ ⓑ ⓒ ⓓ	99. ⓐ ⓑ ⓒ ⓓ
10. ⓐ ⓑ ⓒ ⓓ	40. ⓐ ⓑ ⓒ ⓓ	70. ⓐ ⓑ ⓒ ⓓ	100. ⓐ ⓑ ⓒ ⓓ
11. ⓐ ⓑ ⓒ ⓓ	41. ⓐ ⓑ ⓒ ⓓ	71. ⓐ ⓑ ⓒ ⓓ	101. ⓐ ⓑ ⓒ ⓓ
12. ⓐ ⓑ ⓒ ⓓ	42. ⓐ ⓑ ⓒ ⓓ	72. ⓐ ⓑ ⓒ ⓓ	102. ⓐ ⓑ ⓒ ⓓ
13. ⓐ ⓑ ⓒ ⓓ	43. ⓐ ⓑ ⓒ ⓓ	73. ⓐ ⓑ ⓒ ⓓ	103. ⓐ ⓑ ⓒ ⓓ
14. ⓐ ⓑ ⓒ ⓓ	44. ⓐ ⓑ ⓒ ⓓ	74. ⓐ ⓑ ⓒ ⓓ	104. ⓐ ⓑ ⓒ ⓓ
15. ⓐ ⓑ ⓒ ⓓ	45. ⓐ ⓑ ⓒ ⓓ	75. ⓐ ⓑ ⓒ ⓓ	105. ⓐ ⓑ ⓒ ⓓ
16. ⓐ ⓑ ⓒ ⓓ	46. ⓐ ⓑ ⓒ ⓓ	76. ⓐ ⓑ ⓒ ⓓ	106. ⓐ ⓑ ⓒ ⓓ
17. ⓐ ⓑ ⓒ ⓓ	47. ⓐ ⓑ ⓒ ⓓ	77. ⓐ ⓑ ⓒ ⓓ	107. ⓐ ⓑ ⓒ ⓓ
18. ⓐ ⓑ ⓒ ⓓ	48. ⓐ ⓑ ⓒ ⓓ	78. ⓐ ⓑ ⓒ ⓓ	108. ⓐ ⓑ ⓒ ⓓ
19. ⓐ ⓑ ⓒ ⓓ	49. ⓐ ⓑ ⓒ ⓓ	79. ⓐ ⓑ ⓒ ⓓ	109. ⓐ ⓑ ⓒ ⓓ
20. ⓐ ⓑ ⓒ ⓓ	50. ⓐ ⓑ ⓒ ⓓ	80. ⓐ ⓑ ⓒ ⓓ	110. ⓐ ⓑ ⓒ ⓓ
21. ⓐ ⓑ ⓒ ⓓ	51. ⓐ ⓑ ⓒ ⓓ	81. ⓐ ⓑ ⓒ ⓓ	111. ⓐ ⓑ ⓒ ⓓ
22. ⓐ ⓑ ⓒ ⓓ	52. ⓐ ⓑ ⓒ ⓓ	82. ⓐ ⓑ ⓒ ⓓ	112. ⓐ ⓑ ⓒ ⓓ
23. ⓐ ⓑ ⓒ ⓓ	53. ⓐ ⓑ ⓒ ⓓ	83. ⓐ ⓑ ⓒ ⓓ	113. ⓐ ⓑ ⓒ ⓓ
24. ⓐ ⓑ ⓒ ⓓ	54. ⓐ ⓑ ⓒ ⓓ	84. ⓐ ⓑ ⓒ ⓓ	114. ⓐ ⓑ ⓒ ⓓ
25. ⓐ ⓑ ⓒ ⓓ	55. ⓐ ⓑ ⓒ ⓓ	85. ⓐ ⓑ ⓒ ⓓ	115. ⓐ ⓑ ⓒ ⓓ
26. ⓐ ⓑ ⓒ ⓓ	56. ⓐ ⓑ ⓒ ⓓ	86. ⓐ ⓑ ⓒ ⓓ	116. ⓐ ⓑ ⓒ ⓓ
27. ⓐ ⓑ ⓒ ⓓ	57. ⓐ ⓑ ⓒ ⓓ	87. ⓐ ⓑ ⓒ ⓓ	117. ⓐ ⓑ ⓒ ⓓ
28. ⓐ ⓑ ⓒ ⓓ	58. ⓐ ⓑ ⓒ ⓓ	88. ⓐ ⓑ ⓒ ⓓ	
29. ⓐ ⓑ ⓒ ⓓ	59. ⓐ ⓑ ⓒ ⓓ	89. ⓐ ⓑ ⓒ ⓓ	
30. ⓐ ⓑ ⓒ ⓓ	60. ⓐ ⓑ ⓒ ⓓ	90. ⓐ ⓑ ⓒ ⓓ	

Radiography

Fill in a circled letter to indicate your answer choice.

GENERAL

1. ⓐ ⓑ ⓒ ⓓ
2. ⓐ ⓑ ⓒ ⓓ
3. ⓐ ⓑ ⓒ ⓓ
4. ⓐ ⓑ ⓒ ⓓ
5. ⓐ ⓑ ⓒ ⓓ
6. ⓐ ⓑ ⓒ ⓓ
7. ⓐ ⓑ ⓒ ⓓ
8. ⓐ ⓑ ⓒ ⓓ
9. ⓐ ⓑ ⓒ ⓓ
10. ⓐ ⓑ ⓒ ⓓ
11. ⓐ ⓑ ⓒ ⓓ
12. ⓐ ⓑ ⓒ ⓓ
13. ⓐ ⓑ ⓒ ⓓ
14. ⓐ ⓑ ⓒ ⓓ
15. ⓐ ⓑ ⓒ ⓓ
16. ⓐ ⓑ ⓒ ⓓ
17. ⓐ ⓑ ⓒ ⓓ
18. ⓐ ⓑ ⓒ ⓓ
19. ⓐ ⓑ ⓒ ⓓ
20. ⓐ ⓑ ⓒ ⓓ
21. ⓐ ⓑ ⓒ ⓓ
22. ⓐ ⓑ ⓒ ⓓ
23. ⓐ ⓑ ⓒ ⓓ
24. ⓐ ⓑ ⓒ ⓓ
25. ⓐ ⓑ ⓒ ⓓ
26. ⓐ ⓑ ⓒ ⓓ
27. ⓐ ⓑ ⓒ ⓓ
28. ⓐ ⓑ ⓒ ⓓ
29. ⓐ ⓑ ⓒ ⓓ
30. ⓐ ⓑ ⓒ ⓓ
31. ⓐ ⓑ ⓒ ⓓ
32. ⓐ ⓑ ⓒ ⓓ
33. ⓐ ⓑ ⓒ ⓓ
34. ⓐ ⓑ ⓒ ⓓ
35. ⓐ ⓑ ⓒ ⓓ
36. ⓐ ⓑ ⓒ ⓓ
37. ⓐ ⓑ ⓒ ⓓ
38. ⓐ ⓑ ⓒ ⓓ
39. ⓐ ⓑ ⓒ ⓓ
40. ⓐ ⓑ ⓒ ⓓ

DARKROOM

41. ⓐ ⓑ ⓒ ⓓ
42. ⓐ ⓑ ⓒ ⓓ
43. ⓐ ⓑ ⓒ ⓓ
44. ⓐ ⓑ ⓒ ⓓ
45. ⓐ ⓑ ⓒ ⓓ
46. ⓐ ⓑ ⓒ ⓓ
47. ⓐ ⓑ ⓒ ⓓ
48. ⓐ ⓑ ⓒ ⓓ
49. ⓐ ⓑ ⓒ ⓓ
50. ⓐ ⓑ ⓒ ⓓ
51. ⓐ ⓑ ⓒ ⓓ
52. ⓐ ⓑ ⓒ ⓓ
53. ⓐ ⓑ ⓒ ⓓ
54. ⓐ ⓑ ⓒ ⓓ
55. ⓐ ⓑ ⓒ ⓓ
56. ⓐ ⓑ ⓒ ⓓ
57. ⓐ ⓑ ⓒ ⓓ
58. ⓐ ⓑ ⓒ ⓓ
59. ⓐ ⓑ ⓒ ⓓ

FILM

60. ⓐ ⓑ ⓒ ⓓ
61. ⓐ ⓑ ⓒ ⓓ
62. ⓐ ⓑ ⓒ ⓓ
63. ⓐ ⓑ ⓒ ⓓ
64. ⓐ ⓑ ⓒ ⓓ
65. ⓐ ⓑ ⓒ ⓓ
66. ⓐ ⓑ ⓒ ⓓ
67. ⓐ ⓑ ⓒ ⓓ
68. ⓐ ⓑ ⓒ ⓓ

ANIMAL POSITIONING

69. ⓐ ⓑ ⓒ ⓓ
70. ⓐ ⓑ ⓒ ⓓ
71. ⓐ ⓑ ⓒ ⓓ
72. ⓐ ⓑ ⓒ ⓓ
73. ⓐ ⓑ ⓒ ⓓ
74. ⓐ ⓑ ⓒ ⓓ
75. ⓐ ⓑ ⓒ ⓓ
76. ⓐ ⓑ ⓒ ⓓ
77. ⓐ ⓑ ⓒ ⓓ
78. ⓐ ⓑ ⓒ ⓓ
79. ⓐ ⓑ ⓒ ⓓ
80. ⓐ ⓑ ⓒ ⓓ
81. ⓐ ⓑ ⓒ ⓓ
82. ⓐ ⓑ ⓒ ⓓ
83. ⓐ ⓑ ⓒ ⓓ
84. ⓐ ⓑ ⓒ ⓓ
85. ⓐ ⓑ ⓒ ⓓ

IMAGE PRODUCTION

86. ⓐ ⓑ ⓒ ⓓ
87. ⓐ ⓑ ⓒ ⓓ
88. ⓐ ⓑ ⓒ ⓓ
89. ⓐ ⓑ ⓒ ⓓ
90. ⓐ ⓑ ⓒ ⓓ
91. ⓐ ⓑ ⓒ ⓓ
92. ⓐ ⓑ ⓒ ⓓ
93. ⓐ ⓑ ⓒ ⓓ
94. ⓐ ⓑ ⓒ ⓓ
95. ⓐ ⓑ ⓒ ⓓ
96. ⓐ ⓑ ⓒ ⓓ
97. ⓐ ⓑ ⓒ ⓓ
98. ⓐ ⓑ ⓒ ⓓ
99. ⓐ ⓑ ⓒ ⓓ
100. ⓐ ⓑ ⓒ ⓓ
101. ⓐ ⓑ ⓒ ⓓ
102. ⓐ ⓑ ⓒ ⓓ
103. ⓐ ⓑ ⓒ ⓓ
104. ⓐ ⓑ ⓒ ⓓ
105. ⓐ ⓑ ⓒ ⓓ
106. ⓐ ⓑ ⓒ ⓓ
107. ⓐ ⓑ ⓒ ⓓ
108. ⓐ ⓑ ⓒ ⓓ
109. ⓐ ⓑ ⓒ ⓓ
110. ⓐ ⓑ ⓒ ⓓ
111. ⓐ ⓑ ⓒ ⓓ
112. ⓐ ⓑ ⓒ ⓓ
113. ⓐ ⓑ ⓒ ⓓ
114. ⓐ ⓑ ⓒ ⓓ
115. ⓐ ⓑ ⓒ ⓓ
116. ⓐ ⓑ ⓒ ⓓ
117. ⓐ ⓑ ⓒ ⓓ
118. ⓐ ⓑ ⓒ ⓓ
119. ⓐ ⓑ ⓒ ⓓ
120. ⓐ ⓑ ⓒ ⓓ
121. ⓐ ⓑ ⓒ ⓓ
122. ⓐ ⓑ ⓒ ⓓ
123. ⓐ ⓑ ⓒ ⓓ

RADIATION SAFETY

124. ⓐ ⓑ ⓒ ⓓ
125. ⓐ ⓑ ⓒ ⓓ
126. ⓐ ⓑ ⓒ ⓓ
127. ⓐ ⓑ ⓒ ⓓ
128. ⓐ ⓑ ⓒ ⓓ
129. ⓐ ⓑ ⓒ ⓓ
130. ⓐ ⓑ ⓒ ⓓ
131. ⓐ ⓑ ⓒ ⓓ
132. ⓐ ⓑ ⓒ ⓓ
133. ⓐ ⓑ ⓒ ⓓ
134. ⓐ ⓑ ⓒ ⓓ
135. ⓐ ⓑ ⓒ ⓓ
136. ⓐ ⓑ ⓒ ⓓ
137. ⓐ ⓑ ⓒ ⓓ
138. ⓐ ⓑ ⓒ ⓓ
139. ⓐ ⓑ ⓒ ⓓ
140. ⓐ ⓑ ⓒ ⓓ
141. ⓐ ⓑ ⓒ ⓓ
142. ⓐ ⓑ ⓒ ⓓ
143. ⓐ ⓑ ⓒ ⓓ
144. ⓐ ⓑ ⓒ ⓓ
145. ⓐ ⓑ ⓒ ⓓ
146. ⓐ ⓑ ⓒ ⓓ

Surgical Nursing

Fill in a circled letter to indicate your answer choice.

GENERAL

1. ⓐ ⓑ ⓒ ⓓ
2. ⓐ ⓑ ⓒ ⓓ
3. ⓐ ⓑ ⓒ ⓓ
4. ⓐ ⓑ ⓒ ⓓ
5. ⓐ ⓑ ⓒ ⓓ
6. ⓐ ⓑ ⓒ ⓓ
7. ⓐ ⓑ ⓒ ⓓ
8. ⓐ ⓑ ⓒ ⓓ
9. ⓐ ⓑ ⓒ ⓓ
10. ⓐ ⓑ ⓒ ⓓ
11. ⓐ ⓑ ⓒ ⓓ
12. ⓐ ⓑ ⓒ ⓓ
13. ⓐ ⓑ ⓒ ⓓ
14. ⓐ ⓑ ⓒ ⓓ
15. ⓐ ⓑ ⓒ ⓓ
16. ⓐ ⓑ ⓒ ⓓ
17. ⓐ ⓑ ⓒ ⓓ
18. ⓐ ⓑ ⓒ ⓓ
19. ⓐ ⓑ ⓒ ⓓ
20. ⓐ ⓑ ⓒ ⓓ
21. ⓐ ⓑ ⓒ ⓓ
22. ⓐ ⓑ ⓒ ⓓ
23. ⓐ ⓑ ⓒ ⓓ
24. ⓐ ⓑ ⓒ ⓓ
25. ⓐ ⓑ ⓒ ⓓ
26. ⓐ ⓑ ⓒ ⓓ
27. ⓐ ⓑ ⓒ ⓓ
28. ⓐ ⓑ ⓒ ⓓ
29. ⓐ ⓑ ⓒ ⓓ
30. ⓐ ⓑ ⓒ ⓓ
31. ⓐ ⓑ ⓒ ⓓ
32. ⓐ ⓑ ⓒ ⓓ
33. ⓐ ⓑ ⓒ ⓓ
34. ⓐ ⓑ ⓒ ⓓ
35. ⓐ ⓑ ⓒ ⓓ
36. ⓐ ⓑ ⓒ ⓓ
37. ⓐ ⓑ ⓒ ⓓ
38. ⓐ ⓑ ⓒ ⓓ
39. ⓐ ⓑ ⓒ ⓓ
40. ⓐ ⓑ ⓒ ⓓ
41. ⓐ ⓑ ⓒ ⓓ
42. ⓐ ⓑ ⓒ ⓓ
43. ⓐ ⓑ ⓒ ⓓ
44. ⓐ ⓑ ⓒ ⓓ
45. ⓐ ⓑ ⓒ ⓓ
46. ⓐ ⓑ ⓒ ⓓ
47. ⓐ ⓑ ⓒ ⓓ
48. ⓐ ⓑ ⓒ ⓓ
49. ⓐ ⓑ ⓒ ⓓ
50. ⓐ ⓑ ⓒ ⓓ
51. ⓐ ⓑ ⓒ ⓓ
52. ⓐ ⓑ ⓒ ⓓ
53. ⓐ ⓑ ⓒ ⓓ
54. ⓐ ⓑ ⓒ ⓓ
55. ⓐ ⓑ ⓒ ⓓ
56. ⓐ ⓑ ⓒ ⓓ
57. ⓐ ⓑ ⓒ ⓓ
58. ⓐ ⓑ ⓒ ⓓ
59. ⓐ ⓑ ⓒ ⓓ
60. ⓐ ⓑ ⓒ ⓓ

COMMON SURGICAL INSTRUMENTS

61. ⓐ ⓑ ⓒ ⓓ
62. ⓐ ⓑ ⓒ ⓓ
63. ⓐ ⓑ ⓒ ⓓ
64. ⓐ ⓑ ⓒ ⓓ
65. ⓐ ⓑ ⓒ ⓓ
66. ⓐ ⓑ ⓒ ⓓ
67. ⓐ ⓑ ⓒ ⓓ
68. ⓐ ⓑ ⓒ ⓓ
69. ⓐ ⓑ ⓒ ⓓ
70. ⓐ ⓑ ⓒ ⓓ
71. ⓐ ⓑ ⓒ ⓓ
72. ⓐ ⓑ ⓒ ⓓ
73. ⓐ ⓑ ⓒ ⓓ
74. ⓐ ⓑ ⓒ ⓓ
75. ⓐ ⓑ ⓒ ⓓ
76. ⓐ ⓑ ⓒ ⓓ
77. ⓐ ⓑ ⓒ ⓓ
78. ⓐ ⓑ ⓒ ⓓ
79. ⓐ ⓑ ⓒ ⓓ
80. ⓐ ⓑ ⓒ ⓓ
81. ⓐ ⓑ ⓒ ⓓ
82. ⓐ ⓑ ⓒ ⓓ
83. ⓐ ⓑ ⓒ ⓓ
84. ⓐ ⓑ ⓒ ⓓ
85. ⓐ ⓑ ⓒ ⓓ
86. ⓐ ⓑ ⓒ ⓓ
87. ⓐ ⓑ ⓒ ⓓ
88. ⓐ ⓑ ⓒ ⓓ

SUTURING

89. ⓐ ⓑ ⓒ ⓓ
90. ⓐ ⓑ ⓒ ⓓ
91. ⓐ ⓑ ⓒ ⓓ
92. ⓐ ⓑ ⓒ ⓓ
93. ⓐ ⓑ ⓒ ⓓ
94. ⓐ ⓑ ⓒ ⓓ
95. ⓐ ⓑ ⓒ ⓓ
96. ⓐ ⓑ ⓒ ⓓ
97. ⓐ ⓑ ⓒ ⓓ
98. ⓐ ⓑ ⓒ ⓓ
99. ⓐ ⓑ ⓒ ⓓ
100. ⓐ ⓑ ⓒ ⓓ
101. ⓐ ⓑ ⓒ ⓓ
102. ⓐ ⓑ ⓒ ⓓ
103. ⓐ ⓑ ⓒ ⓓ
104. ⓐ ⓑ ⓒ ⓓ
105. ⓐ ⓑ ⓒ ⓓ
106. ⓐ ⓑ ⓒ ⓓ
107. ⓐ ⓑ ⓒ ⓓ
108. ⓐ ⓑ ⓒ ⓓ
109. ⓐ ⓑ ⓒ ⓓ
110. ⓐ ⓑ ⓒ ⓓ
111. ⓐ ⓑ ⓒ ⓓ
112. ⓐ ⓑ ⓒ ⓓ
113. ⓐ ⓑ ⓒ ⓓ
114. ⓐ ⓑ ⓒ ⓓ
115. ⓐ ⓑ ⓒ ⓓ
116. ⓐ ⓑ ⓒ ⓓ
117. ⓐ ⓑ ⓒ ⓓ
118. ⓐ ⓑ ⓒ ⓓ

ASEPTIC TECHNIQUE

119. ⓐ ⓑ ⓒ ⓓ
120. ⓐ ⓑ ⓒ ⓓ
121. ⓐ ⓑ ⓒ ⓓ
122. ⓐ ⓑ ⓒ ⓓ
123. ⓐ ⓑ ⓒ ⓓ
124. ⓐ ⓑ ⓒ ⓓ
125. ⓐ ⓑ ⓒ ⓓ
126. ⓐ ⓑ ⓒ ⓓ
127. ⓐ ⓑ ⓒ ⓓ
128. ⓐ ⓑ ⓒ ⓓ
129. ⓐ ⓑ ⓒ ⓓ
130. ⓐ ⓑ ⓒ ⓓ
131. ⓐ ⓑ ⓒ ⓓ
132. ⓐ ⓑ ⓒ ⓓ
133. ⓐ ⓑ ⓒ ⓓ
134. ⓐ ⓑ ⓒ ⓓ
135. ⓐ ⓑ ⓒ ⓓ
136. ⓐ ⓑ ⓒ ⓓ
137. ⓐ ⓑ ⓒ ⓓ
138. ⓐ ⓑ ⓒ ⓓ
139. ⓐ ⓑ ⓒ ⓓ
140. ⓐ ⓑ ⓒ ⓓ
141. ⓐ ⓑ ⓒ ⓓ
142. ⓐ ⓑ ⓒ ⓓ
143. ⓐ ⓑ ⓒ ⓓ
144. ⓐ ⓑ ⓒ ⓓ
145. ⓐ ⓑ ⓒ ⓓ
146. ⓐ ⓑ ⓒ ⓓ
147. ⓐ ⓑ ⓒ ⓓ
148. ⓐ ⓑ ⓒ ⓓ
149. ⓐ ⓑ ⓒ ⓓ
150. ⓐ ⓑ ⓒ ⓓ
151. ⓐ ⓑ ⓒ ⓓ
152. ⓐ ⓑ ⓒ ⓓ
153. ⓐ ⓑ ⓒ ⓓ
154. ⓐ ⓑ ⓒ ⓓ
155. ⓐ ⓑ ⓒ ⓓ
156. ⓐ ⓑ ⓒ ⓓ
157. ⓐ ⓑ ⓒ ⓓ
158. ⓐ ⓑ ⓒ ⓓ
159. ⓐ ⓑ ⓒ ⓓ
160. ⓐ ⓑ ⓒ ⓓ

161.	ⓐ	ⓑ	ⓒ	ⓓ	174.	ⓐ	ⓑ	ⓒ	ⓓ	183.	ⓐ	ⓑ	ⓒ	ⓓ	196.	ⓐ	ⓑ	ⓒ ⓓ

161. ⓐ ⓑ ⓒ ⓓ
162. ⓐ ⓑ ⓒ ⓓ
163. ⓐ ⓑ ⓒ ⓓ
164. ⓐ ⓑ ⓒ ⓓ
165. ⓐ ⓑ ⓒ ⓓ
166. ⓐ ⓑ ⓒ ⓓ
167. ⓐ ⓑ ⓒ ⓓ
168. ⓐ ⓑ ⓒ ⓓ
169. ⓐ ⓑ ⓒ ⓓ
170. ⓐ ⓑ ⓒ ⓓ
171. ⓐ ⓑ ⓒ ⓓ
172. ⓐ ⓑ ⓒ ⓓ
173. ⓐ ⓑ ⓒ ⓓ

174. ⓐ ⓑ ⓒ ⓓ
175. ⓐ ⓑ ⓒ ⓓ
176. ⓐ ⓑ ⓒ ⓓ
177. ⓐ ⓑ ⓒ ⓓ
178. ⓐ ⓑ ⓒ ⓓ

SURGICAL TERMINOLOGY

179. ⓐ ⓑ ⓒ ⓓ
180. ⓐ ⓑ ⓒ ⓓ
181. ⓐ ⓑ ⓒ ⓓ
182. ⓐ ⓑ ⓒ ⓓ

183. ⓐ ⓑ ⓒ ⓓ
184. ⓐ ⓑ ⓒ ⓓ
185. ⓐ ⓑ ⓒ ⓓ
186. ⓐ ⓑ ⓒ ⓓ
187. ⓐ ⓑ ⓒ ⓓ
188. ⓐ ⓑ ⓒ ⓓ
189. ⓐ ⓑ ⓒ ⓓ
190. ⓐ ⓑ ⓒ ⓓ
191. ⓐ ⓑ ⓒ ⓓ
192. ⓐ ⓑ ⓒ ⓓ
193. ⓐ ⓑ ⓒ ⓓ
194. ⓐ ⓑ ⓒ ⓓ
195. ⓐ ⓑ ⓒ ⓓ

196. ⓐ ⓑ ⓒ ⓓ
197. ⓐ ⓑ ⓒ ⓓ
198. ⓐ ⓑ ⓒ ⓓ
199. ⓐ ⓑ ⓒ ⓓ
200. ⓐ ⓑ ⓒ ⓓ
201. ⓐ ⓑ ⓒ ⓓ
202. ⓐ ⓑ ⓒ ⓓ
203. ⓐ ⓑ ⓒ ⓓ
204. ⓐ ⓑ ⓒ ⓓ
205. ⓐ ⓑ ⓒ ⓓ
206. ⓐ ⓑ ⓒ ⓓ
207. ⓐ ⓑ ⓒ ⓓ
208. ⓐ ⓑ ⓒ ⓓ